W9-CTE-720

Eye
of the
Lotus

Psychology of the Chakras

Richard A. Jelusich, Ph.D.

LOTUS
PRESS

AUTHOR'S DISCLAIMER: The contents of this book are the observations and opinions of the author and are not intended to be a medical diagnosis. Before beginning any healing effort, always consult with a qualified health practitioner.

COPYRIGHT © 2004 by Richard Jelusich. ALL RIGHTS RESERVED. No part of this book may be reproduced in any form or by any electronic or mechanical means including information storage and retrieval systems without permission in writing from the publisher, except by a reviewer who may quote brief passages in a review.

Page Design/Layout: Paul Bond, Art & Soul Design
Editing: Karen Wilkening, Expert Editing Ink
Cover Art and Graphics: Michael Brouillet
Illustrations: Sabrina Dalla Valle
Yoga Photos: Meenakshi Angel Honig
Back Cover Photo: Augustus Anthony Piazza

First Edition, 2004
    Printed in the United States of America
    Eye of the Lotus: Psychology of the Chakras
ISBN: 0-940985-76-4
Library of Congress Control Number: 2004110821

Published by:
Lotus Press
P.O. Box 325
Twin Lakes, Wisconsin 53181 USA
web: www.lotuspress.com
e-mail: lotuspress@lotuspress.com
800-824-6396

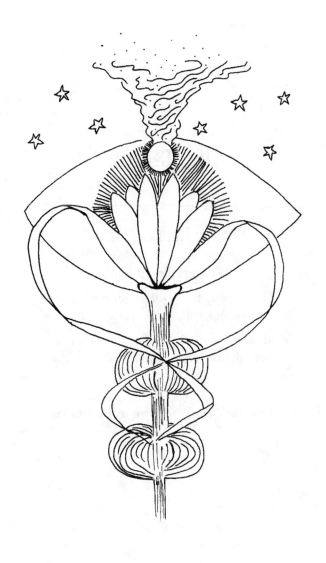

Dedication

This book, its soul, is dedicated to the memory of my father,

Antone Francis Jelusich.

We were best friends.

Thank you, Dad, for cheering me on
from this side for so many years.

And now your spirit, from the other side,
reminds me what is important in life.

I love you, Dad. You are a saint to me.

Table of Contents

Acknowledgements

I wish to acknowledge the many beautiful souls who expressed the courage to change their lives: Thank you for allowing me to counsel with you. It is to you I owe my growing understanding of our nature in Oneness. Without your courage to overcome life's illusions I would not have the opportunity to express my skills in humility and in confidence.

I wish to thank those family members who have shaped my life: my beautiful children, *Richard, Crisann, and Kimberly*; my mother and father, *Lena and Antone*; and my sisters, *Carolyn and Antoinette*. Growing together has afforded us many opportunities to seek the beauty that exists in each of us.

I thank the incredible women who have blessed me in intimacy of sacred relationships. There have been many lessons in teaching me how to receive your gentleness and love.

My appreciation to: *Tom Medvitz and Linda Strom*, who took me under their wing, dispensed invaluable advice, and let me use their copier into the wee hours of the morning; *Donovan and Melissa Coppenrath*, who cared for me as family so I could travel and have time to write this book; My hosts and agents in the cities I have visited and worked: *Bonnie Thorne* (my sister from a past life); *Ida Monea; Lisa Poe; Virginia Fierro; Bonnie Martinez; Anne and Ron Jerome; Hilde McCarthy, Pete Jackson; Rev. Jean Holmes*, my teacher and inspiration; *Dr. Hiroshi Motoyama*, Ph.D., Litt.D., my father in a past life in Japan — You inspired me from the start, and could see in me what I could only vaguely see; *Dr. Jeffrey Thompson*, D.C., one of my heroes in this lifetime, for his passion for helping our fellow human beings to heal themselves. Dr. Gaetan Chevalier, Ph.D., who selflessly supported my efforts at CIHS in obtaining my doctorate.

My profound gratitude to *Karen Wilkening* of Expert Editing, Ink, who applied her considerable skill to shape and polish all the material; *Sabrina Dalla Valle*, illustrator, teacher extraordinaire, and master distiller, who provided the inspired illustrations and cover logo, wrote the chapter on essential oils, provided a safe and nurturing environment for our feelings for each other, and who taught me to remain vulnerable and to accept my abundance; *Michael Brouillet*, graphic artist, who worked with Sabrina to bring Heaven on Earth in depicting the cover art and illustrations in this book; and to *Madhu Honeyman* for contributing the incredibly thorough and loving chapter on Hatha Yoga exercises with the exquisite poses by *Meenakshi Angel Honig*.

As you can see,
the evolution of one's consciousness
is a collaborative leadership:
All of us working together for our
highest and greatest good.
May we all benefit from the
Divine Blessings abundant in each of us.
May we all have the courage
to walk in the Love,
Wisdom, and Will of the Creator.

Note From the Author

It is so easy to just "read" a book and not extract the messages it contains. It takes a certain vulnerability, a willingness to grow and receive more of what I term "**your Self**" to find the revelatory experiences. My hope is that you will use this book to inspire and facilitate a deeper understanding of your Self.

This book is meant to be a jumping-off point for your comprehension of chakras and metaphysics, not a destination. Your chakras are "you" on a higher level of being; they are your higher organs. **It is you, having the experience of your Self**. Pay attention to that experience; it is there for your growth in ways you cannot yet imagine.

Please do not force a definition of your Self into a given specific chakra. You have attributes of every chakra; you live in Oneness with no separation. It is merely the emphasis of a given chakra that causes you to react and have experiences in different ways. A heart chakra person will react and absorb the material in this book in a different way than a throat chakra individual will.

You might tend to identify with a specific chakra, then seek to make the other relevant chakras fit around the one description. It is natural to do this, but to escape the box of "consensus reality," I ask you to keep your heart open and your mind flexible.

We can move into experiences that draw on one or a combination of the influences of our chakras, but the experience is always *fluid* and *dynamic*. There is no "progression" from one chakra to another. A person in his fourth chakra is not further advanced than someone else with a second chakra dominance. This is linear thinking and there is no such thing.

Dominant chakras are *life issues*, not "today" issues. It does not do to look for the quick fix, but rather to understand that the evolution of consciousness is rooted in the effort, not the goal. Your issues are yours for a given lifetime, and you may overcome them all, but the potential weakness (lower aspect of a chakra) is what gives you the opportunity to be strong. I will explain in this book how *your strength is your weakness, and your weakness is your strength*.

If you are here on the planet, you are in some type of illusion. The search for Oneness is the very essence of our attempt to perceive beyond the illusion into truth, through love. In your life you will encounter many challenges, opportunities, and circumstances to meet and overcome your illusions. The manner in which you overcome them will be succinctly your own, and the tenets in this book will provide you with the background and methodology as to *why* and *how* the change is achieved.

This book is best read in stages, and perhaps several times. You'll find there are levels to your own perception of reality; the fruits contained in different chapters are not ready to be enjoyed until they are ripe in the mind and heart of the reader.

Always look to your inner trust to externalize the God-within. If there are things in this book you disagree with, it is for a very good reason. Trust your Self, that you are connected to Oneness; one with all Love, Wisdom, and Will.

It is my honor and privilege to be of service,

Richard Jelusich, Ph.D.

List of Illustrations

Introduction

The challenge of explaining the chakras and their influence on our lives is in their nature: pure metaphysics. After many years of spiritual counseling, teaching, and healing, I formulated a view of the "whole human being" from the perspective of the four archetypes (mental, physical, emotional, and spiritual) flowing together in congruity, along with the inter-working of the chakra system, to assist in this explanation.

Early on, I began to understand that *each chakra has a specific influence on our basic consciousness*; the way we perceive and react to our environment. I also noticed that one chakra would be more "dominant" than the others. We are the sum of the interactions of our archetypes, along with our dominant chakras, and the basic life disposition those dominant chakras cause us to behold as our *reality*.

The difficulty became how to explain the influence of the quality of the soul, through the chakras, as an emanation into this dimension of consciousness. How do you explain the esoteric disposition and life orientation of another human being as it describes that person's life purpose, strengths and weaknesses? And how do you put metaphysical information into practical words to help someone have a productive and meaningful life?

I realized that the effectiveness of my consultations and healing work relied on how well I was willing to trust my intuitive perceptions to see individuals as they "truly are," subject to my own limitations.

By its nature, metaphysics cannot be experienced or measured directly through our five senses, but rather must be perceived through our hearts and emotions. The experience of our higher selves is unique and is not transferred to another by thoughts, but by impressions of our *life-force*, the countenance of the sum of our many-lives experiences emanating the quality of who we are.

By that token, another person is impressed through the quality of our being on a metaphysical level of awareness, but not the cognitive level. In other words, most of our true communication is accomplished on a subtle level much more so than on the physical level. As you read this book *you'll see how the quality of these emanations of character come from our chakras,* how others react to our state of being, and likewise we to theirs.

Truly, all reality is subjective. It is we who decide the nature and extent of our reality. We react to a given situation until we change the cause that changes the effect. If conscious evolution is sprinkled into our reality by the power of our will to destroy any illusion that separates us from Oneness, our reality shifts to accommodate the grander view of our true nature.

To teach that to readers and my healing students is not so easy, for I am asking you to grasp with your heart what your mind may not yet comprehend. More than one student has asked me, "How do you know when you have the right feeling?" The answer is twofold: 1) You are connected to all things, inseparable from the Oneness, and hence available to all the spiritual power to alleviate the suffering caused by illusion, and 2) through *trust,* you grasp what you cannot perceive with your five senses. You must trust your Self and your inner ability to discern.

It is essential that you trust your feelings when evaluating the subject matter contained in this book. Your mind and your heart must be partners if there is to be true growth.

To bring the Hermetic* Principle "As above, so below" into reality, you must first recognize that the only separation between you and your higher Self is a perception of separation: an illusion. It's just that it is a *really good illusion.* To break the illusion requires the trust I speak of. To bring Heaven on earth or, as above, so below, you must trust that the Oneness not only exists, but also that it is absolutely viable in your life. By living in that awareness, you empower your life and your soul's purpose.

You are having an experience of your Self. Higher parts of you, your transcendent nature, are infusing into your everyday life. These higher aspects are the emanation of your Divine possibilities, accessed through *intuition.* You are constantly taking psychic relationships to the higher emanations of others to work out your life's experiences.

We live in Oneness, where there is no separation between us. It is this fact that allows us to work the intricacies of consciousness, our life's mission and goals, karmic influences and freewill choice with one another. The energies of consciousness are constantly weaving in and out in a dance of reality vs. illusion.

Our paths in life are always to reduce and eliminate the illusion. When illusion is destroyed, suffering is also reduced. When reality and illusion meet, there is a period of tribulation where your soul seeks to infuse more of its presence into your personality.

The way to change the cause of a life's issue is to determine the cause (the illusion) and overcome the need for it. The trick to changing an illusion is to recognize that there is an illusion in the first place. Sounds like a Catch-22, but the way it works is that when you're ready, the illusion presents itself in the form of a *crisis*.

Put another way, when reality rubs against illusion, it creates a friction that we know as tribulation or suffering. The suffering brings due process of the possibility of overcoming the illusion, and if you are willing to become vulnerable enough to change, you make an act of will. The power of the will moves your life forward through the process of learning the life's lesson.

Through a great love of your Self as a being of Divine origin, you begin to perceive the true metaphysical workings of the universe, the Oneness, and your part in it. The more you cherish the inner strength available to you, the more you become available to it. *The more you realize you are living in a really good illusion, the more you can be free from it.*

As we live in Oneness without separation, the illusion of space between us, our thoughts of "I think" and "I believe," are continuations of the illusion that we are separate from anything anywhere. Yet, life continues in an evolution of understanding, an ever-growing state of consciousness where we gain a better, more holistic understanding of the universe and our place in it.

By offering a point of view of the whole human being that includes a description of the chakra system and its influence on our experience, I hope to illustrate the Oneness in which we

live. I am sensitive to the fact that we tend to want easy explanations for our conditions and existence, yet I know there is no
such thing. *This book offers another point of view where you may
find some resonance to help explain why you are here, your strengths
and weaknesses in life, and what it takes to make you whole and
complete.*

You'll find that in understanding your dominant chakra,
you'll know what you must do to overcome your inherent dominant chakra's weaknesses. In working on your weaknesses, you
become strong. You cannot help someone from a position of
weakness; you are here to evolve your soul first. After you have
done that, you can help as many people as you wish, but you
must do it from a position of strength.

You'll find that there are little nuggets of truth in each
chakra section, and you may find that bits and pieces of various
sections fit you. So please use those pieces that work, discard
the rest, and don't try to cubbyhole your Self into any one section. We are a combination of *all* chakras, functioning as they
do to infuse and inspire our lives with their higher attributes.

Please do not assume that you must be one dominant chakra
or the other. All chakras are open, and we are composed of the
inter-dynamic fluctuations of our various chakras in every given
moment. Dominant chakras are a focus of life's energy and experience, brought forth through our several incarnations, life's
paths, karma on many levels, and freewill. One may have a
dominant chakra and exhibit traits from other chakras from
time to time because we are composed of the whole human experience.

It is in our nature to want to put identities and psychologies
into a cubbyhole that will neatly fit how we see ourselves. In
reality, we are never the same physical being, nor are we the
same mentally or emotionally. Always evolving, ever unfolding,
we are the new "I" (eye of the unfolding lotus flower) in every
moment. Thus, to lock oneself into a single chakra would be to
deny the very Oneness in which we exist. It is better to consider oneself inseparable from the whole, and to recognize that
we are merely experiencing an attraction towards a dominant
chakra.

The more you understand about your Self, the more self-empowered you will be in understanding life and your part in it, and the more you will choose your reactions, instead of bobbing like a cork on the sea of emotions. Your higher Self led you this far; let it continue to lead you until you and your higher Self are one.

As a dear friend of mine once said, "We are not learning anything, we are merely remembering what we already know." Indeed, if we truly live in Oneness, we are not separate from what we seek. You have as much access to your spirituality as anyone else. No soul has a greater path than you, no person is loved by God any more than you are, and no person is any closer to Source than you.

This book is a basic premise of the chakras, plus exercises, resources on light and sound methods, essential oils, meditations, prayers, methods for balancing the chakras, and a section on unique Hatha Yoga poses created by Madhu Honeymann, an accomplished yoga instructor. I also provide a variety of techniques to care for and balance your chakras. I urge you to try them out and see which works best for you.

My next book, *Your Chakric Relationships: Why We Pick the People We Do*, will discuss in detail how we interact with each other energetically. It is a guide on how to respond to and optimize your relationships by gaining a thorough understanding of the fundamental energetics taking place, with an emphasis on how and why we take *inverse relationships* (mirroring) to others to bring about our own challenges and growth.

It is my sincere desire that you will use this information to empower your life, to live as a fully-conscious and awake whole human being, and to enjoy the Oneness in which you live. Remember who you really are - *you are a magnificent and eloquent being of light, and nothing less.*

The following Seven Hermetic Principles, upon which the entire Hermetic Philosophy is based, are referenced several times in this book:

I. The Principle Of Mentalism: "The All Is Mind; The Universe Is Mental."

II. The Principle Of Correspondence: "As Above, So Below; As Below, So Above."

III. The Principle Of Vibration: "Nothing Rests; Everything Moves; Everything Vibrates."

IV. The Principle Of Polarity: "Everything is Dual; Everything Has Its Pair Of Opposites; Like And Unlike Are The Same; Opposites Are Identical In Nature, But Different In Degree; Extremes Meet; All Truths Are But Half Truths; All Paradoxes May Be Reconciled."

V. The Principle Of Rhythm: "Everything Flows Out And In; Everything Has Its Tides; All Things Rise And Fall; The Pendulum Swing Manifests In Everything. The Measure Of The Swing To The Right Is The Measure Of The Swing To The Left; Rhythm Compensates."

VI. The Principle Of Cause and Effect: "Every Cause Has Its Effect; Every Effect Has Its Cause; Everything Happens According To The Law; Chance Is A Name For The Law Not Recognized; There Are Many Planes Of Causation, But Nothing Escapes The Law."

VII. The Principle Of Gender: "Gender Is In Everything; Everything Has Its Masculine And Feminine Principles; Gender Manifests On All Planes."

Chapter One

Definition of the Chakras

Chakras regulate the flow of life-force energy (chi) between the physical and the higher dimensions, and they are the filters through which you perceive life: They are portals for your consciousness to this dimension.

The chakras are more or less vertically aligned with your spine *(see Illustrations #1-a and #1-b)*. There are seven main chakras, twenty-one minor chakras, and in my experience, tens of thousands of chakras located throughout the entire human body *(see Illustration #1-c)*.

"Chakra" is a Sanskrit word that means vortex, or wheel. The chakras are inter-dimensional energy vortexes that regulate the flow of life-force energy between and among dimensions in a two-way movement. Most often they are depicted as spinning wheels of light, or with many petals representing their dual manifestation in the physical and higher realms.

Every chakra is an illumination point of consciousness flowing into this dimension from higher dimensions. The chakras have been called our organs on a higher level, and ourselves on a higher level of being.

There are higher dimensional chakras as well *(see Illustration #1-d)*. Four of them, chakras eight, thirteen, twenty, and sixty-four, are discussed later in this book. There may well be an infinite number of higher dimension chakras not located on the existing human body.

The "shushumna" is the main channel of energy, or column of light, that runs up and down your spinal column *(see Illustration #1-e)*. It distributes life-force between and among the chakras, and also serves to connect the higher aspects of your

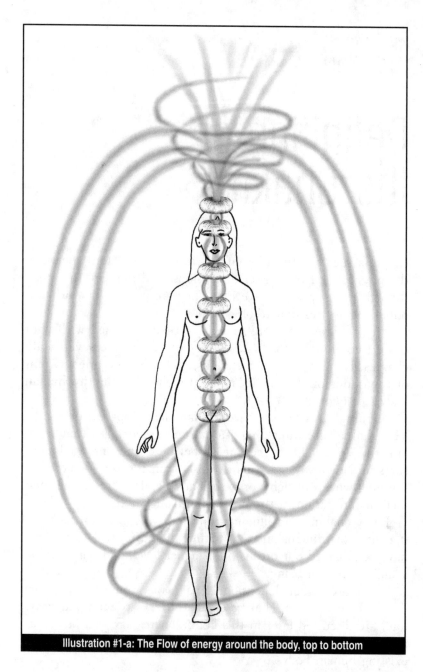

Illustration #1-a: The Flow of energy around the body, top to bottom

existence with the lower aspects. It can be visualized as extending infinitely upward through your crown chakra into all

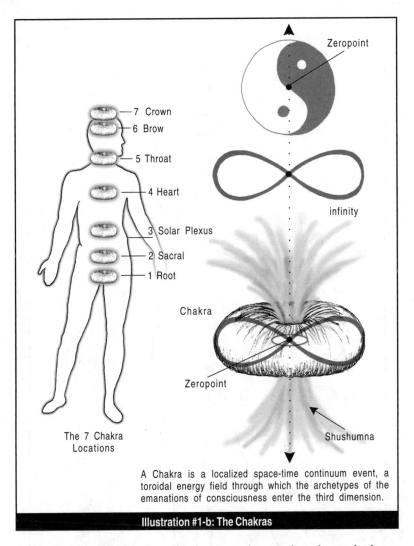

Zeropoint

7 Crown
6 Brow
5 Throat
4 Heart
3 Solar Plexus
2 Sacral
1 Root

infinity

Chakra

Zeropoint

Shushumna

The 7 Chakra
Locations

A Chakra is a localized space-time continuum event, a toroidal energy field through which the archetypes of the emanations of consciousness enter the third dimension.

Illustration #1-b: The Chakras

higher realms, and infinitely downward into the physical plane. It shines the column of light that is the core, or signature, of human existence through the lenses of each chakra.

The difficulty in representing chakras with graphics or even geographically on the body is that they are there, *yet not there*. The inter-dimensional quality of the chakras locates them as *energy nexuses* on the body, but they exist on other levels as well.

In fact, the best way to think of chakras is not dual in the

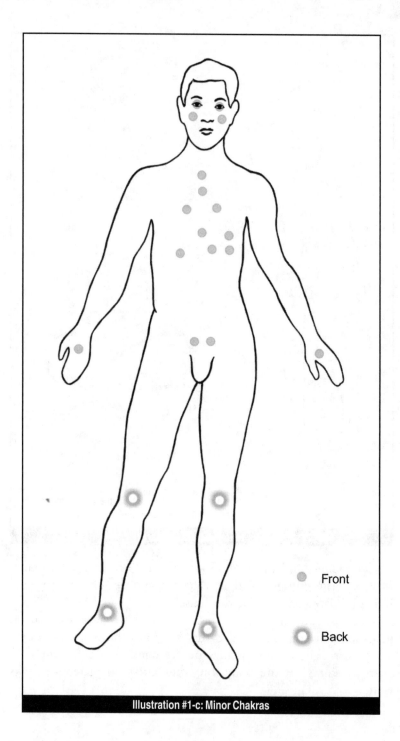

Illustration #1-c: Minor Chakras

Front

Back

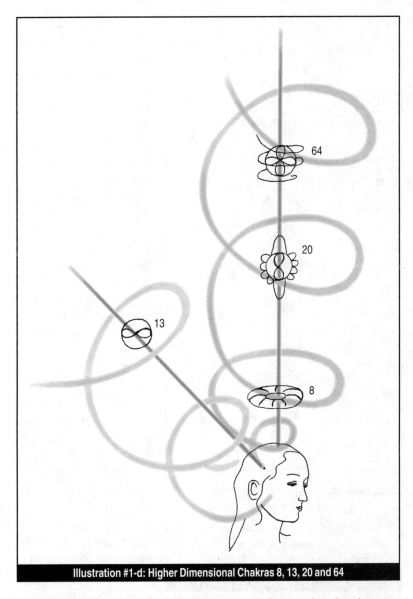

Illustration #1-d: Higher Dimensional Chakras 8, 13, 20 and 64

sense of physical and higher dimensional, but as localized quantum events where everything and nothing exists in the same moment, and that our availability to infinite levels of reality is perceived through the colored (influence) lenses of each chakra.

For most humans the externalization of reality is perceived

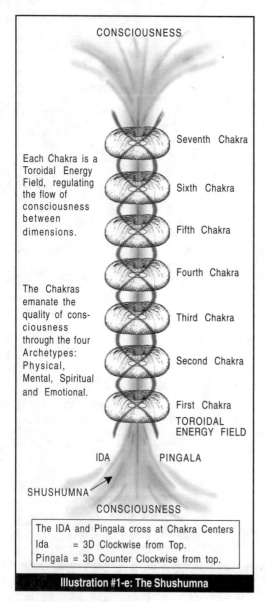

CONSCIOUSNESS

Each Chakra is a Toroidal Energy Field, regulating the flow of consciousness between dimensions.

The Chakras emanate the quality of consciousness through the four Archetypes: Physical, Mental, Spiritual and Emotional.

Seventh Chakra

Sixth Chakra

Fifth Chakra

Fourth Chakra

Third Chakra

Second Chakra

First Chakra

TOROIDAL ENERGY FIELD

IDA   PINGALA

SHUSHUMNA

CONSCIOUSNESS

The IDA and Pingala cross at Chakra Centers
Ida   = 3D Clockwise from Top.
Pingala = 3D Counter Clockwise from top.

Illustration #1-e: The Shushumna

consciously through the five senses, what *Brave New World* and *Perennial Philosophy* author Aldous Huxley called the "touchstones of reality." Your senses provide the way through which you reach out into this dimension and decide what is real and what is not real. For most of Western society this has not included any concept that we exist simultaneously on different vibrational levels.

Western society tends to use a reductionist or dualistic method of philosophizing its existence in the universe (e.g., "I and God") in what is called a "bottom up universe," where everything can be reduced to its most elemental aspects, like molecules and atoms.

The Eastern mind tends to see the universe from the top down, where everything emanates from a higher to a lower vibrational level. There is no separation or seam between you and God, only levels of illusion that there is any separation at all. *It is with that understanding of the universe that this book is aligned.*

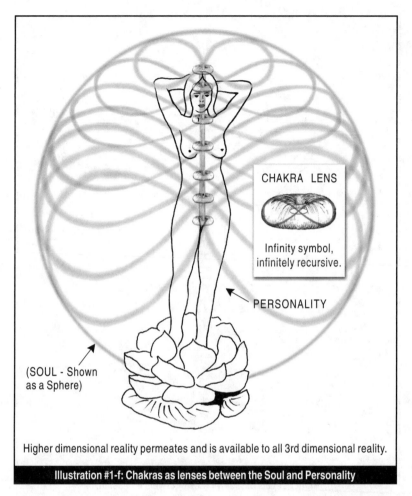

CHAKRA LENS

Infinity symbol,
infinitely recursive.

PERSONALITY

(SOUL - Shown
as a Sphere)

Higher dimensional reality permeates and is available to all 3rd dimensional reality.

Illustration #1-f: Chakras as lenses between the Soul and Personality

The chakras represent a qualitative influence on the mental, physical, spiritual, and emotional archetypes of being human. They affect the manner in which our four archetypes interact with the physical world and our understanding of spiritual phenomena.

The chakra sits between the "personality" and the "soul" (*see Illustration #1-f*). The infusion of the soul into our personality is where most of us are working, though actually there are three levels: *personality, soul,* and *monad* (*see Illustration #1-g*).

The *personality* is what you observe in most human beings. In our spiritual endeavors we are attempting to become more soul-

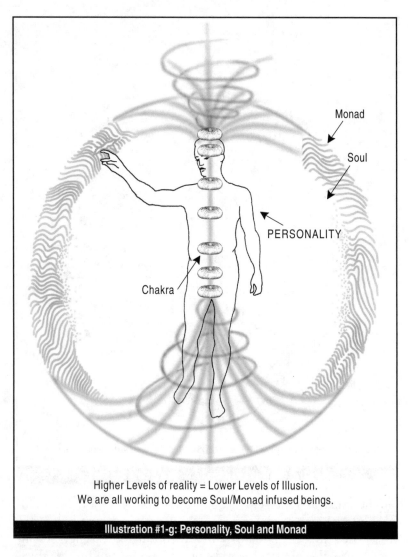

Higher Levels of reality = Lower Levels of Illusion.
We are all working to become Soul/Monad infused beings.

Illustration #1-g: Personality, Soul and Monad

like and are thus working to infuse a greater soul-quality into our personality. The personality is our waking level of consciousness: the most basic skill sets required to navigate this temporal and spatial linear dimension.

The *soul* level is the next higher state of consciousness: the level to which we are aspiring through myriad means and religions. The soul level represents the transcendence of the limitations this dimension represents. As we attempt to infuse that soul-quality into our personalities, the nature of our character changes completely, because our soul-character is very different from the character of the personality. An example of a soul-infused personality would be someone like Paramahansa Yogananda, or any of the saints.

The *monad* is the highest possible expression of a human quality, while still retaining some understanding of being human. An example of a monad-infused personality is a Jesus the Christ, or a Buddha. The light of our monad shines through the soul; the light of the soul shines through our personality. All are seamlessly linked in a Oneness that we only dimly perceive.

When the illusions of our lives are met with reality, it creates a friction or resistance that we know as tribulation or suffering. As we overcome our illusions we go into the higher aspects of our given dominant chakras, we dispel the illusion itself (releasing the need to re-learn the lesson), and we infuse a greater portion of our soul into our personality.

The more soul-like we become, the more our personality changes to match that of the soul, and the more illusion and suffering are reduced in our lives. Or, the more illusion that is destroyed, the more soul-infused we become.

The soul shines its light through our given chakras into our personality, influenced by the dominant chakra, and given the circumstances of karma, mission statement and freewill, affects our lives accordingly. As we gain experience and deal with the little urgencies of life, we are given opportunities to evolve our soul-quality through the understanding and realization of truths that destroy our illusions and our dwelling in the lower aspect of our dominant chakra. Many times we are called upon to embrace a truth with our intuition before our conscious mind can discern it.

"Dominant" chakra is similar to dominance in right- or left-handedness, or right- or left-eye dominance. Even though you have two hands one is likely to be dominant and the one you favor when writing or throwing. As you have two hands, you have seven chakras, and all are functioning. You can go through issues in each chakra throughout life, but will tend to emphasize or take a relationship to a *dominant* chakra.

You use the strengths and weaknesses of all your chakras

during the course of a lifetime, but will tend to emphasize the dominant chakra because of its inherent influence on all states of being.

Chakras have both a higher and a lower aspect, covered thoroughly in a later chapter. The nature of both aspects is a function of the development of your consciousness. The nature of the *lower aspects* of the given dominant chakra set up situations and circumstances you encounter in order to provide the opportunity to grow towards the higher aspect of your chakras. The *higher aspects* represent the fulfillment or attainment of increasing levels of awareness, development, and soul-infusion into your personality.

Your chakras are functioning all the time, whether you know it or not, and whether you believe it or not. Our minds think and plan, conceive and control, but the chakras are flowering and flowing energy day and night, whether you are asleep or awake, happy or sad. It is the constant state of consciousness that flows and exists without respect to the minutes of the day and the emergency of the moment. Most people are unaware of their own multi-dimensional nature.

The chakras sit above the physical plane and influence your mental, spiritual, emotional, and physical aspects as the light of your soul shines through them. The chakras are still you, but on a higher dimension. As the light of the soul shines through your chakra, your personality is fueled into enacting its purpose in a given lifetime.

The soul creates a deep yearning in our hearts to express what cannot be uttered. We feel a connectedness, an intimacy with our spiritual nature, but have not the words to adequately express the exquisite sense that there is "something more." Nonetheless, the energy of the soul is infusing its quality into our personality daily: *The way in which you respond to your earthly environment is a reflection of the perceptions you have of your own soul-quality.*

A dominant chakra colors that perception according to the characteristics of the chakra. Depending on the dominant characteristic, the personality is affected according to those characteristics for your *entire lifetime.*

The following table illustrates the chakras and their primary effects on the personality. Remember that these effects are not just physical, but also mental, emotional, and spiritual.

Chakra	Name	Characteristic	Effect
1	Root	Survivability	Gateway to mere existence in physical form
2	Sacral	Creationist	Creativity, burdens, responsibility, sexuality
3	Solar Plexus	Charismatic Leader	Power of the Self, individuation, truth
4	Heart	Empath	To give, receive, and be love
5	Throat	Communicator	Elucidation and illumination
6	Brow or Third Eye	Prophet	Higher communication
7	Crown	Zero-Point	Gateway to higher dimensions

Certainly you've encountered someone in your life for the first time and had an instant "vibe" from that person, an instant chemistry. *That is an example of the approximately 95% of communication that is energy.* You are accurately sensing the true disposition of the individual.

One of the greatest disservices we do to ourselves is to underestimate the power of our intuitive abilities. As everyone (by default of the Oneness) is psychic, we all can avail ourselves of our intuitive abilities. The difficulty is that there is no direct physical evidence. Even dowsing, divining, using pendulums, and muscle testing are not the direct experience itself, but externalizations of doubt. However, you can "know" the truth of something, without having to test for it. As human beings we tend to grossly underestimate who we are and what we represent. "Ye are gods," Jesus said. "Greater things than these shall ye also do."

The energy that is "you" emanates from you at all times, asleep or awake. The energy from others reaches you as well, at all times, no matter where you are. It is this interchange that you react to when engaging in relationships with others, be they intimate, familial, social, work-related, etc.

Most human beings unconsciously take *psychic* relationships to each other based on the dominant chakra, karma, and mission statement. The ones who take a *conscious* relationship have been trained in their respective spiritual practices, or have a working understanding of metaphysics.

The difference we make in our lives is the effort we put into accessing the consciousness that is available through our chakras. Our chakras are still "us," our soul is still "ourselves," but the level is higher and qualitative. That means the energy cannot be quantified, as in "I am 25% more psychic today than I was yesterday," or "I love my father 50% more now than yesterday."

Accessing any given chakra's attributes does take effort and focus, but the availability of "you" to "your Self" is much more simple than you might expect. However, we in Western society are so acculturated into an analytical framework that it is difficult to trust our innate ability to access a part of ourselves that already exists.

Applying effort to access more of your chakras' strengths through trust and exercise changes your life. Many hidden benefits accrue:

- Your life becomes more centered, focused, and grounded.
- You move into the higher aspects of your given dominant chakra and your very presence is healing to others.
- The old habits and traits that beleaguered and slowed you down no longer have any attraction because you have moved beyond the need to experience them.

You are here in a given lifetime to accept your Self, not to heal others. By accepting who you are and what you represent, by "acknowledging" (acceptance of knowledge) you become whole and complete. In that way, from a position of strength, others will tend to want to heal merely because you exist. You cannot heal from a position of weakness, nor can you love unconditionally.

Through strengthening the chakras and their associated energies, you attain self-composure, you maintain poise and balance in life, and it is much harder for you to go "off center."

An important distinction to make is the difference between what a given chakra dominant person is to "do," versus what you came here to "learn." By "learn" I mean to externalize to consciousness the aspect of your being that may be suppressed about *feeling*.

For example, a throat chakra dominant person is incarnated *to be* a teacher and communicator; one who articulates, illuminates, and elucidates through many forms of communication. However, the throat chakra person is here *to learn to feel*, and to feel in the physical presence emotionally/intuitively.

Specific examples are covered in each chakra's chapter, but for now I've recreated the previous basic chakra chart and added what the individual is here to "do" and to "learn" in the following chart.

What we came here to *learn* is related to our ability to fully externalize our gift of what we came here to *do*; our own way of

Chakra	Name	Characteristic	To "Do"	To "Learn"
1	Root	Survivability	Gateway to physical form	Corporeal presence
2	Sacral	Creationist	Creativity, visionary	Create by acceptance and love of Self
3	Solar Plexus	Charismatic Leader	Represent truth through individuation	Qualitative reality, individual power
4	Heart	Empath	To give, receive, and be love	To communicate
5	Throat	Communicator	Elucidation and illumination	To feel
6	Brow or Third Eye	Prophet	Inception of higher communication	To be in the heart
7	Crown	Zero-Point	Gateway to higher dimensions	Metaphysical nature

first bringing Heaven on earth for ourselves. The Hermetic Principle "as above, so below" means you must bring the higher manifestation of your soul and its strengths through your dominant chakra before you can be of assistance to others. It is the same with each chakra. The more you remove any impediments between your soul and personality, the more soul-like you become, and the more you manifest the possibility that your soul-group can evolve as a whole.

Spiritual Impediments

Why do I only progress at a certain rate when I can sense so much more? What is holding me back?

Spiritual impediments are deliberate safeguards put in place by your higher Self to prevent you from holding what you cannot grasp, or, holding a vibration that is too high. An example would be giving your car keys to a three-year-old child. Not an advisable action because the child does not have the maturity to drive a vehicle, no matter how strong his will. It is not safe for him or for anyone around him, even though he may assert that he is absolutely ready to do it.

Though we perceive dimly and yearn strongly for states of consciousness to come, they must unfold in their own time, as the petals of the rose. A guiding force or Divine Presence asserts a level of restraint, or middle path, where we may aspire to our heart's yearning in a safe manner.

There are exceptions to every rule; an individual can have a sudden spiritual opening, or epiphany. Generally, though, spiritual impediments are those imposed limitations to spiritual growth that are in place to prevent us from growing more rapidly than our physical minds can assimilate.

There are people who burn the lenses of their chakras through unsafe practices practices - from the overuse (beyond practitioner's recommendations) of psychoacoustic music/ brainwave entrainment to performing kundalini exercises without proper supervision. There are case histories about those who have unwisely continued spiritual exercises to their detriment. If you experience sudden spiritual growth and feel you are losing your perspective, stop your spiritual practices until you feel safe to continue. It is unwise to continue spiritual practices such as kundalini-raising exercises without proper instruction, and can result in injury. In fact, unwise actions in this manner can result in a karma that must be satisfied in the next life - suffering yet to come.

Likewise, there are ultimates in life. *Ultimate fears create ultimate challenges.* It is my opinion that we set forth an ultimate challenge for a given dominant chakra, and I've summarized them in the following chart.

Chakra	Greatest Fear; Hardest Thing You'll Ever Do in This Lifetime
1	I don't physically exist. To accept your corporeal existence.
2	I cannot create anything greater than what came before. Nothing I do is enough. To accept and love your Self as much as anyone or anything.
3	What could be true is true. To accept your power; that you are that powerful.
4	That I am not pure. To accept the purity you have earned from past lives, well-lived: To be love itself.
5	No one knows me for who I truly am. Nothing I communicate or teach matters. To unite as above, so below: To unite Heaven and earth.
6	To never touch the earth plane. To unite universal mind, physical mind, and heart.
7	I don't metaphysically exist. To accept your metaphysical existence.

Remember, your chakras are you, and through them flows the higher consciousness that is available to you at all times. It could not be otherwise, for if you truly live in Oneness, you cannot be separate from what you seek.

To access something you already have requires great trust and vulnerability to let go of the conventions, or lower truths, you've learned to date. They've served you well and brought you thus far, perhaps even to this book.

Greater truths are gifts you give to your Self by understanding you are the Creator of your circumstances, and by taking responsibility for them. You must also accept the opportunity to hold the higher truth fully with your heart even if your mind does not yet understand.

It is in the process of *allowing* your Self to be evolved that true transcendence of consciousness takes place. When you live in this qualitative state of being that transcends quantitative thinking, then you can enter into a sincere and intimate trust of Oneness.

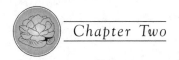

Chapter Two

Your Chakric Relationships

We all take psychic/energetic relationships to each other long before the mind thinks a single thought *(see Illustration #2-a)*. We are in constant energetic contact with each other through communication that is neither verbal nor physical.

The truth is that everyone is psychic, though most of us are unaware that such subtle energies even exist. These energies cannot be measured directly. They are often called "subtle" energy, in that energy presence is pervasive, and not third dimensional. It is these energies that one tunes into when performing spiritual counseling, whether in person or remotely. Since subtle energies cannot be directly measured, it is very easy to discount their existence. The chapter called *Qualitative vs. Quantitative Reality* will help to explain this.

We observe the effects of gravity, though no one has ever seen a gravitational line of force. It would be easy to say that you do not believe in gravity because you've not seen it, though when you awake tomorrow morning you'll still stick to the planet regardless of your belief.

Similar to gravity, you are subject to other energies that cannot be seen. The difference is that gravity, electricity, and magnetics, while invisible, can be measured. Subtle energies can only be measured indirectly.

Science has begun to study the phenomena of subtle energy; to seek to explain what yogis, swamis, gurus, and evolved human beings have been telling us for thousands of years. Science can observe indirectly that these phenomena exist by taking measurements of bodily functions and known energies (light, electricity, etc.).

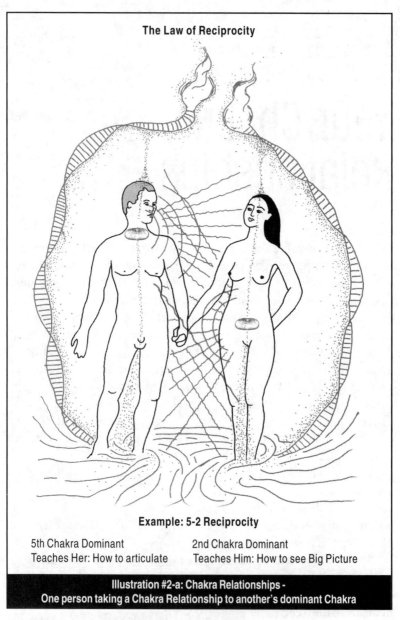

The Law of Reciprocity

Example: 5-2 Reciprocity

5th Chakra Dominant
Teaches Her: How to articulate

2nd Chakra Dominant
Teaches Him: How to see Big Picture

**Illustration #2-a: Chakra Relationships -
One person taking a Chakra Relationship to another's dominant Chakra**

There are three levels of energy that emanate from the human being; the first two can be measured.

1. *Biochemical*: Relates directly to the human body, nervous and electrical system.

2. *Biomagnetic:* Relates to the electromagnetic field that surrounds and permeates the human being.
3. *Quantum field:* Relates to the emanation of the human character through simultaneity. This level cannot be measured quantitatively.

There are scientific devices that measure the amount of light (photons) emitted from the body. Research at the California Institute for Human Science (CIHS) has shown that chakra centers emit 100 to 1000 times more light (measured in biophotons) than elsewhere on the body.

Another device, called the AMI (Apparatus for Meridian Identification), measures the functioning of the meridians (energy channels) of the body through small electrical pulses applied to the termination of the meridians on the fingers and toes. By measuring all the pulses together, a map of the overall energy system (and chakras) is created, depicting the overall health of the individual, while pointing out deficient or excessive energies in the meridians. The AMI is used widely in Japan for medical diagnosis.

Preliminary research done by Dr. Hiroshi Motoyama (founder of CIHS) in Japan has shown that a person emits very small amounts of visible light. The amount is so small that a photon counter is needed. Dr. Motoyama found that photon emission is higher at certain acupuncture points compared to a region of skin with no acupuncture point.

According to unpublished research done by Dr. Motoyama in Japan, there is some indication that emission at certain acupuncture points is increased for people with psychic abilities. Furthermore, this research showed that there is a possible link between specific acupuncture points and the chakras of the Yogic Tradition.

Even with science, we know *indirectly* that chakras exist. It is very difficult to ascertain directly. How do you discern something that is inter-dimensional? You must have spiritual evolvement and trust of your inner feelings to know what mystics, yogis and swamis have been teaching for thousands of years: that chakras are real and they are you, just on a higher level that cannot be seen or heard with the physical senses.

We do know chakras exist, as they are a part of our nature, but to reach a level of understanding takes spiritual practice, a trust of one's inner feelings and inner confidence.

As we take psychic relationships to each other at all times, it is this psychic connection that creates our chakric relationships. In this way, we take relationship to each other to work out our life's karma, mission statement, and freewill choices. You are in chakric relationships to others at all times, whether you are in a restaurant, movie theater, elevator, at work, etc. Non-physical communication is ongoing whether you are asleep or awake, aware or ignorant.

In taking those chakric relationships, we engage in the principle of interaction based on externalizing our life's purpose and maturing the nature of our character through decisions. Poor decisions can result in life's lessons repeating until the lesson is learned. This goes back to our Hermetic Principle of *cause and effect*.

The chakras sit above the mental, physical, spiritual, and emotional states of being. They are the filters through which we "see" and "experience" life. The chakras color everything we do, think, feel, and perceive. The chakras are you, just as your blood and nervous system are you. They exist on a higher level of consciousness, and are in ceaseless connection with every facet of your corporeal existence.

Everyone takes a chakric relationship to others. Everyone is at an evolving level of understanding and awareness. The difference lies in taking responsibility for your own awareness of the dynamics. *The more aware you are, the more self-empowered you can be, and thus the less suffering you incur.* And correspondingly, the more aware you will be of why others interact with you the way they do.

Reflect on those you have around you - family, colleagues, friends, and associates. Recognize that you are in an energetic relationship to all of those people, and that in some measure they are reflecting back to you your own nature through the filter of your dominant chakra.

Chapter Three

Your Dominant Chakra

Corporeal dominances are something we all have - a dominant hand, eye, brain hemisphere. We tend to favor our dominant features when undertaking tasks. If you are right-handed you'll tend to write and perform most functions with that dominant hand. And, even though you could write with your left hand, you may not tend to because it does not feel as comfortable, or the script won't be the same.

After a while our dominances become unnoticed functional parts of everyday life. We don't give it much thought, but on some level they are a choice we've made to cope and interact with our world. And the manner in which we choose to interact defines the interaction through the feedback to our mind and emotions, shaping our experiences and *our opinion of our experiences*.

As humans we have seven main chakras that are functional, dynamic, and constantly regulating the flow of life-force energy into this dimension at varying levels of efficiency and openness. When we incarnate, through a higher-level agreement or contract, we enter into physical reality with one of these *dominant* chakras, that is, chakras two through six.

Dominance in a chakra means the soul's primary influence, through the shushumna, emanates the greatest part of its reality through the lens of one chakra over the others. This is so to the extent that the dominant chakra remains throughout your lifetime.

The quality of your soul infuses itself to varying degrees based upon your dharma (right action or right behavior). In doing so, you manifest qualities related to the chakra that is dominant, with all other chakras generally playing a subordinate, relative role.

Your mental, physical, emotional, and spiritual disposition is set against the backdrop of your dominant chakra. That chakra becomes the psycho-spiritual stage upon which your experiences of life are played out. Your mind is impressed with the qualities of the chakra that is dominant to the extent that your orientation towards life in all its aspects relates along the lines of the attributes of that chakra.

A chakra does not tell you what to think, but orients your thinking to a disposition relative to the dominant chakra's strengths and weaknesses. It does this by impressing a higher level of qualitative consciousness through the light channel of the shushumna, and by imbuing that consciousness directly through the lenses of the chakras themselves.

The consciousness that emanates through to the physical plane has the coding of all your past lives, along with the sum of your actions, development of character, spiritual evolution, karmic debts, and current mission statement. And although these emanations from a higher level of consciousness are your consciousness, there is still the mystery of being an individuated soul while existing in Oneness. It is a grand paradox that we all must live through, life after life.

The chakras are the final nexus, or interchange, for the energies that externalize in physical form in the third dimension. The chakra centers in your body feed the meridian system, nervous plexuses, emotional, mental, and astral bodies.

An interesting note is that your auric field is the aggregation of all your subtle body energies taken together. That is, your aura is a rough approximation of the more refined mental, emotional, and astral energy fields accumulated into one energetic representation, usually seen as colors but also able to be "smelled" and "heard" by intuitives.

It is those energy fields that emanate you, not the other way around. The vibratory sequencing of the character of universal form is from a top down perspective: everything in the universe develops into physical form after having first exhibited itself and externalized as reality on higher vibratory levels first. Then the process of coalescing into physical form takes place.

When you look at an aura photograph you are seeing the energies that hold your physical form in place. *Your aura emanates you - you do not emanate your aura.*

There is a dynamic, interdependent flow of energy between and among chakras and your corresponding energy fields. The idiosyncratic or unique effects upon you are determined by your dominant chakra, in combination with your karma and mission statement.

And so that uniqueness will be different for chakras two, three, four, and so on. The person whose dominant chakra is three, or solar plexus, will not manifest or respond to his environment in the same way as a person whose dominant chakra is four, or heart, for instance. The impression on your mind is so holistic and complete that you would not know of the influence until later spiritual development in life.

Chakras have a quality of being the great doorway to higher levels of your own consciousness. They are still you, a part of you. The quality they represent is at once physical and non-physical. They are ever-evolving, ever-unfolding, ceaselessly interacting between your physical presence and your higher levels of being. The impression of any chakra, especially the dominant chakra, upon the mind is so great that the mind is daunted by the power the chakra represents. The reaction of the mind is to grapple with the conscious-reality that the trans-dimensional chakra represents. The physical mind does the best it can to cope with the incredible energetic realities; the truths that exist in their purest forms, through the energies inherent in the multi-dimensional chakras.

The mind, because it is linear, attempts to control in the physical plane that which exists freely on the higher planes. It is very difficult to describe, react, and apply in a physical realm that which exists in the higher realms of consciousness. It is better to hold the energy than to try to understand it.

With effort in evolution of consciousness comes a disposition of inner knowingness, a calm contentment of what is, rather than what should be as dictated by the physical mind. As you progress in your spiritual understanding you overcome the weaknesses or lower aspects in your dominant chakra. There is no need to control towards a predetermined outcome, only to guide towards a goal: It is more important to apply effort along the way than it is to reach the goal.

The mind is linear - the chakra is not. The mind attempts to make linear sense out of a nonlinear event. The mind attempts to do in the physical plane what the chakra (as consciousness) is doing in the higher planes. Since there is no limitation of space or time in higher levels of being, the mind can become confused when attempting to utilize the chakra's strengths in third-dimensional reality.

There's an old saying: "The only way to destroy an illusion is to realize there is one." Sounds like a Catch-22, but with the evolutionary aspect of all human beings upward and outward in awareness, we overcome our illusions by presenting ourselves with the necessary lessons through circumstance, conditions, and opportunities that we, in fact, author.

Experiences we set for ourselves on the stage of our dominant chakras give us the perfect opportunity to rise above the situation; to evolve beyond the circumstance if we so choose. We do this by making not only informed decisions with our mind, but also evolved decisions from our hearts.

It is necessary to understand that true spiritual growth does not result from a high intellect and discerning mind alone, but through the inner yielding that can only be a highly intimate relationship with the Self to be vulnerable to growth. This type of growth cannot be predicted and is not tangible, but it shifts you to higher levels of consciousness.

That intimate encounter of Self requires complete confidence and complete humility in each and every moment. You must be confident of what you feel, yet remain humble in applying the results of your feeling.

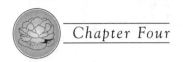

Chapter Four

Five Dominant Chakras, Not Seven

This book focuses primarily on dominant chakras *two through six*. You may wonder about considering chakras one and seven as dominant. In my work I have not observed anyone whose dominant chakra is either the first or the seventh. The patterns I've noted in many years of spiritual counseling indicate that chakras one and seven are "gateways" to and from the physical dimension, but this is yet to be corroborated.

I have been asked about the *distribution of dominant chakra characteristics*. The following table is based on my observations:

Dominant Chakra	Aspect	Percent of the Total Population
2 Sacral	Creationist	40 %
3 Solar Plexus	Charismatic Leader	28 %
4 Heart	Empath	4 %
5 Throat	Communicator	28 %
6 Brow	Prophet	.002 %

Chakras one and seven are presented and discussed, but not as dominant to one's experiences. Chakras eight, thirteen, twenty, and sixty-four are discussed following the chapter on the seventh chakra.

Both chakras one and seven serve as entry points of consciousness into physical form, and rather than behave as a lens to the mental, physical, spiritual, and emotional states of being in what it is to be human, these two chakras are the gateways

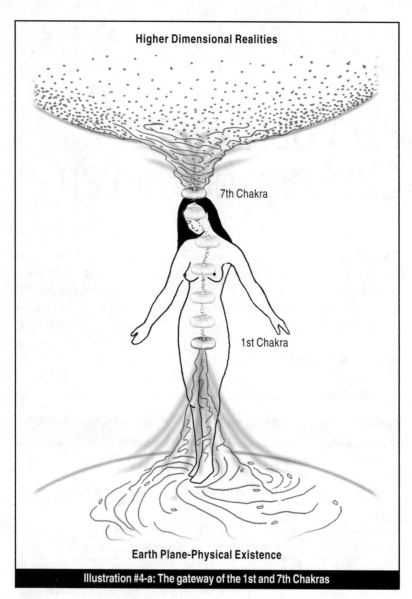

Higher Dimensional Realities

7th Chakra

1st Chakra

Earth Plane-Physical Existence

Illustration #4-a: The gateway of the 1st and 7th Chakras

themselves (*see Illustration #4-a*).

Imagine a door from one room into another. The door serves the purpose of representing the barrier between rooms. But it is better to think of that door as the union, or joining, of the two rooms that makes movement between them possible. It is the function of the union, the act of uniting together, that is the

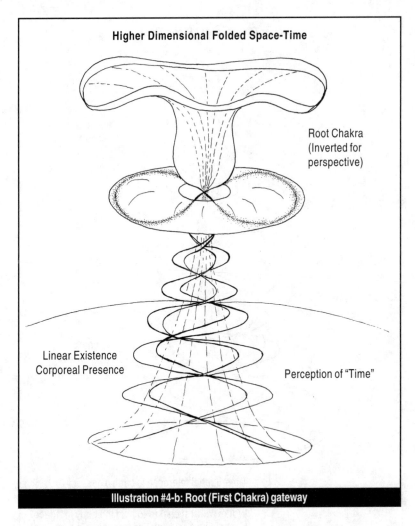

Higher Dimensional Folded Space-Time

Root Chakra
(Inverted for
perspective)

Linear Existence
Corporeal Presence

Perception of "Time"

Illustration #4-b: Root (First Chakra) gateway

key to understanding how chakras one and seven function for the whole human being.

As you may know, the whole human being consists of not just what can be seen and experienced in the third dimension or physical plane, but rather one who exists seamlessly in a Oneness where there is no separation. The gateways of chakra one and seven are holding the union, or meeting, of these planes seamlessly. As we evolve in consciousness the mists of illusion dissipate and we come to realize that this is so.

The base or root chakra represents a grounding into the

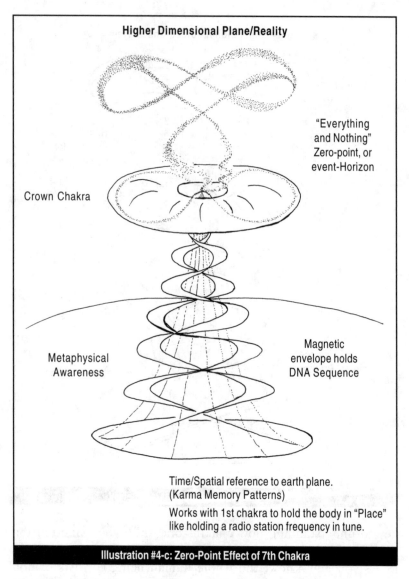

Higher Dimensional Plane/Reality

Crown Chakra

"Everything
and Nothing"
Zero-point, or
event-Horizon

Metaphysical
Awareness

Magnetic
envelope holds
DNA Sequence

Time/Spatial reference to earth plane.
(Karma Memory Patterns)

Works with 1st chakra to hold the body in "Place"
like holding a radio station frequency in tune.

Illustration #4-c: Zero-Point Effect of 7th Chakra

physical plane. It has been put forth by others that the root chakra represents sexuality and base desires, but these are not my observations.

It takes a whole chakra (the root) just to have a physical existence: the root chakra is most effective in representing survivability and existence, or just merely having a physical presence in the third dimension *(see Illustration #4-b)*.

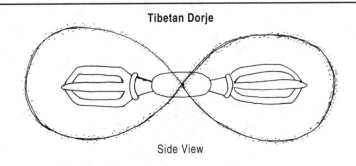

Tibetan Dorje

Side View

Energy Dynamic of a Dorje (also called Vajra)

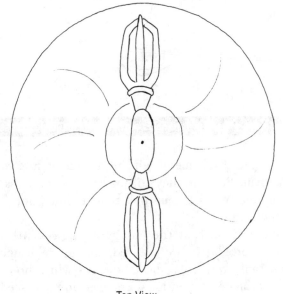

Top View

Toroidal Energy Field
Grasping the Dorje places one's hand over the zero-point, touching
everything and nothing in the same moment.
The field appears flattened into a doughnut shape, but is actually spherical.

Illustration #4-d: Tibetan Dorje and toroidal energy field

The seventh or crown chakra represents the "God spot," or
the point where everything and nothing exists *(see Illustration
#4-c)*. Similar examples (representative of zero-point physics)
are black holes; super condensed stars that may once have been

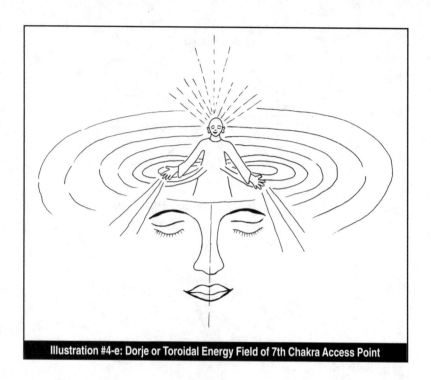

Illustration #4-e: Dorje or Toroidal Energy Field of 7th Chakra Access Point

millions of miles in diameter but are now condensed to the size of a basketball. Because they still have the same mass, they exert such a great gravitational pull that nothing, not even light, escapes their pull.

It is my opinion that the energy of the seventh chakra is similar to a toroidal (donut-shaped) energy field, operating in much the same way as a black hole (or white hole), in that much of the higher dimensional energies are coalesced into the physical plane through the lens of the seventh chakra. Nothing can escape the zero-point region because it represents the totality of reality.

In Tibet, the use of the dorje (*see Illustration #4-d*) or vajra represents the same application in zero point physics, where closing one's hand over the dorje represents grasping the spot where everything and nothing exists, the seamless integration in the Oneness through the destruction of the illusion of separation.

The access point through the seventh chakra represents the point where everything and nothing exists, (*see Illustration #4-*

e) and it is the grasping of this point that allows the transcendence of the limitations of a physical existence into the seamlessness of the Oneness that *includes* a physical existence.

There is no "progression" in successive lifetimes from a lower chakra to a higher one. A person who incarnates in this lifetime in his heart chakra is not further advanced nor more a part of the Oneness than another person who incarnates with a second chakra dominance.

In the higher dimensions, there is no linearity; there is no 1-2-3 or A-B-C. One thing does not follow another. Rather, it seems to be a pervasiveness where everything and nothing exists at once, and there are no moments, just a "beingness."

No one lives in a doorway or gateway, but rather in rooms. Chakras one and seven are true gateways of consciousness, but not a dwelling place of the conscious mind.

In contrast, chakras two through six represent rooms or "places of dwelling" that originate the most major aspects in the ways human beings respond to and interact with the physical dimension.

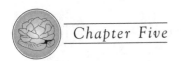

Chapter Five

Subcategories of Dominant Chakras

There are subcategories, or themes, as the subtleties of the dominant chakra differentiate and externalize through the individual. These subcategories should be considered "job descriptions" or specializations of the given dominant chakra.

Not everyone specializes into a subcategory, and some of the categories repeat for more than one chakra. These labels are just pronounced qualities of the given chakra dominant person that will affect an entire lifetime.

Specializations of the Dominant Chakra

Second Chakra

The Lusty Human Being

The Mystic

The Pioneer, the Explorer

The Visionary

The Way Shower, The Person of Two Worlds

The Harmonizer, The Conductor

Harmony through Chaos

The Warrior

The Emotional Anchor

Third Chakra

The Protector of Those Who Cannot Protect Themselves
The Defender of the Innocent
The Person of Ultimates
The Pairs of Opposites
Harmony Through Conflict
The Good King
The Beneficent Dictator
The Spiritual Leader

Fourth Chakra

The Healer
The Hub at the Center of the Many-Spoked Wheel
The Person of Symmetry
Relationship with the Fairy Kingdom
The Preserver
The Conservationist
The Ecologist
The Emotional Anchor

Fifth Chakra

The Destroyer (of illusion), the Sword of Michael
Frequency Matching
The Teacher
The Person out of Time

Sixth Chakra

The Prophet
The Person Out of Time
The Autist
The Hermit

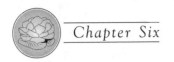

Chapter Six

Higher and Lower Aspects of Each Chakra

Each chakra has a higher and a lower aspect. You will operate from a given chakric disposition according to your level of clarity and accomplishment as a soul meeting your challenges in this lifetime.

A *higher chakric aspect* means that the qualities most optimal for a given chakra are present and in operation. You are aware of your higher nature and exude those given qualities. You would have learned to treat your Self as much with the higher aspect as you would towards others.

A *lower chakric aspect* is fraught with illusions and suffering inherent in pacing through the lessons you have chosen to learn within the dominant chakra. The lessons you learn become repetitive. Their nature is determined by the law of cause and effect, and you will achieve the same effect until the cause is changed.

You go through the lower aspects of your given chakra until you learn the life lesson and produce a more optimal effect. Once the effect is changed, there is usually no need to repeat it, unless for some reason you willingly cycle back into the lesson once again, or there is some karmic reason why the lesson must be repeated until your individual or group karma is satisfied.

Following is an overview of the higher and lower aspects of the main chakras *two through six*. You will find a more detailed discussion in each chakra chapter.

Second Chakra

Higher Aspect: The Creationist; the Visionary; one who sees the big picture; one who helps others and oneself with optimal development and performance in life.

Lower Aspect: The Martyr and Victim; hopelessness, the state of no power, loss of faith. "Nothing ever turns out well no matter what I do; my best is never good enough."

Third Chakra

Higher Aspect: Charismatic Leader, or one who stands in the authority and authenticity of Self.

Lower Aspect: The Manipulator, or one who is being manipulated; one who is expert at procrastinating one's own development, especially through the illusion of being busy or being distracted by addictions. One who sometimes maintains relationships with less powerful people to avoid growth. "If I seek my power it will destroy my relationships."

Fourth Chakra

Higher Aspect: The Empath, or one who exists as love itself. You heal others merely by your presence. You have accepted the purity that you've earned in previous lifetimes.

Lower Aspect: The human emotional pincushion; one who takes on the emotional problems and suffering of others as though deserving to suffer; one who feels not qualified for or deserving of love.

Fifth Chakra

Higher Aspect: The Communicator, or the multi-dimensional teacher who accepts "students" who are drawn to you. You recognize your communicative abilities are 95% non-verbal, but energetic on many levels.

Lower Aspect: Continuously ungrounded and mentally/emotionally/spiritually unfounded. Bobbing like a cork on the sea of life, only reacting to life's issues.

Sixth Chakra

Higher Aspect: The Prophet. One who grounds new paradigms on the earth plane; one who is the inceptor of the evolving group consciousness and plays the lead in the process.

Lower Aspect: One who is in constant analysis of any given situation. One who experiences an un-groundedness that is neurological and consists of mentalisms and mental abstractions. One who has the most difficulty getting into heart-based reality.

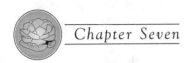

Chapter Seven

First Chakra - Survivability

The first or "root" chakra, located at the base of the spine, is concerned with existence and physical being. Merely having a physical presence on this planet takes a whole chakra to define one's stature as a human being.

In my practice I have not seen anyone who qualifies as a first chakra *dominant* individual. It seems that the first chakra is a secondary influence with a primary protocol, meaning the first chakra emphasizes what it is to be in a physical body in a temporal and linear dimension. For some, having a physical body can be a severe experience when their vibratory rate encounters the reality of third dimensional existence.

I have seen several clients who have a first chakra effect on their dominant chakra that caused serious issues with grounding, relating to leg and foot problems. Some have come onto this earth plane of existence with much distress in the mental, physical, emotional, and spiritual areas of their lives because of grounding issues.

Several clients have exhibited problems that I psychically saw in each category, including but not limited to:

- *Mental* – Locked into a lower state of consciousness, survival, quick changes of mind, sudden decisions based on perceived constriction of incoming ideas and thoughts.
- *Physical* – Circulatory issues in the legs, scoliosis, knee issues, cramping in lower legs and arches, raised/fallen arches, foot problems. Problems in the areas of the perineum, genitals, urinary tract.

- *Emotional* – Fight or flight syndrome when emotionally challenged. Issues with remaining incarnate; can suffer suicidal tendencies.
- *Spiritual* – Somatic life, cut off from God/universe.

Think of the first chakra as a gateway to the physical dimension, where one contacts the earth plane while in physical manifestation of the body. The first chakra is the gateway for the experience of being in this dimension. It takes a whole first chakra just to be here.

Philosophers wrestle with the problem of experience: *Is our eye having an experience of sight and reporting it to our mind? Is the eye merely passing information, so that our mind may have the experience? Or is there something behind our mind that is having the experience of our eye's vision and our mind's conception of what is?*

You can see that philosophers grapple with what many of us take for granted – that we are physical beings having continual dynamic metaphysical experiences. This begs the statement that we truly do exist on *all levels*, but to embrace that statement means we must yield to our qualitative nature. This is the most difficult tenet of metaphysics; that we exist in a Oneness, where there is no separation. In fact, it is the other way around: we are metaphysical beings having the illusion of a physical experience.

It is a great paradox, for how can you live in Oneness and yet experience individuality? Only through an intimate, revelatory experience, an epiphany, can you know the truth of the paradox. It cannot be learned any other way.

The search for meaning and understanding begins with vulnerability to your higher nature, recognizing that there is a continuity that is endless, ceaseless, and seamless.

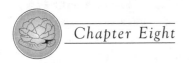

Chapter Eight

Second Chakra - The Creationist

Of all seven chakras, the second is the most closely connected to the five physical senses. It is what I call the *visceral chakra* – the main portal of consciousness through which the input of the five senses (seeing, hearing, tasting, smelling, touching) creates the perception and judgment of our physical world.

This chapter is longer than the others because so many of us have issues related to the second chakra, regardless of which chakra may be dominant. As our sense of life and living, creativity, love and lust, sexuality and sensuousness, perception and meaning are products of our five physical senses, we must play the experience on the life stage through our karma, mission statement, and freewill.

The second chakra is associated with creativity, burdens and responsibilities, sexuality and sensuality. It is the "salsa" of what it is to be a human being.

Imagine the creative consciousness that flows through the second chakra in this way: You are in a spaceship, orbiting at a comfortable distance around the sun. No matter which orbit you take, equatorial, polar, or any other, the view is that the sun (your second chakra) is a brilliant sphere of light radiating outward in all directions. The power of creation through the second chakra emanates through the individual with such magnitude that the sense of responsibility also creates the fear of letting go, the fear of creation, and more.

Now imagine that your physical mind is like the earth, a small sphere located a great distance away from the sun. The mind only receives a small portion of the available light, but knows that the light from the sun (second chakra) is emanating in all directions. Since the mind is linear and the chakra is multi-dimensional, the mind attempts to imitate the chakra, but is limited to linear expression. Your second chakra is ever-unfolding, self-evolving, always creating; no matter what your mind is doing. This is our great dilemma - the physical and non-physical planes meeting in the *linear* desires of the mind to make sense out of our *multi-dimensional* existence.

The resolution of these two seemingly separate states of being is the essence of our evolution.

The greatest fear of second chakra individuals is that they cannot create anything greater than what has come before. Their life path is colored by a desire to control the outcome of what they create. It takes many forms and examples, as many as there are second chakra dominant people. Often, they equate creativity with how hard they must work.

The lesson here is that true creativity is effortless, especially if you live in effortless congruity with higher Self through an intense trust and faith. The more willing you are to trust in your own higher chakric aspect, the more effortlessly your life path flows. Knowing that you can create whatever is needed to meet the challenges of life is at once the easiest and the hardest part of having a dominant second chakra.

Another difficulty for the person whose dominant chakra is the second arises from having goodness of heart; you seek to externalize the powerful aspect of creativity by seeking to help others. You can assume too many responsibilities in order to validate your existence, assuming the illusion that because you can create, you *must* create for others. This is due to the strong mysticism emanating from the second chakra, the visionary, who can see others as they could be, whole and complete. This is the essence of a life-long lesson in creating for your Self as much as creating for others – the resolution of the *illusion of separateness*.

The sun is constantly reinventing itself as a nuclear process of fission, never the same, constantly changing and creating light, heat, and radiant energy. It has existed for three billion years and will exist for another three billion years. Our lifespan makes that of the sun infinitely long by comparison. Thus, the relationship to its creative aspect seems limitless. The limitless nature of this creative process is flowing through the second chakra individual twenty-four hours a day, ever-evolving and self-unfolding, and thus externalizes through the linear mind in various creative ways, according to karma, mission statement, and freewill of the individual.

Those in their second chakra are oriented towards life with an infinite amount of creative life-force through the mental, physical, spiritual, and emotional aspects of their being. They are composed of tremendous creative abilities, as well as the ability to assume great burdens in life. This can be a problem. Some who have this disposition may feel a certain urgency to create, to be and to do. They can feel the pressure of responsibility to create and to know the right answers, and often are very hard on themselves. There is a driving force that causes the individual to seek outlets for the creative expression. The personality of this individual may be constantly involved in Self-evolution.

The second chakra individual inspires others, who are shown an inner spirit ray (inspiration), because the second chakra individual represents infinite possibilities and alternatives. The more soul-infused the second chakra personality, the more effect there is on the spiritual growth of those around him.

Second chakra people make great architects, interior designers, engineers, artists, visionaries, poets and romantics.

Second Chakra Responsibility

In a constant effort to create, the good heart of the second chakra individual may take on increasing responsibilities, like a juggler with three balls in the air who says, "Throw me another." A fourth ball is added and you say you can handle more until you are juggling so many things you come to implosion, and entropy ensues, starting the cycle of reinvention.

The intense creative consciousness that comes through the second chakra causes a disposition in the mind and thoughts to be in a creative aspect continuously - so much so that you tend to validate your Self based on how many responsibilities you carry. If you are not continuously creating or taking on responsibilities, you may feel a lack of purposefulness or fulfillment in life.

The Law of Shelves

Imagine you have a child. You decide to put up a shelf in her bedroom. What's the probability that she'll place "stuff" on that shelf? 100%? What if you put up two shelves? Three? More stuff, right? The point is that as a second chakra individual, you tend to place as much responsibility on your Self for creation as there is room to do so. It does not matter how many shelves there are, the universe will fill them.

The positive benefit of this law is that if you decide your life is that of effortless creation, there will always be enough that flows through you to see to the needs of others, if you keep your Self emotionally whole and complete first. The concept of "enough" is what is *Divinely appropriate*, not what your linear mind thinks is appropriate.

The negative benefit is that the second chakra individual will always have a tendency to add more things (multiple shared priorities) to their lives, thus creating chaos with too many things to do. As with any chakra, these are life issues: not meant to be totally overcome, but rather to continue to work on in order to develop character. Part of the life issues of the second chakra individual is to continually work to reduce their shared commitments to a manageable number.

One of the bigger mistakes second chakra individuals make is that when creative power flows through you, you think you must create by your Self, and not in collaborative leadership with the infinitude of the universe. You assume you have to do it alone, when it is always a partnership (really, the Oneness). The more you release your Self into that partnership, however, the more harmoniously your life flows, because you've partnered your linear mind with your higher Self, through trust.

Second Chakra Sexuality

Some individuals may be highly sexual, as a strong spiritual concept of sensuality through the second chakra may transcend the prevalent belief system concerning sexual conduct. Heightened sexuality relates to the consciousness of creativity that externalizes through the second chakra. In fact, you can be a polyamorist to the extent of having the capability of being in unconditional love and having more than one intimate relationship at the same time. To the polyamorist, you are truly in love with each individual you are intimate with, and may have great difficulty letting go of prior relationships even if they ended badly.

Such individuals may also cross gender lines and express an androgynous (male and female together) orientation toward sexuality. It is because they perceive the whole individual on higher levels of existence. The danger for second chakra individuals is losing themselves in possible illusions or in the grandness of their vision. They need to keep aware of their personal boundaries to preserve their sense of integrity.

Sexuality and metaphysics, especially for those who are healers, can be a very difficult blend to reconcile because it brings into question morals, ethics, and religious orientation. We all have a sense of right and wrong, and sexuality is a natural expression of our desires and longing for Oneness. It is all too easy to place a burden of guilt (which a second chakra person so easily bears) on one's sexuality by labeling as "right" and "wrong" one's sexual orientation, desires, and feelings.

In my work, I have found that our higher spiritual nature, because of its androgyny, does not make a distinction between male and female, sexual orientation (hetero, gay, lesbian, bisexual), or sexual conduct, other than whether love is at the root of the relationship. Moral and ethical questions are for the individual to decide, as no one but you holds the keys to the evolution of your soul.

So many people suffer needlessly because they have taken upon themselves the presumption of guilt through their desires. Is the guilt because of what others think? To be liberated one must let go of guilt and shame.

I've counseled many people who exhibit a strong second chakra sexuality but do not know what to do with its power. Some feel that unleashing it (though they sincerely desire to) would too quickly transcend the emotional and social barriers they have been living by. These same individuals often have difficulty expressing their desires to their partners for fear of rejection, ridicule, and other blows to their self-validation.

Remember, the second chakra is the visceral chakra; the

chakra most closely connected to our sensuality (meaning *of the senses*). The sexual urge, through the second chakra, seeks creative expression. Channeling it through healthy emotional boundaries, through healthy relationships, and especially through a fierce love of self-integrity, is the best way to grow in understanding your own sexuality.

Energetic healers have suffered needlessly because their gifts have been misinterpreted as sexual in nature when the energy of the second chakra was misread to be in a lower, sex-magic realm. That may happen because of energetic projections by the patient onto the healer. Of course, healers must have impeccably healthy emotional energy boundaries or they have no business being in the profession. The discussion of our energetic relationships with each other, including sex-magic, will be covered at length in my next book, *Your Chakric Relationships*.

Second Chakra Attributes

The second chakra dominant individual incarnates to create, to bring something from nothing. You come to be the visionary and the creationist, to illustrate to the world the new way of doing things and the new way of experiencing the world with the five senses, sensuously. It is a world of infinite possibilities; the ever-unfolding and self-renewing energies prominently urging the personality, through the soul, to expand your horizons and to be the example of what your passions can accomplish.

Through those passions, endless creativity flows in countless ways, always illustrating to humanity the infinite creative potential of your nature, and the power to completely reinvent your Self.

The second chakra dominant individual also comes here to teach faith and to inspire others, often through deep and serious tests of your own where you must lose your faith, sometimes losing everything else as well, only to reinvent your Self and rise like the Phoenix through the ashes of your lower understanding.

The same energy disposition of creativity that is your strength is your weakness, as well. You must in some way prove that as the second chakra disposition is ever-unfolding and self-evolving, so too are you. You must inspire your Self. And that is only accomplished through trusting and having faith in your Self. Sometimes we must re-invent ourselves several times in one lifetime, if only to prove that as souls *we can.*

The energy of the mystic is solely related to the second chakra: The second chakra dominant person is the mystic, imbued with the ability to intuitively, accurately see how others, but rarely your Self, can be as whole and complete. Many relationships are built on these intuitive assumptions made about your partners. But whether your partner is ready, willing, or able to be whole and complete is another question.

Second chakra individuals came here to learn something different – to accept, to love, and to trust in your Self. The urgency of the second chakra induces the creativity to externalize to the outward world, often at the expense of Self, in the mistaken assumption that doing well for others evolves your soul. This is one of the key errors that a second chakra person makes: that because you can create so very well, you must create for others, and that what you create will naturally be accepted by others. This error is the core of many relationship problems.

It is a mistake to build your validation on how much you can accomplish for others. But it is a matter of how much love you are willing to *receive* that defines the evolution of your soul as a second chakra individual. This is a very easy, yet very costly mistake to make, if you assume that duty to humanity takes care of duty to Self. It does not. *You must accept as much love as you give to keep the energy equal.* The vulnerability involved in this decision is the fulcrum upon which much suffering weighs: All abundance, abandonment, and abuse issues come from the consciousness through the second chakra.

Is it a wonder that strong second chakra individuals constantly reinvent themselves? And it's not uncommon for them to do it several times in one lifetime.

One of the second chakra's attributes is to remember your power of *choice* - that freewill is always available. Heaven on earth for you would mean that as your energy is always creating, it is always available to tap into. But Heaven on earth also means that nothing happens until there is an act of will to join the two. Your mind sleeps, thinks and contemplates, becomes filled with doubt, but must ultimately recognize that no matter what it is doing, the second chakra is ever-creating and available through the ability to be vulnerable to your Inner-Creator. Remembering that you are the infinite Oneness in which you exist, releases limitation.

How could it be otherwise? And could you say this of all people? Perhaps, but different chakra dominant people have different influences and perceptions of this dimension. You cannot love unconditionally from a position of weakness, but many second chakra people are weakened with disease, emotional disorder, poor relationships, self-loathing and more, because they make the fundamental mistake of working harder at the relationship without working on themselves and their ability to receive love. Until this is addressed, their souls will progress only very slowly, and many lessons will ensue to create the opportunity to receive love and allow self-acceptance.

Higher and Lower Aspects of the Second Chakra

The difference between chaos and focus can be measured by inner faith. The higher and lower aspects of the second chakra are a natural consequence of faith, trust, a fierce love of one's Self, and the will to choose passion, inspiration, healthy emotional boundaries, focus, and a simple life. Higher aspects reflect a life well-lived through the dominant chakra characteristics.

Higher aspects of the second chakra:

1. The Creationist
2. The Visionary, Explorer, Pioneer
3. The Labyrinth, the Walk of Faith
4. The Healer
5. The Fierce Lover
6. Infinite Alternatives
7. The Wayshower

8. Master of Many Trades, Jack of None/Simultaneity
9. The Harmonizer
10. The Lusty Human Being
11. The Warrior

Lower aspects reflect fear, manipulation, and ignorance, which result in much suffering involving physical, mental, emotional, and spiritual issues.

Lower aspects of the second chakra:

1. Chaos
2. Loss of Identity, Integrity, Inspiration
3. Apocalyptic
4. Reverse Chaotic, Manipulator
5. The Victim, Martyr
6. False Humility, Self-effacing
7. Passive-Aggressive, Codependent
8. Squandering One's Power
9. Self-destruction, Self-loathing, Hopelessness
10. Remorse, Regret, Resentment, Guilt
11. Abuse, Abundance, Abandonment
12. Vampiric Energy
13. Control

Higher Aspects of the Second Chakra Explained

1. The Creationist

The creationist is one who brings about something from nothing. A perfect example of this in everyday life is a woman. At one moment she is as herself, but when she becomes pregnant, she will bring something from nothing, if you will - a baby. The child is not the mother, not the same person, even though he/she came from the mother's body. Where there was nothing but the mother, there is created something new.

We breathe in and out, and we are made in the image of the Creator. That means the universe breathes in and out. Your creativity is a rhythmic association with the breath of the universe coming through your higher organs; your chakras. When the universe breathes in, you are inspired. When the universe breathes out, you are creating, externalizing your soul's desires into this dimension.

As you learn to breathe this creativity through your inner trust, you act in concert with your higher Self; your life manifests the infusion of your soul-quality into your personality. You become more soul-like.

If the second chakra could only be described by a single word, it would be *creativity*. The ever-unfolding, self-evolving aspect of the second chakra that surpasses the linear concept of time and space is ever-present in us all. Accessing that ability is something we all can do. Trusting in that ability is another matter.

This is why some of the greatest creationists have been the least understood people in history. They brought forth something from nothing in their passion and desire to create the same beauty that inspired them from above to manifest in this dimension. As above, so below: Heaven on earth.

You will see in this and succeeding chapters that each chakra dominance presents unique tests for bringing Heaven on earth. Second chakra dominant creationists must have absolute faith in their ability to create something from nothing.

As a creationist, you may, through the Law of Reciprocity, bring people into your life who have lost hope, who are very linear, or who are in a very low level of creation (creating the same problem over and over).

You are present in this lifetime to bring forth the something from nothing that the rest of us cannot yet see, even if it has been right in front of us. You are the puzzle-master, who, like the visionary, sees the whole picture and offers the "something" the rest of us has been trying to find.

One of the interesting things about the metaphysics of this is that the rest of us created the opportunity for the creationist to exist, to show us the something from nothing, to show us the answer. All too often we disconnect ourselves from the very answer we seek - we separate our own higher ability to create from the answer in front of us, and do not realize that we are the inception itself.

Explained later, soul-groups create the creationist, the truth-giver, the teacher, and so on. Most do not realize it, but that is the reciprocity of our universe. *We are all creating something from nothing.*

2. The Visionary, Explorer, Pioneer

The visionary sees the whole, the complete process, and is not destined to get involved in the details. Many potentially great visionaries get mired in the details of their vision, often with control issues, due to the mind's fear that it cannot create anything greater than what has come before. In certain cases visionaries can become so stuck that they live their lives through others, through vicarious association, and thus do not reach their soul's potential in the given lifetime.

As a visionary, you must learn to delegate, just as the king does not go into the bakery to bake bread, and the CEO does not go into accounting to run the reports. You must remain at the top, responsible to your Self. You may ask, "What do you mean 'delegate'? I have no one to delegate to!" Well, you must delegate to your Self the personal boundaries that prevent squandering resources on unnecessary or off-center goals. You must delegate the authority to receive, to put a value on what you do. Your goal is to be totally in your power, and you cannot be so if you are too busy serving everyone else's goals and needs.

Were you to seek out a guru and ask to be a healer, the wise one would tell you to first heal your Self. In that moment, you would have to decide to love your Self so fiercely that you would not surrender any of your power, for you cannot assist anyone from a position of weakness. Neither can you love unconditionally from a position of weakness. You must first be in your strength, which is defined by your appropriate healthy personal boundaries. Only you can decide what those boundaries are. Remember that surrendering your power to others, even through good actions, will put you outside of your center and into a state of weakness.

To be in a healthy relationship, the second chakra individual must have freedom of independence, and also a watchful eye that codependence doesn't result from being given so much freedom that it is abused.

The visionary is akin to the pioneer or explorer - one who must blaze a fresh trail. The pioneer is only effective when discovering new ways and new ideas. Your soul's purpose as a visionary and a pioneer is to bring back to society the new ideas, the new ways and the new territory of awareness. This is often done through creative expression such as art and music. However, you must be in that element of creation that is the unknown territory of the physical/emotional/mental/spiritual existence in order to bring higher levels of awareness to humanity. It is then up to humanity to partake (or not) of your visionary experience.

Beethoven was unappreciated in his time; few liked his music. Undaunted, he created his masterpieces of music anyway, as if to say "you don't know what great music is; I'm doing this anyway." When he died, it was estimated that 20,000 people came to his funeral - an impressive number in the days before modern transportation. He became appreciated only after his passing.

This happens so many times with visionaries - appreciated for your gifts only long after your deeds are done. A non-receptive, unappreciative public does not give you due regard for your vision; such is the life of a visionary. You must give to your Self, receive, and accept your Self above all, and then you can help give the vision to as many people as you wish.

3. The Labyrinth, the Walk of Faith

The popular labyrinth image that we see today is modeled after the labyrinth on the floor of the Chartres Cathedral in France, created in 1210 AD (*see Illustration #8-a*). It consists of eleven courses, or successive concentric rings, as a maze. You enter from the outside ring and take the circuitous and winding path, turning back and forth, navigating successive inner rings of the labyrinth to ultimately reach the center of the maze.

Original supplicants to the faith made the long journey on their knees! Instead of our knees, we must navigate the laby-

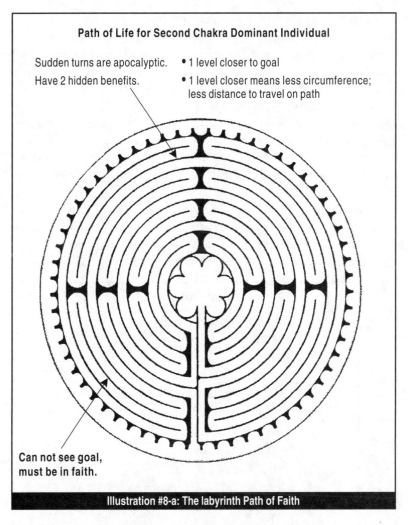

Path of Life for Second Chakra Dominant Individual

Sudden turns are apocalyptic.
Have 2 hidden benefits.

• 1 level closer to goal
• 1 level closer means less circumference; less distance to travel on path

Can not see goal, must be in faith.

Illustration #8-a: The labyrinth Path of Faith

rinth of our life's path with our hearts, through faith and passion.

For a second chakra individual the path through life is very similar. Your goal may be in sight, but often you must traverse the outer course of your labyrinth when it appears the center is off to the left or right. This causes great consternation because it can appear that your goal, while in sight, is tangential to your efforts. It can be frustrating because you may not know how long to stay the current course, feeling no closer to the goal (the center), feeling "off track."

Abruptly, you turn onto a new course. Such is the life of second chakra individuals - a life of faith where you can see the whole picture for others but most times not for your Self. The realization is not immediate that upon turning, you have reached the next course or inner ring towards the goal. That is a level of achievement especially difficult for second chakra personalities, because you tend not to give your Self validation for the arduous course from which you have graduated. You would not see it as an accomplishment because the perfectionist within you would only regard it as a means, not a fulfillment in itself.

The length of time on each circuitous course provides the experience necessary on your life-path before the next inner course (and higher level of consciousness) can be entered. Though this metaphor of the labyrinth can be applied to any-

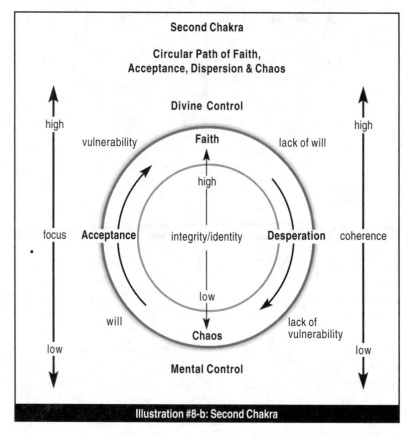

Illustration #8-b: Second Chakra

one, it is particularly applicable to the second chakra individual.

Mystery is what gives your faith elbow room to work. As a second chakra individual, you cannot know how things will turn out to any certainty for your Self, but you can know very well for others.

Some case histories include people who have nearly died and had near death experiences (NDE's), but have been allowed to remain to teach faith to others because of their transitional experience. In this instance, second chakra individuals must embrace with their hearts what their minds cannot yet comprehend or control.

This is a life of faith, where you will pick relationships in which your second chakra will show others the big picture, how they could be as whole and complete. Yours is a life of inner knowing; a fierce tenacity to trust your heart, even when there is neither physical evidence nor concurrence from others to support your feelings.

Some have lost faith and entered into chaos, hopelessness, or into controlling natures from fear *(see Illustration #8b)*. There is a cycle where one may descend into chaos by trying to control the outcome with the mind only, then arise out of it by surrendering to the feelings through the higher Self. As a second chakra individual you must live a life of faith and trust, especially because others may not.

4. The Healer

It is the incredibly strong psychic sense of the whole vision of the second chakra individual that makes a good candidate to be a healer. You tend to see the whole picture, and through the goodness of your heart, attempt to help others to complete the picture of their lives.

There is an extremely delicate balancing act between helping others and helping your Self. On the one hand, if you overextend your helping, you can substitute loyalty for integrity, surrendering your power and supplicating your desires to someone else's goals because you did not have healthy boundaries to love your Self enough.

On the other hand, you can pull in too tightly and stunt

your own spiritual development because you did not perceive your ability to conceive of the entire project, the vision, which is your inherent strength. In this case, the strength of the second chakra becomes the weakness. The very ability to see the whole vision is so great that you assume you have no part in it because of its greatness.

Because of the disposition to see the whole picture, second chakra healers intuitively, automatically know what it takes and what the whole picture looks like, because you "see" the other person as whole and complete. This includes the whole human being - mental, physical, emotional, and spiritual.

One of the difficulties of having a second chakra dominance is that you can see the whole picture without years of studying the "how to" text. This is especially true with energy healing, where trusting your intuitive abilities is absolutely crucial to effective healing. The second chakra healer can "see" the difficulties, but initially dismisses what is accurately seen because it seems too easy, or because it should only come with great study. In fact, the more you are willing to trust your feelings in a healing environment, the more accurate you can be.

Of course, study is important, as is experience. However, if you are to embrace the second chakra fully, absolute trust in feelings is essential. It is at this point that you may ask, "How do I know what I feel is accurate?" Trusting your feelings is a state of being; the mind becomes your partner to your intuitive abilities, not your enemy. Heaven on earth is uniting the physical and metaphysical, mind and intuition. The more you bring these two together, through trust, the more your awareness improves.

Why a Second Chakra Person Makes the Perfect Healer

"All the right wounds." I know several second chakra healers who are superb at what they do because they have all the "right wounds" - the right experiences - to become great healers. These individuals have been through the Trials of Sisyphus. They have accomplished significant self-healing and graduated to a high degree of self-love through the trials of much pain

and inner personal persecution, along with many years of perceived inadequacy and inequality.

It seems these individuals have had the necessary visceral opportunities to experience, as consistent with the second chakra, through their five senses, ultimate forms of sensory input. This orients you to be in a place of having been there first, as the "way-show-er" would be - the one in the soul-group who, as visionary, must experience sensation on the earth plane first, to set the sensory pathway for those to come.

With the tremendous and apocalyptic events that can befall the second chakra individual, the stage is well set to understand the sufferings and the future direction of humanity.

It is the second chakra individual who sits at the end of the beginning for those who wish to follow what you already experienced. These are the true healers.

I have noticed, after years of doing "flower readings," three hand signs or symbols of a healer. (A flower reading is a group event where people bring a flower and I do a reading/healing on each flower, not consciously knowing who brought which one.) Often in these readings I notice a special symbol in the palm of the hands of second chakra healers. Upon physical inspection and verification, most individuals show patterns, in one of three configurations, in the palms of their hands:

- *The letter "M" or "A"* - Signifies "Master."
- *The Star* – The star pattern in the palm of the hand signifies an influence of Quan Yin, or a higher guidance of another evolved being.
- *The Sword* – The sword of Michael the Archangel. Note that a sword means business: it cleaves one thing from another. In this case, it means that the healer is here to destroy illusion.

Often accompanying the symbol in the hands of a healer is a mottled look to the palm. The coloration of the hand is varied, due to tremendous energy flowing through the minor chakra centers in the hands (and often the feet), denoting a person of some considerable energetic healing capabilities.

In recent years, scientific research has determined that the magnetic field measured around the hands of trained energetic healers is hundreds of times stronger than untrained healers.

5. The Fierce Lover

Fierce lovers give 110 percent of their love to their relationships. The danger in doing this is that it can be at the expense of identity and integrity. As a fierce lover, you will give your all; total commitment. But you will have difficulty finding others who are willing to commit equally. The lesson is that you must first commit to your Self; you must love your Self as fiercely as you love others.

Many women have faced the difficulty of total commitment to a relationship that suddenly changes course. You wake up one morning, look at the calendar and say, "Where did the last two years go? What have I been doing?"

The focus of your attention has been on the fierce and passionate love you have given, flowering and flowing forth from your second chakra, in the illusion that doing for others is doing for your Self. You have given your power away. This is a subtle and easily misunderstood circumstance.

Working hard to make a great relationship is honorable. Doing it from a position where you love your Self so much, where you would do nothing to denigrate your character, makes for the greatest relationship because it includes *you* in the process. In this way, you are not leaving your Self out of the creative process of building a relationship between two people.

When a minister marries a couple, the greatest thing said is: "May you each retain your own individuality." Your integrity, once solid, gives you a basis for your identity, the notion of who you are and what you represent. Fierce lovers often lose a sense of Self, working so diligently at making the relationship "work" that they leave themselves and their spiritual health out of the picture. This opens the door for many problems with mental, emotional, spiritual, and physical health.

Some fierce lovers deliberately focus on the other person's life and well-being, because fundamentally you do not want to face your own second chakra issues of self-validation, self-worth, abandonment, or abuse. The fear of not receiving love can cause you to become controlling, where you attempt to "guarantee" a relationship that works.

This is very unhealthy because not only does it impede your spiritual growth, it also impedes the growth of your partner, for it is a lower-level, fear-based relationship that will ultimately cause suffering.

6. Infinite Alternatives

A life-path of the second chakra aspect can be to represent infinite alternatives to the world. Often, through the Law of Reciprocity, you can be raised by rigid and inflexible parents or engage in intimate relationships of the same sort until you recognize your second chakra dominance to continually create. After all, the consciousness of the second chakra represents an ever-unfolding, always-creating state of being, no matter what your mind is doing. The trick is to focus on your continual ability to reinvent and create through the second chakra.

If you consider that the second chakra represents infinite creation, that same creative aspect is infinitely unfolding and ever-evolving. The personality of the second chakra can be overwhelmed by the *infinitude of alternatives* (especially emotionally), but the soul-infused personality can offer these same infinite alternatives to others. You become a font of possibilities.

The strength here is that the second chakra represents infinite creation. Sometimes the rigidity imposed on you by others is the force that pulls the slingshot back far enough so that you will release your Self into a life that represents these infinite alternatives. Of course, nothing happens until you give your Self permission to be free. But look at the example of the slingshot: It is pulled back a few inches until the rubber is taught. The pebble within experiences no movement as long as the tension is there, but what tremendous tension there is. Once let go, the pebble flies a distance much, much farther than the initial few inches that it was held in tension. The tension served as the potential power to propel the pebble very far forward, but only when the pebble was released.

You have to be your own releaser: the tension of being held back is something you experience, especially if you are here to offer infinite alternatives to the world. The fear of being released is that you will move forward very fast, into unknown territory of your feelings, as there are no longer self-imposed impediments to your alternatives.

You must first give the power of choice, the power of alternatives, to your Self. Once you have done so, the rigidity by which you have lived your life - the external impositions and rules - have been replaced by your own "Inner Knower." From that position, your second chakra is accessed through trust. By example, others have the opportunity to offer themselves choices, *because you have.*

But do not forget that just because you have made an optimal decision for your Self and the infusion of your soul-quality, it does not mean that others will too. They also must decide for themselves, even if you are correct (and sometimes *especially* when you are correct), the course of their evolution. You can represent healing to the world, but you must let the world decide for itself. God provides, man decides.

7. The Wayshower (Way-show-er)

The wayshower is like the person who has one foot in the boat and one foot on the dock. Metaphysically this means that the person has one foot in each dimension, through the second chakra. The function of the wayshower is to help others get from this dimension to the next (in their consciousness) by holding the awareness that such realities exist. The problem is that most others do not share the vision, because they either cannot, or because of fear, will not.

For the wayshower, the good news is that you have one foot in each dimension; the bad news is that you have one foot in each dimension. How can both be true? Because your strength is your weakness. Having your reality in two dimensions is a strength because you are not fully anchored in either direction, hence not totally influenced by it. However, the weakness is that not being fully in either dimension can make you feel clumsy and unsure. If, for example, your most recent past life was not on earth, your polarity as a wayshower can be greatly exacerbated, accentuating the difference between you and society.

But, one person must go first into the higher levels to be the visionary. There must be a signpost for others to follow. The problem with being a wayshower, like that of the visionary, is that you can have that most unappreciated of lives, perhaps being born way ahead of your time. No one is *really* born ahead of their time, but you can shoulder a tremendous second chakra responsibility of being the visionary, or wayshower, when no one around you is, or if they lack the vision.

Mozart, Beethoven, Kepler, Schauberger were all wayshowers who were ridiculed and unappreciated in their own time. They bridged the gap of understanding and awareness, some died poor, some in unmarked graves. It can be a most difficult path because the wayshower does have knowledge of the other dimension: it is in you, a part of you, whether you want it or not.

8. Master of Many Trades, Jack of None/ Simultaneity

In coping with the consciousness coming through the chakra, second chakra personalities often labor under the assumption that you should be able to accomplish many goals at the same time. You are probably a list maker who has several concurrent projects in varying states of completion. It is not uncommon for people of "simultaneity" to exhibit different states of physical externalization through your organizational skills. One may be highly efficient and organized, while another may have "piling systems" of organized chaos, with stacks of papers, memos, magazines, etc. everywhere.

A person of simultaneity feels so because of an ability to psychically perceive the whole picture. Attempting to make that psychic picture fit in the third dimension of limitation, the linear mind cannot make all of the non-linear qualitative aspects of consciousness fit into a quantitative state. You perceive so much, but often get caught in the same great vision when attempting to bring all of it into physical reality at once.

Many second chakra people have the ability to multi-task, and to do everything rather well. The *old* saying is: "Jack of all trades, master of none." I have reworked this phrase to: "Master of all trades, Jack of none," because the second chakra individual's driving force is sheer creativity.

It can also be said that you may be a master at starting tasks, but not of finishing them. This one little detail has been the cause of much guilt for second chakra people. Your life can be organized chaos, like so many plants that have taken over the backyard in an explosion of creativity.

I have found that it does not matter so much that there is a little chaos in your life. It is the amount of attachment to the feelings about that chaos that matters most. I have seen many second chakra individuals who are intensely creative, but who are not the most organized or neatest of folks.

There is another downside of this higher aspect that second chakra individuals must overcome: If you are master of many trades, you become a "moving target," and it's very difficult to love a moving target. You can be absorbed in so many tasks that you are emotionally unavailable to receive love from others, and therefore you are not in your higher aspect. You can see how it is possible to use the excuse of "staying busy" to conveniently avoid dealing with receiving love from others.

We know that society likes to impose a single attribute on people. A second chakra individual might endure a great amount of personal persecution due to society imposing the "pick one thing and do it well" mindset. Parental influence and peer pressure exert tremendous energy on you to force an unnatural adaptation of your immense creativity into a single mold. It is in your nature to do many things well, and not to adopt a single personality.

Many second chakra individuals suffer because you attempt to focus on one thing only, when it is not in your nature to do so. While it is your tendency to create, the pitfall is in creating unmanageability.

Galileo, Copernicus, and Emmanuel Swedenborg are examples of such people. As with any chakra, there must exist a harmonious balance between creativity and functionality to achieve a meaningful and productive life. If you are given to such creativity and the undertaking of simultaneous tasks, it is in your best interest to make the number of tasks manageable.

A healthy exercise is to take an inventory, at regular intervals (daily, weekly, monthly, as you see fit), of how many tasks, obligations, and projects you have committed to. Reduce the number: If it is 20, make it 12, if it is 10, make it 7, if it is 5, make it 3, and so on. It is not enough to do this exercise once: You must do it regularly for life, because it is a life issue of the second chakra, not just a "today issue."

9. The Harmonizer

When a symphony orchestra is warming up, it makes a cacophony of noise. It is disjointed, chaotic, and uncontrolled.

The conductor walks in, raises a baton, and seventy-two instruments play together in congruity. The harmonizer is a second chakra person who helps to harmonize the energies of others by helping them to create balance. The danger is that you can spend your time improving the lives of others without improving your own.

Harmony means to make discordant energies flow together in congruity. No two musical instruments sound alike, not even two of the same type of violin. All our planets, though different, orbit around the sun in a synchronous orchestration of movement. As a harmonizer, you put things in their natural order, and have a wonderful sense of balance, poise, and elegance. Poise is grace and power. Elegance is poise with the power of the will.

Harmonizers draw harmony from chaos, and because of the Law of Reciprocity, tend to draw chaos and chaotic people into your life. One of the lessons you will learn is that of equanimity; the ability to remain calm when all around is chaotic. It teaches you that you always have a choice; that you can choose to be calm in a room full of chaos. This is a major lesson for the second chakra person.

Even if you have the ability to harmonize the lives of others, you still have a freewill choice to remain in chaos despite your best efforts. You only have control over your own freewill, not that of others.

10. The Lusty Human Being

Writer and lecturer Louise Hay said, "Sometimes the bowl of our love is scoured out deeply by great pain so that we can know great joy." The life of the lusty human being often starts with great pain and great trials because this brings about the conditioning and experience necessary to allow the creative flow of the second chakra through the five senses.

Lusty human beings will sometimes have experiences that none of the rest of us would want to have. But if you are one, you are often very brave, insisting that you don't just want to hear of someone else's exploits, you want to experience it for *your Self*. This applies even if the experience is very painful. It is one of the ways second chakra individuals know they are alive and viable, through their five senses, in this dimension.

In Western society, the word "lust" is most often associated with sex, and though the term does include sex and sexuality, it is meant to mean the sensual existence, as applies to those who exist with a very strong association with their physical senses.

So often these individuals are observed reacting to their environment, say, a beautiful sunset, and emoting heavily. You turn to the person next to you and exclaim your exuberance: "Would you just look at that sunset!!" only to find that person bland and uninterested. Lusty human beings often have difficulty finding others who share the depth of their senses. You share some of the problems of the visionary in getting others to be aroused to their passions.

The worst thing the lusty human being can do is to ignore your passion. This is made more poignant in a relationship, where expressing your feelings may be difficult or even frowned upon. To give up your passion is to starve your senses, as you live your joy (and sorrow) through your second chakra.

As a second chakra individual, you must live in your passion, ignore the rejection, and follow your heart. It is vitally important for you to express that infinite love and creativity in your heart. Doing so raises your vibration, infuses more of your soul-quality into your personality, and provides the best opportunity for the evolution of your soul-group. You may not find many people as "lusty" as you are, but better to fully express your soul than to wait for society to catch up to you. If you wish to be truly alive, you must follow your passion.

11. The Warrior

The warrior is one who fiercely believes in something worth fighting for and worth protecting. As a warrior, you selflessly project your Self into the world, into the fray, to stand for what is true and noble, often uncompromising in your passion to defend what is worth defending.

The warrior stands for a belief or a paradigm (truth or set of truths). Warriors can give their lives to their causes. The worst thing that can happen to you is that you become so consumed holding up the banner for what you are defending that you forget the reason for the banner. You can also spend so much time defending the cause that you lose part of your identity in the process.

The problem warriors face concerns loyalty to the very causes you defend. Because you represent the ability to take on great burdens, you tend to take on major causes *because you can*. Just because you can do a thing, does not mean that you must!

A warrior, by definition, fights for a cause or to defend the nature (in principle) of the cause. As a second chakra individual you can get very involved in issues of loyalty or in defending a loyalty, but you may tend to forget the reason or the foundation of the cause. Warriors are dedicated, fierce, and loyal, but your shortcoming is that you are all of these qualities for others, not for your Self.

The warrior, as the second chakra, requires the renewing strength of inspiration, revisiting the creative aspect to recharge your passion to be the warrior. You must consistently remind your Self of the cause and why you have invested in it, or remorse, regret, and other self-deprecating afflictions can ensue.

Warriors train over and over, for the preparation of war, praying that it never comes. So it is with the second chakra warrior, who spends time contemplating how to best be in world service, selfless service, committed to a relationship, and sometimes unappreciated for your valor.

Chameleon Warrior

The chameleon changes its coloring to match its immediate surroundings. It attempts to blend into the twig, but it is not the twig. It attempts to blend into the leaf, but it is not the leaf. So too, you attempt to blend, through fear, into surroundings that are not your Self, in an illusion of defenselessness to an attacker that never comes. You may spend too much time in the lower aspect in fear of events that have not yet transpired. The higher aspect of the warrior allows you to blend into your surroundings so as not to take on responsibilities that are not yours.

There is a tremendous feeling of responsibility that comes with the second chakra, and many feel that because you can create, you must also create a lot of responsibility. Staying in your higher aspects as the warrior, you will instead choose your battles and responsibilities carefully, and remember the cause.

Lower Aspects of the Second Chakra Explained

1. Chaos

Chaos is the spreading out or diffusion of the coherent light of creativity. Creativity is like a laser beam - phase-coherent light that is tightly bound by the integrity of Divine inspiration. The beam (focus) disperses when individuals are fraught with doubt and trepidation because they cannot foresee or control the outcome of their initial inspiration, or when they have assumed too many multiple shared priorities, or when they insist on acting without the inspiration of Divine will. When the chaos becomes a continuum, the momentum of the creative spark is lost.

The second chakra can also represent such creative capacity as to be overwhelming, with too many alternatives. Some individuals have difficulty making commitments in relationships, either because they are in chaos, or because they feel there are such infinite alternatives that no one person can satisfy them.

The way out of chaos, the way to gather back the creativity, is to be totally present in each moment, knowing that you may control only that moment in time and no other. Using inspiration, your inner connection provides that intimate and sacred feeling that the visceral chakra is connected to the earth plane, and is creating anew (see Illustration #8b). Remembering that you have freewill to choose, and choose again, is to remember this dimension is an illusion, where the only importance is in the present moment.

Second chakra people can become obsessed by the goal, but

it is more important to remember that it is the *effort* that defines the nature of the development of your character. It is important to plan and have goals, but not at the expense of the moment.

In that moment of inspiration are borne all of the possibilities and alternatives, and those are borne in every moment thereafter. *It is in the living of each moment that we find our power and our inspiration*; the God-within externalizes in all present moments through trust, faith, and our willingness to let go of control and be inspired.

Chaos also results in hopelessness. You chart a course on a downward, involutionary spiral (as opposed to an upward, evolutionary spiral) if you rely only on your mind and not your intuitive resources, or better put, your access to Divine inspiration.

Chaos can be used as a tool to prevent growth by avoiding responsibility to your Self. But chaos can also be a terrible scourge of your emotions and spirit, in that it effectively hides spiritual faith, the Divine connection. Some people in chaos suffer greatly because the pain of separation from their creativity is so great that they cannot perceive their inner connection clearly. The dim connection causes much suffering and grief because not enough soul-quality has been infused into your personality through faith and the will to live a focused life.

Chaos can be used as a way of preventing the taking on of success. The fear of success can be accentuated in that by guaranteeing you are in chaos, you never have to deal with achievement.

Many people miss the important point that in healing, the next step is to deal with the success of being healed, the success of overcoming deficiencies in your life, the success of success. This is another key to the second chakra: knowing that you are infinitely creating beyond what your mind can think, with that intuitive part of you that is accessing all possibilities and alternatives, *including success*.

As with other chakras, balance is a moment-to-moment endeavor. It is in the power of the moment that the nature of your character is defined. To overcome chaos, the second chakra person must practice equanimity, the ability to choose calm, even when it is chaotic all about. Equanimity is a choice; it enables you to stay focused, even if no one else is.

This is similar to choosing faith through the will to connect to the Inner Knower, even when there is no physical evidence to support the choice. It can be no other way if you are to unfold your life's purpose as a creationist.

2. Loss of Identity, Integrity, Inspiration

The loss of identity is not a first-cause in a second chakra individual, but is the result of the dispersion of your energies though emotional overwhelm, false assumptions and expectations, taking on too many responsibilities or loyalties and "getting lost in the details." Your sense of personal identity is meant to include a type of sacredness, or holiness, a sense of being precious, of the integrity of Self and self-preservation. The opposite is self-destruction.

"Integrity for loyalty" is a condition of the second chakra where you become more loyal to your promises and responsibilities to others than to your Self. You sacrifice your integrity for loyalty.

When you lose your sense of inspiration, you lose your integrity. When you lose your integrity, you lose your identity, as in the example of waking up in a relationship and wondering where "you" have been.

That sacredness and preciousness of Self is due regard for the integrity the second chakra individual has as creator, bringing forth something from nothing. When your energies are squandered, the second chakra becomes chaotic and loses focus. When the chaos becomes significant enough, you go through issues of identity, purposefulness of direction, loss of inspiration, and the world becomes very black and white, with little or no perceived options.

The relationship of identity to the second chakra is a function of maintaining your sacredness of personal space and integrity; maintaining what it is to be whole and complete without parceling your Self out for the perceived benefit of others.

This can be exceedingly difficult because these conditions creep up slowly and are not readily identifiable. It can occur to the extent that you may already be in trouble before you recognize that you have been overwhelmed for some time.

This is similar to the condition where you lose a sense of Self in service to others. Without a firm, sacred foundation in the tradition of spiritual practices, a fierce love of Self (the God-within), and healthy emotional boundaries, service to others becomes one-sided and unfulfilling.

You may enter into "vicarious consumption" where your identity is defined through the lives of others, such as when a woman marries a doctor, and then "Mrs. Doctor" lives her life through the accomplishments of her husband. This may be OK as long as she does not surrender her personal identity, unique-ness, and growth. Otherwise, it is a very unhealthy second chakra lower aspect.

To achieve a strong sense of identity, second chakra indi-viduals must practice perspective through inspiration (PTI). You must be in a position of *vulnerability to your Self*. It may sound simple but it's very difficult to do. PTI means placing your Self in a position of vulnerability to be inspired (watching a sunset, reading poetry, meditation, etc.) where you are seek-ing an elevation of your perspective.

Walking through the forest could be an example. Suppose while walking through all the trees (details of life) you lose your way. The wise thing to do is to climb the nearest little hill until you are above the trees. From that vantage point (perspec-tive) you can see where you came from, where you are, and where you're headed.

Doing this in your life periodically keeps you on the path to your goals, and you also will not suffer in relationships from liv-ing vicariously through the experiences of others. When doing PTI, you become aware of your own goals and aspirations, and whether they are in alignment with those around you.

To retain identity and integrity, you must also create healthy emotional boundaries. A boundary has both an obvious and a hidden benefit. The first is that it is like a fence, keeping oth-ers at a safe distance. The second is that the same fence gives you a yard, a place to *be*. Too many second chakra people have unhealthy emotional boundaries because they confuse their creative abilities for others with preservation of Self.

Ask your Self these questions, especially in relationships of any intimacy:

- Am I giving my power away?
- Is this person taking my power?
- Have I too many multiple shared priorities?
- Have I spread my Self too thin?
- Are these my goals, or my partner's?

Having healthy emotional boundaries is not easy. It is easier to be the harmonizer, to keep the peace, at the loss of your identity, but it is very costly to Self and will impede your spiritual growth.

3. Apocalyptic

The apocalyptic second chakra person experiences sudden life changes. Things seem to be going well, and then suddenly something occurs that radically changes your life. The way to tell whether this is a second chakra phenomenon is to observe the consistency of the changes. If many radical changes occur over the course of your life, at the very least you are suffering from the second chakra challenges of reinventing your Self, self-approval, and self-validation.

It is true that some apocalyptic second chakra people maintain the chaos of such change activity in order to avoid taking responsibility for their own lives. This apocalyptic behavior can couple with that of the victim or martyr to create a continual cycle of trauma/drama leading to the possibility of emotional and physical disorders. It is also true that there may be karma or a mission statement that guarantees you a level of traumatic challenge.

This is a difficult lower aspect because of the disorientation of sudden change, and because there is no guarantee that it won't happen again.

4. Reverse Chaotic, Manipulator

Deliberate Chaotic Character
Some individuals choose chaos as a defensive weapon by offensively keeping others off-balance. By projecting imbalance, you avoid taking personal responsibility.

Creating chaos to maintain control and to divert attention from real healing is very self-destructive. It indicates you suffer from lack of inner trust and faith and perhaps feel there are issues so great that they may never be overcome. This plays into the fear of absolute overwhelm, with so many creative thoughts of consciousness leaking through from higher dimensions. You may have a sense of hopelessness, in that the linear mind cannot comprehend the immensity of the higher consciousness coming through the second chakra.

Those who the chaotic character keeps off-balance cannot perceive the real person or tune in to the real issue, creating a tremendous waste of time and energy. You can leave a conversation with a chaotic character not knowing where he stands, or what the real agenda is. His second chakra orientation is to be elusive, yet controlling; to take the focus off himself, and at times to assign blame and guilt to anyone but himself.

5. The Victim, Martyr

Second chakra people who live in this lower aspect maintain a form of chaos where they are suffering needlessly from problems they create. It is true that sometimes this individual does not know the answer, is daunted by the immensity of the task of getting well, feels a sense of hopelessness with the amount of healing required, and feels totally alone in their suffering.

"I would heal, but there is always something that gets in my way." You must be willing to accept healing, without yet knowing the benefits of healing. You must surrender your fear, your control, and be vulnerable to your infinite capability to create, from within.

The victim/martyr falsely sees that his suffering brings the recompense of healing for others. If Christ died on the cross to relieve our sins, he did so not to take our karma but to offer an example of a life lived fully in the higher aspect of his dominant chakra, the second. *Christ's message was not about how much pain you can take on, but how much love you can hold.* Holding that love means you must hold it for your Self first, then you can give it to others, by your example. It means being totally responsible for not suffering needlessly.

Metaphysical teacher Louise Hay says, "Fill the cup of your love first. That which overflows, give to others." Do not be a victim/martyr because you think it is helping others; that is a manipulation against your Self that will starve you of the love you must accept. Have enough self-love to never engage in any self-destructive behavior.

6. False Humility, Self-effacing

False humility is neither pernicious nor contrived by your design. It is the illusion that you must be so humble as to leave your Self out of emotional, mental, spiritual, and material abundance.

If you were on the operating table about to go under from the anesthetic, and you heard the surgeon say, "Well now, I think I remember how to do this!" you'd probably not feel very confident. You would want that surgeon to be the best at what he does.

So it is with your Self. When your second chakra is dominant, a lower aspect can be that you assume being humble is enough. It is not. You must first see your Self as powerful, infinite, composed of all will, love, and wisdom. *Then you can be humble.*

The Buddhists believe that you must first empty your cup before you can fill it. That means you must first destroy any illusion that separates you from the Oneness in which you live. That is not to say you should be arrogant or self-important, but with healthy emotional boundaries, you should acknowledge your Self as sacred, a holy being of light, not separate from what you seek.

It is OK to be very powerful and to be humble at the same time. There is a saying: "You must be absolutely humble and absolutely confident in the same moment."

Those who follow the Bible refer to the phrase, "Blessed are the meek, for they shall inherit the earth." However, many believe there are thousands of translation errors in the Bible, as it was translated from Aramaic to Greek, to Latin, to Old English, and to modern Old English. There is a version of the Bible translated directly from Aramaic to English by Harold Ramsa,

Ph.D., in which that same phrase translates as, "Blessed are the *courageous*, for they shall inherit the earth." Quite a different meaning.

You must be courageous enough to accept your Self as a reflection of the Divine: Remember Heaven on earth. Please do not make the assumption that being falsely humble is the same as being holy.

7. Passive Aggressive, Codependent

Many passive-aggressive and codependent relationships are borne of the second chakra disposition to create and to hold responsibilities. It is a way of seeing life, like holding a huge fire hose, through which pours the creative aspects of the universe - for someone else, however. But it is so very limiting to live your life through the experiences of another because you fear to hold the experience for your Self.

Passive aggression is manipulation of the other to obtain your desires, and subtle manipulation of the relationship to reach your ends, without looking like it is you making the power decisions. It is born of the second chakra fear that you cannot create what you desire, so you'll create through your partner's efforts. So many marriages are like this!

Codependence is a relationship in which one person is psychologically dependent in an unhealthy way on a partner who is addicted to something or has self-destructive behavior. All of this comes from the second chakra fear of the codependent that he cannot create for himself, on his own.

It is possible for you to engage in such relationships with others who have no desire whatsoever to heal themselves, and wish to continue the relationship for as long as possible.

Both of these conditions are so wholly debilitating as lower aspects of the second chakra that they can continue for years until one of the two participants changes his or her behavior. As in stories of abuse, these problems have long been brewing as unresolved issues with each person and in their relationship to each other. The relationship continues in its current form until one of them decides to heal and self-empower.

8. Squandering One's Power

Squandering one's power can best be described as losing your focus through chaos. If you consider that the incredible force of the second chakra is urging the creative consciousness of the individual onward, you have an idea of what the second chakra person is dealing with. Of course, there are many ways to squander your power:

- Taking on too many multiple, shared priorities
- Vampiric relationships
- Giving your power to another through surrender of integrity
- Creativity with no discipline
- Self-loathing through perfectionism

Dissipation of energies out of the second chakra can be as mild as delightfully distracting, to very serious, as in cancer of the cervix and other diseases that destroy one from the inside out. If there is enough dissipation in one chakra, the energies can be taken from the referent chakra to compensate, creating even more problems.

To regain your power is a decision of the moment, but only that. *You must choose your power in every moment.* Often, you become aware of a problem with squandering power only after the suffering it induces has been recognized, acknowledged, and acted upon.

9. Self-destruction, Self-loathing, Hopelessness

A self-destructive behavior usually comes about from the dissipation of the energies in the second chakra towards the perceived benefit in helping others without regard to Self or self-preservation. Just working harder to deal with the issues in a relationship where you are doing most or all of the work will put you on the path of self-destruction.

The squandering of your energies produces a chaotic state of consciousness where a degree of self-loathing can be experienced, even nurtured, as you assume tremendous guilt and remorse for not having created the perfect moment, the perfect relationship, the perfect project, etc.

The self-destruction comes about when your guilt and remorse accumulate to form the chaotic state that not only disperses the energies of the second chakra, but also affects the well-being of others. Self-loathing is the inner anger you feel when you can sense the perfection of events, the fruition of desires, but cannot manifest them in the world. Self-loathing is the fruit of the perception of unfulfilled desires. It is psychically, mystically "seeing" others as whole and complete, watching them suffer because they are not, and you becoming angry with your Self because there is nothing you can do to prevent it.

It is self-loathing that creates serious diseases through the second chakra, including cancer, multiple sclerosis, muscular dystrophy, and more. It is not letting your Self off the hook emotionally, and destroying your Self from the inside out.

The energetics are exacerbated by any lingering issues of guilt, separation, abundance, abuse, or abandonment from childhood. These longstanding issues, if not dealt with and healed, add fuel to the self-destructive tendencies and misplaced intentions of becoming ever more loyal in service to others at the expense of your Self and your integrity. Working harder will not assuage the feelings of destructiveness if the energies of the second chakra are not focused through their inherent *strength of creativity*.

You must maintain a focus on your ability to ever-create anew - the foundation of what the second chakra represents. The difficulty is that this focus relies heavily on trust and faith, also the higher aspect hallmarks of the second chakra dominant individual. When the perfection you mystically perceive does not come to be, it is all too easy to become self-loathing.

This is how many women create issues in the female reproductive organs, hip joints, lower back, urinary system, multiple sclerosis, muscular dystrophy, cancers, endometriosis, ovarian and uterine cysts, and much more. In many men, it can be the colon, prostate or genitals. In either, it can be most anything in the geographic area of the second chakra, but can also relate to depression and other emotional problems. All are manifestations through the second chakra lower aspects.

The external results of self-loathing and self-destruction include any phenomena coming from the second chakra, not just physiological health issues. Issues that are destructive but non-physical include bi-polar disorders, OCD's (obsessive-compulsive disorders), clinical depression, loss of hope, loss of faith, and lack of creativity.

Such self-destructiveness is the result of the frustration at the mental/emotional level of not seeing the whole picture you might believe the creationist should. Remember that the life of the second chakra dominant person is a life of faith, where you may not know the outcome for your Self, but mystically, intuitively will know it for others.

If you say, "I'll suffer quietly for everyone," there is no recompense for you, because no one else holds the keys to your enlightenment. Others in your life are there as reflections of your soul. They stopped giving out medals a long time ago for how long you can hold onto pain. Let go of your self-loathing; instead love your Self.

Hopelessness is a condition that is the opposite of faith. It is better to have faith than to have hope. Hope is placing your trust in an experience that is separate from you. It is not enough to say, "God will save me." You must, by your actions, "save your Self" by acting in faith. Faith means trusting your Inner Knower, that qualitative part of you that is your connectedness and which binds you to the Divine mechanics in all things.

You engage in hopelessness when you've lost the desire or ability to trust that you have the power to produce a favorable outcome *that includes you in the process*. It is easy to lose hope, because hope does not include the power of your collaborative leadership in the creative process through the second chakra. It is a lower aspect because of the assumption of separation from creativity and the ability to choose among alternatives.

To overcome hopelessness, you must be willing to be vulnerable to your own inner trust. There is a natural rhythm and harmony in the universe, a flow that is like music. And you don't appreciate music with your head - you do it with your feelings and emotions. When we listen to music, no thought is required. We either like it or not, instantly, because the music goes straight to our emotions. *When you tune into the Divine music that effortlessly plays through you, you are setting the stage to trust what you feel and apply what you know.* It is in the will and action that the nature of your character is defined.

10. Remorse, Regret, Resentment, Guilt

Regret, remorse, resentment, and guilt are thieves. They rob you of the present moment by rooting you in the past. In one of my lectures, I invited a woman to stand at the front of the group with me. I asked her to grasp my forearm with one of her hands, and to exert a slight pull. While she pulled lightly on my arm, I asked the group, "Who has hold of whom?" They responded that she had hold of me. But I told them, "No, I have hold of her," because as long as she was pulling on my arm, she could do nothing else with that hand.

So it is in life.

As long as you hold onto your past, it has a hold on you. You are like the boat in life; you make the wake wherever you go. But your boat makes the wake - it does not make you. *You make your past - it does not make you.*

Letting go of guilt can be so very difficult. Any of you who are parents and have used "tough love" with your children know exactly how hard. Rejection, or the fear of rejection, can create tremendous guilt. The fear of rejection is rooted in the desire for approval and validation that what you do is meaningful and productive. The second chakra person often has issues with the fear of rejection and the guilt that comes from non-action to change the lower aspect behavior.

You have to validate your Self as a creator, not wait for someone else to give you permission or approval. I know we all like our accolades and acknowledgements and that sometimes they are slow coming, *but in the end only you can approve of your Self.*

Guilt is one of the worst/best ways to manipulate the second chakra person. You will tend to hold your Self an emotional hostage, due to the desire to see the great vision, to do things perfectly, to please others instead of Self. Some relationships are built on this pattern, and once it is enacted, it takes very little energy on the part of the manipulator to add guilt to the second chakra person to keep the unhealthy relationship going for a very long time. It takes a great act of courage and will to break such debilitating patterns.

Do not be bound in guilt or remorse. They are powerful negative and limiting forces that root you in the lower aspect of the second chakra and cause you to lose faith, hold anger, and give up your dreams.

Only you can forgive your Self; only you can relieve your Self of guilt, remorse, regret, and resentment.

There is the story of Sri Yukteswar, Paramahansa Yogananda's mentor, who had an ashram in India. Many people would come to his ashram to study. One man said that he was apprehensive about joining the ashram because he had been a thief in order to feed his family. Sri Yukteswar told him not to worry so much about his past, but to concentrate on the moment.

Don't we all have the "coulda, shoulda, woulda's"? We can find many reasons why something cannot be done. You can kill anything if you throw enough doubt on it. Give up your past. *Concentrate on the now.*

11. Abuse, Abundance, Abandonment

All abundance issues come from the second chakra. All of them. Abundance is delegating the authority to your Self to receive. Many suffer abundance issues because they do not place a value on themselves or on their time.

Too many times people with strong second chakra dominance or issues overuse humility, or do not see themselves as personally abundant. *In order to be abundant, you must place a value on who you are and what you do.*

And please remember, abundance is not just material or physical. It is also mental, emotional, and spiritual abundance. You can only receive it if you allow your Self to. It is the permission you give your Self to receive that makes the difference.

Ever-evolving, self-unfolding: You've heard it before. Who could say that those who have been abused, either early in life or currently, have been in some way willing participants in the evolution of their souls by taking on such suffering? This book does not have all these answers, but rather attempts to help you avoid the lower aspects of each chakra, to avoid and overcome the suffering that living in illusion brings.

The abuse stops when you stop, unless you are a child, or are infirm. Some count their value by the amount of negative attention they receive, thinking that negative attention is better than no attention at all. This lower aspect of the second chakra can only result in more suffering, because it offers no positive, upward path. It is like the addictions a third chakra person can suffer. It relieves the pain, but not wholly, because it does not offer the whole, spiritual solution.

Who could say that abandonment is a good thing? Some say it is neither bad nor good, but what we do with the experience that defines the nature of our character. Consider the middle child. You've heard of the middle-child syndrome, where there is an older and younger sibling, and thus the middle child misses out on attention. Let's say the parents study all the books, talk to all the psychologists, and apply all their wisdom in raising that middle child with lots of love and attention.

If that child does not perceive love from the parents, then it does not matter how much or how well the parents show it. To the middle child, it does not exist. We can be affected, in our consciousness through our second chakra, to perceive abandonment even when perhaps there are no outward signs of its existence in our lives. *It is our perception that counts, not the reality.* This is precisely the type of problem that exists in most suffering - the perception does not match the reality.

Ultimately, you must come to love and accept your Self, whether others give you love or not.

12. Vampiric Energy

You know what a vampire does; he sucks the blood (life) from his victims. No discussion of the second chakra lower aspects would be complete without this subject. Modern-day vampires suck the life from their victims by attaching to their energy. I must tell you that there are many more male vampires than female, and that the energetic attachments (cords) can be very long-lasting, even after a relationship ends. You do not have to be physically near someone who has attached to you, for him to continue to steal your energy. This is a violation of the sacredness and privacy of the second chakra individual.

I have seen and removed cord attachments that have been in place well over twenty years. Sometimes there are telltale red marks on the skin where the tissue has been discolored by the flow of energy away from the victim. Imagine having 10 to 15 percent of your life-force energy being taken at all times, until you remove the cord. (And so many people are unaware of this dynamic: Those with no metaphysical background may be stretched to acknowledge that energetic vampiric relationships are ongoing in everyday life.)

If you suspect that this may be the case for you, use your inner trust first, then seek a qualified energetic healer. I have noticed dramatic, instant changes in the lives of people who have had these debilitating attachments removed by a healer.

13. Control

Sometimes trust is a large challenge for the second chakra individual, because of the control issues that ensue when you feel the awesome power of responsibility for creation. It is difficult to trust that others will be able to bring to fruition those things for which you endeavor. Thus, control becomes an issue when you feel you are the only one who can accomplish a task with the total vision and perfect outcome that you as a creationist perceive.

The lower aspect of the second chakra that is in control is due to that greatest of fears: that you cannot create anything greater than what came before. This is how some second chakra people get into relationships where they want guarantees of the outcome and longevity through commitments, and on the other hand, how other second chakra people have such difficulty making commitments.

Some second chakra individuals can become very analytical, which in itself is not a problem, unless it is at the expense of their feelings. In this manner of the lower aspect the analytical, controlling individual is very separate from their own inner harmony. That is why the word "anal" is in "analysis".

Smothering Relationships through Control Issues

Smothering is a condition where second chakra people give so much love and attention that it is not in proportion to the amount of love they are willing to receive. It is a way of avoiding being vulnerable to love, or receiving the gift of love from another.

In a fear response, you over-attend to the perceived "needs" of your partner. Smothering a partner in one-sided love and affection assures an imbalanced relationship. Perhaps seldom done intentionally, it is nonetheless a very unhealthy relationship.

This does not leave your partner without personal responsibility, else there would not have been an engagement in a relationship with a smothering personality in the first place. Individuals being smothered must eventually set limits and seek their own identity, or they will suffer a continuation of the exchange.

Second Chakra Perfectionism

The perfectionist tendencies of the second chakra dominant individual occur because of the "mysticism" associated with that chakra. Most all second chakra individuals become recovering perfectionists, due to the mystical, visionary tendency to see people and the world in their highest potential.

It is a natural impression upon the physical mind from the chakra disposition that you view the possibility of a perfect outcome. When events transpire, according to the freewill of others, that are not as optimal as you have seen, it is easy to take on a negative attitude. To feel, "nothing I do is good enough" is a typical statement, due to the perfectionist mind, driven by the creative second chakra.

Many second chakra people, in deference to their innate ability to sense mystically, head in the other direction, literally, to be in their minds as *analysts*. It is a natural consequence of the basic fear of the second chakra, externalized as a control phenomena.

The mental aspects of this disposition include the desire to know everything, such that you will seek every class, workshop, and lecture in your desired study to attain the knowledge you seek. (Note the word "anal" in "analysis.")

Often, there is a feeling of perfectionism; you set goals in succession to validate your exceptional amount of creative energies. You will often take many classes yet *still* not feel qualified. It is because the heart must yearn for what the mind cannot grasp, and the mental state is overshadowed by the second chakra consciousness to bring through creativity. Knowing the entire contents of the dictionary would not make you wise any more than going to church makes you holy. It is what you *do* that defines you.

Second Chakra Relationship Dynamics

One of the most fundamental issues regarding second chakra people in relationships is their mystical tendency to psychically, accurately (whether they are aware of it or not) see others in perfection. Making the leap between seeing what a partner is capable of, and the reality of whether your partner is ready, willing, and able to become that potential, is a very dangerous leap of assumption. The assumption leaves out the freewill of your partner to *not* achieve perfection.

When you psychically see other people's potential, you often don't take into account that they may not be ready to heal or grow. Sometimes, the desire for approval is so strong, that you disavow your feelings in favor of continually working to improve your partners, even if they have no intention of improving themselves. Many relationships are built on this fundamental problem.

Second Chakra Reciprocity-Focus in Relationships

The *reciprocity-focus* of the second chakra person is to stay focused like a laser beam when things are going well so that you do not scatter your resources, and to stay flexible when your horizons dwindle and your world becomes black-and-white.

Second Chakra Decisions/Commitment in Relationships

When you desire to make decisions, especially emotional decisions, give your Self a time limit (e.g., "If nothing happens in two months, then I will do such and such.") In this way, you can have no remorse because you gave your Self an option instead of just losing time.

Likewise, commitments in relationship should come up for review in the light of new circumstances. Do not victimize your Self by a commitment you made under old circumstances. Above all, it is important to be honest with your Self.

If second chakra individuals over-commit, as in the smothering of a relationship by giving one-sided love, this has the effect of rendering them emotionally unavailable, because they are giving but not allowing themselves to receive love.

When second chakra individuals have difficulty making commitments, either:

1. They have not matured enough emotionally to commit

2. They do not want to be emotionally overwhelmed and have not yet developed healthy-enough emotional boundaries

3. They do not want their alternatives limited to one person. They feel the pull of their second chakra to create and experience many alternatives, and do not want to be limited in their "sensuousness."

What a Second Chakra Individual Needs

The second chakra person needs *freedom to create* and to be individualistic. To keep second chakra individuals in a relationship, you must give them a measure of freedom to be themselves.

Were you to feed one of the small animals at the park from your hand, the only way to keep it there is by not closing your fingers, entrapping it. If you wish to keep a second chakra individual in your life, you must create the balance between giving that person great freedom, yet not so much freedom that you appear not to care. The more freedom you allow these individuals, the more they will stay in relationship with you, provided they too are responsible beings to themselves, and that karma, mission statement, or freewill is not an impediment.

Second chakra individuals will always react favorably to being given a space of private, alone time at regular intervals in order to center their infinitely creating personalities.

Healing Issues for
the Second Chakra

Illness is often related to the glands, organs, joints, and tissues of the geographic area of the chakra in question, but is not always limited to these areas. Some issues are from the referent chakras because the primary chakra is stressed.

Physical/physiological issues for the second chakra individual include problems with the lower back, neck, hips, sacrum, genitals, prostate, female reproductive organs, urinary system, lower abdomen, sciatica, water retention (including edema in the legs), the structure, architecture and strength of the legs, and blood circulation. Other issues include, but are not limited to:

- Cancer, muscular dystrophy, multiple sclerosis
- Musculature, legs supporting the trunk of the body.
- Lower thoracic and lumber misalignment and fusion, loss of cartilaginous matter between vertebrae.
- Men: prostrate, erection/ejaculation.
- Women: female reproductive organs, orgasm, hormones, endometriosis, cancer (especially of the breast), cysts, PH imbalance, miscarriage.

Psychological issues can be prolific for the second chakra individual:

- Clinical depression
- Bipolar issues
- OCD's (obsessive/compulsive disorders)

- Controlling and passive/aggressive behavior
- Sexual identity and preference
- Hopelessness, faithlessness, fatalism.

Second Chakra Priorities

- Perspective through inspiration
- Freedom to create
- Healthy emotional boundaries
- The perception of infinite alternatives
- Time alone
- A fierce love of Self
- Reduce the number of multiple, simultaneous obligations.
- Don't try to fix everyone
- Don't assume responsibilities for which you are *not* responsible
- Allow your Self to receive love
- Receive as much as you give
- Live a life of faith and trust
- Live your passion
- Allow your Self to be the true mystic, correctly, intuitively perceiving others
- Hold the vision, the big picture, without getting bogged down in details
- Cherish your Self. Do nothing to denigrate your character.

Evolving the Soul-Group Consciousness

As any chakra dominant person evolves spiritually, the raised level of consciousness has an effect on the entire soul-group, whether others are consciously aware of it or not. There is an elegance in all of us that transcends time and space, a mutual energetic association where we are all psychically linked to one another. Every individual has the possibility of helping raise the consciousness of the entire soul-group by individual dharma (right action, right behavior). *Everyone benefits, in some way, from your right action.*

The second chakra person, the creationist, inspires others by becoming inspired. As you take accountability for your desires and actions and your infinite ability to create effortlessly, you represent a higher aspect, the upward evolutionary spiral that involves the members of the soul-group. By your actions you ground on the earth plane the possibility of alternatives, inspiration, faith, connection to your sensuality, resolution of guilt, and the vision of what is to come.

However, holding the energies of being an evolved, higher aspect second chakra does not guarantee happiness, no matter the chakra dominance. It has been said that many saints attained contentment, but not necessarily happiness. But it does represent the pinnacle of what it is to create, to bring something from nothing, to go from hope to faith, to go from an absolute trust in your Self that transcends opinion and established knowledge.

Chapter Nine

Third Chakra – The Charismatic Leader

The third chakra is the "I am" center of a person's reality. It is the "I am becoming, who I am, who I think I am, who I feel I am" chakra.

Third chakra dominant individuals have incarnated to learn personal power, to learn of their own distinct individuation as a spirit in a physical body with freewill. Most of what you will read in this chapter has to do with the exposition of personal power and that of the individuated soul incarnate. This includes the strong sense of Self and the acknowledgment of your personal power through the understanding of ever-increasing levels of truth.

We all aspire to truth. Third chakra dominant individuals live in the essence of this consciousness, and it drives them, impels them to higher and higher levels. It is this energy that induces others to follow the third chakra individual - the same energy that creates a powerful spiritual leader.

It is not easy to be a third chakra dominant person; your life is the aspiration towards the inculcation of truth, ultimate truth. Telling the truth is not always the safest or even the most prudent thing to do. Throughout all history the one thing to be stomped out most quickly is the truth. Ask Jesus, Joan of Arc, or Jacques DeMolay about what happened to them for telling their truths.

Third chakra individuals are looking for the essence of "the thing itself": a term used by western philosophers to describe the reality of our existence. Third chakra individuals can tend to be blunt and to the point, suffering needlessly because their peers are looking for a softer collaboration. As you so readily, psychically, see the truth of things, the answers color your disposition through a very direct demeanor, unless you have fear and procrastination of personal power.

It can be a difficult chakra to work with, as you can be in power struggles, manipulative behavior, addictions, and serious confidence issues.

The greatest fear you have as a third chakra dominant individual is "what could be true, is true." Power coming through the third chakra is so great that you may surmise nothing could be that good, or that powerful, or that authentic, *especially your Self*. In fact, it is just the case - the illusion of not being in your power when the power is there already.

As it is for the second chakra, your greatest fear is an illusion that your personal power and truth is not as strong as it is, initiating life in the lower aspects. Overcoming these illusions results in the payoff of owning the role of charismatic leader, imbued with the highest level of truth and personal power. This leads to authenticity, veracity, and further exposition of power through truth.

The great Zen Buddhist master Suzuki Roshi said, "All this talk about prayer and meditation. If we would just realize we are Big Mind, we wouldn't have to do any prayer or meditation."

Some third chakra people are born in their power and must learn to use it, whereas the majority of people on the planet must spend time developing and accepting their personal power. Often, third chakra dominant people are unaware of the actual, and especially the potential, personal power they have.

The Three-Legged Stool

- Truth
- Individuation
- Power

The third chakra has as its basis three specific energies or aspects that must be in place for you to be stable in life. Truth, individuation, and power must share an equal position, similar to the three legs of a stool. If any one leg is taken away, the stool will fall. In the development of your character, the very perspective that the chakra commands, dictates that these three aspects be in full congruence throughout your life. The alternative is to suffer if any one (or more) of these aspects is out of place.

As the chakra is the filter through which life is perceived, you must go along with your most dominant perception until, at some point of evolution, you realize that mastership in life, and the affective chakra, is no longer an influence.

A Yogi once said, "You cannot be influenced by anything." What he meant was that once you are in your truth, nothing can affect you. This is particularly so for the third chakra, as its very essence is in the individuation and externalization of truth.

As it is, we each espouse truths that we hold as "true" for ourselves, based on our opinions, facts, and feelings. Reality is an elusive concept when your feelings are brought into focus. As your mind loves its surety in the physical world of things we call "laws" of gravity, magnetics, electricity, and so on, your feelings, on the other hand, can be a nebulous convolution of swirling emotions.

It is the effort to know the truth that transcends the truth. Along the way comes the power to make the changes and destroy illusion as you realize and enact higher levels of truth. This focus is the centerpiece of your endeavors, though, as there are many ways of understanding, there are an equal number of ways of externalizing this focus in life.

As it is important for third chakra individuals to make the truth true for themselves, enacting this truth requires resolving the difference between Self and selfish, driving its own point of small (and some large) self-fulfilling conclusions throughout life. That is, power struggles that require answers to questions, such as "is it OK to be right?" or "is it OK to be powerful?"

It is the motivation for what you do that defines the power of the third chakra individual. The solder who throws himself on the grenade to save his fellows could be the same man who commits suicide by slashing his wrists. What is the difference? The difference is his *motivation.* Your experience and your karma are colored by the perception of your motivation for your actions.

Is it arrogant for a saint to externalize powers, such as sitting in a box of flames without injury? To know God, and to fully externalize God's power and truth is our goal, but if it is your focus in a lifetime, the point becomes by definition intensely personal. As we are here to know God, we must also learn of the Oneness through these different expressions we call chakras.

When you approach the third chakra personality, on some deep level you receive the impression that this is a person of authority and authenticity, for it is the lesson the third chakra personality came to learn. When meeting a third chakra personality you will psychically assume that he is in power.

When third chakra individuals are in their power, others will tend to do whatever they say. Depending on their level of development and awareness, this can take several forms:

1. *Manipulative* – The third chakra personality is in his weakness. This is the negative state of the third chakra, or its lower aspect. Individuals in this negative state can manipulate others with some ease, using the wants and desires of others against themselves.

2. *Manipulative Self* – In the same lower aspect, the third chakra individual can allow himself to be manipulated by others due to his low self-esteem and feelings of low self-worth.

3. *Authoritative* – The third chakra personality is in his strength, tapped into his authenticity. This is the positive state of the third chakra, or its higher aspect. From this position the third chakra personality seeks to bring through the absolute truth with authority, thus the term "charismatic leader."

Third Chakra Characteristics

Anger

Anger is one of the greatest dangers for the third chakra dominant individual. It arises when truth is withheld or deferred by procrastination. Knowingly doing so creates the anger, and it must reside somewhere. You internalize it through the solid and hollow organs in the midsection of the body, including the entire gastro-intestinal (GI) tract, urinary system, liver, gall bladder, spleen, appendix, and thoracic vertebrae.

Anger also arises in a non-personal manner and collects in the third chakra individual like a room collects dust. It is a matter of not personalizing this anger and ridding one's self of it on a regular basis. This anger comes from the innate love of truth and the essence of things, and is a reaction (both conscious and unconscious) to the iniquities in the world. Part of the life-path of the third chakra individual is to dispel and disperse this anger.

There is also an energetic relationship between the third chakra and the thyroid gland in the throat (blood pressure, skin temperature, metabolic rate). If you suffer enough anger through the third chakra, there will be a reaction in one or more of these parts of your body.

Anger can also affect your feeling of powerlessness, assertiveness, and threshold values for "stuffing" anger. These are just a few examples of the many negative affects of holding in your irritation.

Remember that others are taking a relationship to the third chakra individual of authority, "trying you on for size." There are many situations in the world where individuals knowingly manipulate you in order to prevent you from being in your truth and power. The worst manipulation is knowingly lying. There is an old Yugoslavian saying that my father used: "It doesn't bother me that you are lying to me. What bothers me is the fact *you think I believe you.*"

There can be years and years of subtle and not so subtle manipulation in the life of a third chakra individual.

It's Personal

If anger weren't enough, third chakra individuals tend to take situations personally. You personalize issues, focusing on your Self, once again giving great possibility to the internalization of tremendous anger.

As Don Miguel writes in *The Four Agreements,* "One of the

four agreements is *nothing is personal*." In other words, only *you* can make an issue personal. It is your decision. The reason you take things personally is that you are still in the lower aspect of the third chakra, mired in personality and individuality.

How to mitigate taking things so personally? Read the section later in this chapter on "Self, not Selfish" and you'll see how a little arrogance is actually a healthy state of being for the third chakra individual.

The power of the consciousness that flows through the third chakra emphasizes your uniqueness and personal power, thus the drama of developing the sense of "Self." When your consciousness begins to feel the hint of the greatness that is available, lessons in strengthening your character inevitably ensue.

You are here to deliver the truth, and most times, not to sugarcoat it. When faced with conveying truth, you are often up against the qualitative aspects of emotions when making decisions: You came here to learn how to make *emotional decisions*.

The truth, as it is, is an ultimate with respect to your capacity and capability to hold it. As a third chakra individual, you will always exceed the truth, especially if you conceive that there is a level of truth above you that you sense but do not yet know. Hence, you will always tend to exceed your Self, often at any expense, if you perceive there is any truth above what you currently understand. There is an ongoing aspiration that drives you to higher and higher forms of truth, to ultimately reject a truth that is greater than the personality can bear, or to embrace that level of truth to the exclusion of all lesser truths.

You would have no difficulty making decisions for another person or for purely "mechanical" issues: "Should I go to the store, or should I get gas, etc." Where you would have difficulty making decisions is with *emotional* issues. This is because emotional energy does not follow the same pathways as linear thinking.

Emotions are *qualitative* and thoughts are *quantitative*.

A qualitative energy such as emotion cannot be quantified, as in, "How much do I love you?" but rather is a state of being that has a nexus of many feelings at the same time. Throughout human history, emotions have been most difficult to describe and to convey and have been communicated through intermediary devices, such as poetry, art, music, and personal acts.

The struggle in being a third chakra dominant individual is that truth will drive you to reject or accept reality as it is. To suffer would be to live in anything less than the truth you presently perceive as ultimate. To suffer would be to create "mentalisms" through addictive behavior where your mind attempts to capitulate to the strength of the chakra and picks up any or several of its lower aspects.

Third Chakra Reciprocity

Because of what third chakra personalities represent, sometimes you will, through the Law of Reciprocity, pull others into your life in various categories. Some people who encounter you really are looking for truth and the individuation of power. These people want nothing from you other than to improve their lives.

By associating with you, other people infer the qualities that the third chakra represents, depending on their own chakric disposition. (The dynamics of the possible combinations of interactions will be covered at length in the book *Your Chakric Relationships*.)

The reciprocity of the energies is a function of the relative truth you are willing to hold. As with any other chakra dominance, lessons in life are constructed in an upward evolutionary spiral, to represent breaking through the upper limits of your waking consciousness.

Any reciprocity is the inverse relationship that you experience with others, in order to create the possibility of transcending the illusion currently predominant in your life. You are in constant, progressive unfolding of energetic dynamics in the Law of Reciprocity. Having overcome one obstacle only clears the way for the next, and the next, and so on. This type of resistance training prepares you for attaining increasing levels of clarity within the path of your life and mission statement.

We often invite the inverse of what we represent into our lives so that we can then learn from the mirror of opposites. You can draw a manipulative person into your life, so that by being manipulated, you finally become angry enough to stand in your power. If you do not, you will suffer the persecution of self-imposed powerlessness.

The innate psychic understanding of the highest levels of personal truth provides the basis of suffering for you, if you do not live it, and live by it. The manipulation you feel is from surrendering your power. Many are afraid that the power is real, when in fact, *it is real*.

Sometimes you can draw into your life others who could not find the truth with two hands and a flashlight. The truth that flows through you sets the stage for others to come into your life to be presented with ever-higher levels of truth unfolding. As always, this energy has two dimensions: whether you will accept your power or not. If resisted, both parties will spiral into another set of circumstances that will provide the possibility of optimal outcome based on right choice and right action. This set of circumstances will repeat itself in endless variations, also dependent upon the karma, skill sets, mission statement, and freewill of the individuals involved, until the lesson is learned. That does not mean that you, like any other chakra dominant person, will have learned those lessons in this lifetime.

It is only by applying that you gain the experience necessary to evolve your character: It is not enough just to know - the truth must be active.

Am I the Only Person in the Room Who Gets It?

Sometimes as a third chakra person, you will say, "Am I the only person in the room who gets it?" And the answer will be, "Yes, you are." That is because soul-groups will create the space for the truth-giver to appear. The soul-group will co-create the circumstances so that the group may be facilitated by the level of individuated truth that you, as a third chakra individual, represent.

In that situation, the more you are aware of your position relative to the group, the better able you are to facilitate the group's evolution of consciousness. You are there to give the level of truth that the group is able to receive. Remembering that the third chakra is concerned with the *individuation* of the externalization of truth, it is likely that you will work to make the truth available in the broadest common denominator.

However, it also means that even after you give the truth, there may be none to receive it, for others may be unaware such a truth exists, may not be along their paths far enough to embrace it, or both. All third chakra people can do is their best; give the truth as highly as they can perceive it, and allow others to receive it as best they can.

Most often, until you obtain a certain level of spiritual evolution, you as a third chakra dominant person will not be cognizant that you are in the dynamics within that soul-group. To aspire to higher levels of truth is inherent in the third chakra dominant person, but that does not mean you would understand your interactions with others in those terms.

You can step up a level, or, as often is the case of the third chakra dominant person, you can procrastinate or develop addictions to defer the acceptance of personal power.

The Law of Reciprocity assures that you will constitute lessons that enhance and define personal power, individuation of truth, and qualitative decision-making in interactions with others.

Remember that a third chakra person will exceed himself in truth, hence you may always be in situations or circumstances that set the stage to give the truth, or hide from it. If denied, the truth will surface in another way, unless any of the participants must reincarnate to learn the lessons in a different way.

The King Energy

Often the third chakra dominant personality will wonder why others bring their disputes before him. Wondering why others have made you judge, you will represent truth as it shines through the third chakra as an individuation.

Others, perceiving the chakra energy or authority that is individuated, will bring their differences before you because they perceive the authenticity and veracity that are antecedents of the individuation of truth. Others will expect that your answers will be in authority, whether you perceive it so or not.

It may amaze you that others continue in their quest for counsel and the settling of opposites. That amazement is rooted in the growing understanding that you hold truth, more truth, than many of your peers.

This can be more difficult than it seems, because when people have a relationship with you as a third chakra dominant person, they may assume psychically that there is little you require. An example is the king, who, because of his office, may induce the thought in others that there is little that he requires, and that if he seeks love or comfort it's because he as the material manifestor can do so easily. This assumption leaves a gulf of understanding that is not bridged until you come to terms with your own power.

No one questions whether the king is king. As it is third chakra, it is whether and how you will use your power, not whether you have it. Some of the biggest problems occur because you do not see your power, when all your contemporaries do.

Often we do not perceive that we are powerful beings. Only through the experience of living life do we become aware that such power exists, and that we must accept and accrue it. Even more so for third chakra dominant people, because their disposition is rooted in the individuation of power, and because many (not most) third chakra dominant individuals are born in their power. It means that, "what could be true, is true" *is really true*: that you as a third chakra dominant individual, in this lifetime, really do have that much individuated power. It is part of the major lesson you are here to learn.

That power is much more active as a result of the dominance in the third chakra, both to you and to everyone in your life. The fact that the power exists as active is cause for the externalization of your life's lessons that go along with being a third chakra dominant person.

To make an assumption that you do not need certain things does not take into account whether you have evolved to conscious recognition of your own power. And not having done so creates a powerful illusion and misconception for both parties in the dynamics of the interaction.

If you are not aware of your power, and another person assumes that there is little you need, the possibility for suffering on all levels continues until you accept your power. Remember, though, that the truth is relative to an individual's capability and capacity to hold and understand it. And this is one of the keys to understanding the third chakra dominant person.

As you grapple with your sense of individuated power, you are somewhere on the continuum of consciousness in the development of your being through imbuing the quality of your soul into your personality. More than any other chakra, the issue of personal power, its individuation, and externalization are key elements that issue forth from the internalization of truth on the personal level.

In accepting that level of individuated power, the transcendence of your consciousness includes hidden benefits, such as:

- The ability to manifest material needs more easily through the power of the word or effort
- The emanation of authenticity is more coherent
- The relative recognition of individuated truth is greatly increased
- The tendency to preclude procrastination and addictive behaviors with right action or right behavior (dharma)
- The discerning mind becomes the healthy skeptic who questions lower levels of truth, and chooses not to dwell in them
- The veracity of the individual increases to the point of intolerance to "lesser" truths, begging the question of truth vs. harmony
- The tendency to not take things personally
- The focus on ever-ascending levels of truth, even to the extent that it causes the individual to exceed his relationships with others.

Hidden benefits are those subtle (and sometimes not so subtle) changes that occur as a result of inner growth and transcendence to higher levels of awareness. As a result of the transcendence, it does not mean that you are aware of any or all of the hidden benefits. That awareness comes with time and experience, but the 95% of communication that is energy emanates the quality of those hidden benefits to others who take psychic relationship to you in their interactions.

Another aspect of the king energy is that you as a third chakra dominant person can often say, "When will I ever meet my peer?" You can feel that there is such a gulf between the personalization of higher levels of truth that you hold, and the relative truths of people around you, that no level ground is to be found where they can see eye-to-eye. You may seem to be on a constant search for a peer.

Your illusion is that you will reach that level of ultimate truth when the concept of a "level" is strictly confined to a third-dimensional reference.

The truth is that your nature is rooted in the aspiration to higher levels of truth, hence the dilemma of finding someone at your level. That level is constantly shifting and evolving. The person you are today does not hold the truth of the person you are tomorrow; it is a part of the drive of the third chakra.

It can feel like a trap, for you continue to make a good effort to hold higher levels of truth, and as you do so, you exceed the relationships you are in with your partner, peers, associates, colleagues, and so on. If you exercise your power, the relationships can be changed forever. Yet not exercising your power is living in a lower level or lower aspect of your own truth. And the *externalization of inner truth* is the path of the third chakra dominant person.

You may have a succession of relationships where you exceeded your partner's ability to hold an equality of energy. You can simply "outgrow" your partners. It doesn't have to be that way, but the tendency to exceed your Self (and thus the other person) is always present in the third chakra dominant person.

This can be most difficult because you would not necessarily surrender the level of truth you have obtained for the benefit of a harmonious relationship. It begs the question of "where is the middle line?" for you, between your own level of truth that you constantly aspire to, and the harmony of a relationship with a person who does not hold that level of truth.

If you were the king of a country, you would automatically know that each country can have only one king. And if you wish to find another king (someone at your own level), you must go to another kingdom. You would have to go where the other kings hang out.

If you are living in your higher aspect, you will want to pair with others who are peers, who represent the kings of their respective countries (i.e., chakras). You will be best suited to look for individuals who accept the truth of their own dominant chakra, and who can include another third chakra dominant person.

Sometimes, however, when two third chakra dominant personalities get together, the association can be represented by holding the north ends of two magnets close to each other. The closer you try to hold them together, the more they resist. Many times, two third chakra individuals are in a power struggle with each other. Of course, if the two are in the higher aspects of their third chakras, the relationship can be very powerful and beautiful in its exposition of truth and individuation of power.

But in looking for other dominant chakra individuals, you will look for what is best and most powerful, and by the reciprocity of the relationship will draw the individuation of those qualities out of the other individual by your association.

Eventually, the king does find a peer, but the decision remains dynamic and ongoing as to the representation of his own level of truth in the relationship. Can the king keep a peer relationship without evolving out of it? Is the king willing to allow the other person to "do his best" and be tolerant of the other person's level of truth, even if it is not as evolved as the king's?

In seeking equals, third chakra dominant people illustrate the emphasis of their own dominant traits, and they are impelled towards what is greatest and what is best. But because you are king, others assume you can "command" what you will, especially in love and emotions. Remember to speak up, to communicate the desires of your heart to others. Do not be silent, but be the communicative "king."

Truth vs. Harmony

The example of the king represents the ultimate of personal authority and authenticity. Emanations through your dominant third chakra will draw you into situations that will cause you to experience the difficulty of truth versus harmony. This is because it represents your struggle to accept the individuation of your own power through truth, and maintaining a harmonious relationship with others.

You must come to terms with the daunting power of the third chakra, that it impels you towards higher levels of truth. Truth, in itself, is an intimate and revelatory experience, and if your disposition in life is central to the pursuit of that truth, automatic conflicts are created to offer the opportunity to embrace it. It is in the very individuation of that power that makes you develop your character in such an individuated manner.

Form follows function, and you will always externalize to the physical world that which your chakric disposition represents. The light of your soul is shining, by orientation of your dominant chakra, more than the others, through your personality. This sets in motion the disposition of experiences; the way in which you experience the world.

The situations ensue when a qualitative choice must be made because the truth can never be quantified. The difficulty in holding absolute truth is that harmony represents the gathering together of discordant energies into a cohesive whole. It is similar to the harmony of an orchestra. Each instrument is individuated, unique, producing its own sound. Yet when played in harmony, the combined instruments flow together all their representations of truth.

So it is for individuals. You as a third chakra dominant person creates the opportunity for truth vs. harmony because it is your skill set that must be developed through the resistance training of deciding between the two. In so doing, you develop your skill in making qualitative decisions - one of the hardest things the third chakra dominant person will ever do.

Harmony Through Conflict

You as a third chakra dominant person will often draw one or more people into your life who assume you can divine the truth between harmony and conflict, because the representation of the third chakra's energies (when dominant) is that of authenticity. Others assume (though most often not consciously) that you will know the right decision.

Conflict does not mean violence. Think of conflict as yes or no, black or white, up or down, and so on. This concept of conflict is also called "The Pairs of Opposites." The third chakra must stand between the Pairs of Opposites before it can decide the direction to go. It is necessary to have the "Yin" and the "Yang" because they represent the polarization of the opposites; the "as above, so below" where the two must meet, in the middle.

The presence of the third chakra dominant person draws the "middle" of the pairs of opposites into the upward evolutionary spiral, and thus draws the whole plane of current level of understanding of truth vs. illusion. This effect works for two people, a group or larger soul-group, or an entire race of beings. It depends on the lesson, mission statement, karma, and level of spiritual development.

The effect becomes more powerful for all involved if you are in the higher aspect of this chakra. You elevate the evolution of the understanding and the individuation of truth and power by raising the plane of the Pair of Opposites (see Illustration #9-a). Yin/ Yang symbol (Pairs of Opposites), where the energy of the third chakra dominant person pulls the plane of the symbol upward in consciousness (truth).

People engage the third chakra dominant person because of the assumption, energetically, that the level of truth will be gained. The opposite or negative effect occurs in two ways:

1. Others receive the truth from you and refuse to accept it, negating an opportunity for growth. The truth they would "receive" from you is the reflection or reciprocity of the truth they already hold, just illumined for the sake of the current lesson or level of self-empowerment. And if those who receive the truth reject it, they will recreate the lesson again later, perhaps even more vigorously.

2. Others elect to manipulate you into a subordinate position for fear that acceptance of the truth may make them address their own issues. It is sometimes easier to keep another person down than it is to take responsibility for one's own issues. (see Chapter 24 on *psychic manipulation*).

You will create harmony through conflict to address your own inner confidence and self-worth issues. Drawing upon the limitless well of truth, it is the internalization or acceptance with total confidence of that truth that defines your journey into the higher aspect of the dominant chakra.

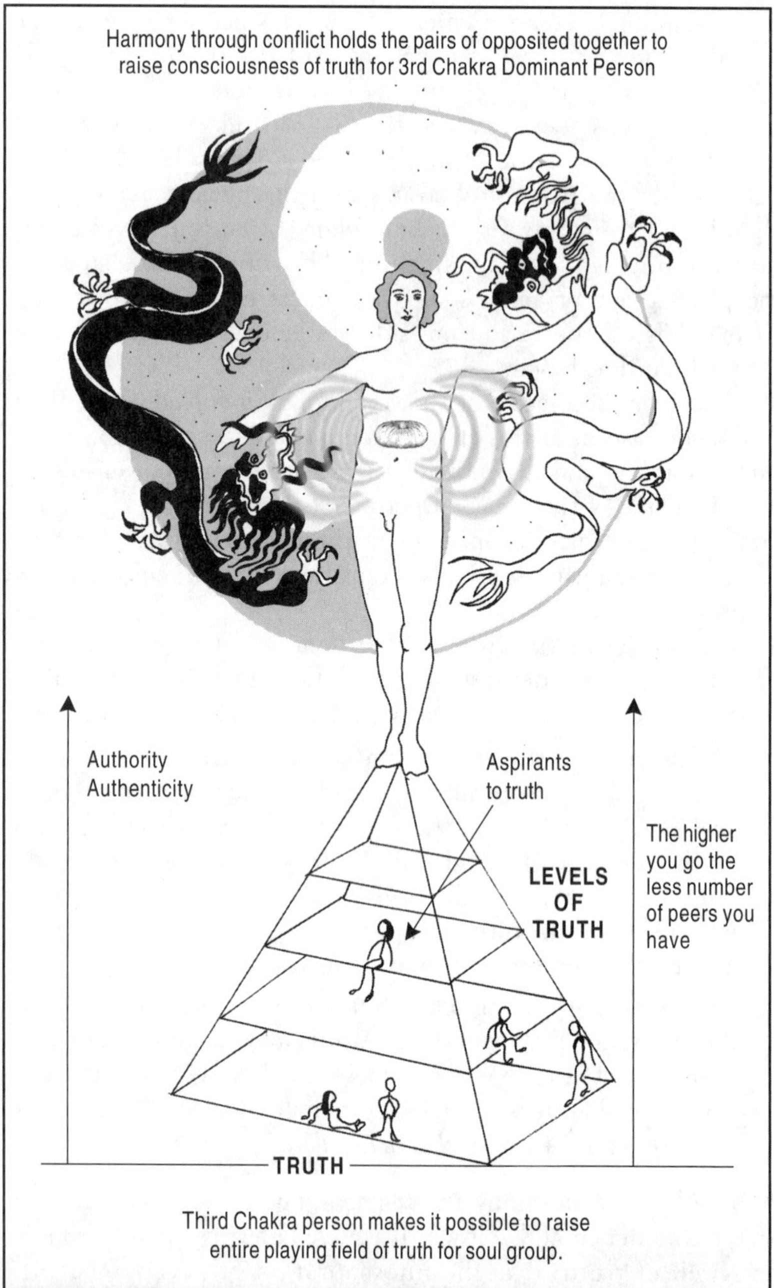

Harmony through conflict holds the pairs of opposited together to raise consciousness of truth for 3rd Chakra Dominant Person

Authority
Authenticity

Aspirants
to truth

LEVELS
OF
TRUTH

The higher you go the less number of peers you have

TRUTH

Third Chakra person makes it possible to raise entire playing field of truth for soul group.

**Illustration #9-a: Illustration of Yin/Yang Symbol
(Pairs of Opposites) and Elevator of Self-Truth**

The Difficulty of Emotional (Qualitative) Decisions

The most difficult decisions you as a third chakra dominant person ever make are those that are emotionally based. Any other quantitative decision (e.g., how many ounces in a pound) is much easier in comparison. It is because of the rootedness in truth as the essence of "the thing itself" as a quality of being that you have such difficulty making decisions of any emotional import. The truth is rooted in your capability and capacity to hold and understand it.

However, since your goal is rooted in highest personal truth, the difficulty becomes one of applying such lofty truths to emotionally-composed situations. Emotions are many times convoluted and especially qualitative in nature. An emotion cannot be quantified (e.g., "How much do you love your mother?"). Bringing emotions into question is something we all face, yet it is more difficult for you because it requires your authority to make decisions reflecting that ultimate truth. To do less is to live in the lower aspect of the third chakra.

Many people struggle with their emotional decisions, more than a few by procrastinating. Procrastination is a way of deferring or avoiding the responsibility of being right, or the bearing of the responsibility of making an authoritative, authentic decision.

Emotional decisions require you to draw upon your inner belief systems, sense of fairness, protection and nurturing of the sense of Self, and your sense of self-truth. You will draw the harmony through conflict and many other circumstances that will test your ability to make emotional decisions.

The third chakra represents the individuation of truth and personal power. The truth that you hold is not necessarily the truth of others. But truth, in itself, has no personality. As absolute, it has no respect for others; it will not bend to suit the purposes of the individual.

While embracing higher and higher levels of personal truth, you have a psychic knowing that there is an ever-increasing awareness in truth available to you, but your physical awareness has not yet achieved those vaguely available levels.

Even so, the impression upon the four archetypes of the third chakra dominant person is to aspire to those levels of truth, regardless. And in knowing that to be so, even on a subtle level, you realize the difference between making an emotional decision in third dimensional reality that must take two things into account:

1. The current level of understanding and acceptance of truth through emotion of the other parties involved, and
2. How much fidelity to inner truth you are willing to hold.

It is more difficult than it sounds, because you will recognize the difference between ultimate truth and waking reality, even if dimly. And, that the truth is relative to the holder, even though absolute. Is it any wonder that many third chakra dominant individuals engage in procrastination or addictions when faced with making emotional decisions even though they are innately powerful people,?

If you, by virtue of your innate ability to manipulate, do in fact manipulate situations so that you are constantly avoiding (thus procrastinating) emotional decisions, you do it so that you are in your power in the way you feel most comfortable, without really addressing the issue. No real progress is made because you are operating from the ego, avoiding your own inner truth and ability to make good emotional decisions. Many third chakra dominant persons fear their power. It is that inverse relationship (your strength is your weakness) that impels us towards surmounting our illusions. It's one thing to be in power - it is another to recognize the right use of power.

The qualitative state is relative to your idiosyncrasies, and thus points directly towards third chakra issues. It is not the same as a second, fourth, fifth, or sixth chakra person. Those individuals must face their trials in terms of their own dominant chakras, and those orientations do not create the same dynamics.

Remember, however, that whatever the dominant chakra may be, you can always experience tests related to your other functioning chakras, although the tendency will be to favor the dominant chakra. Forays into other chakras are always possible.

Making Emotional Decisions – The Thirty Second Rule

In order to help you make emotional decisions, there is an exercise called "The Thirty Second Rule:" For a *full* thirty seconds, ask your Self the following repeatedly, "What am I feeling now? What am I feeling in this moment?" At the end of thirty seconds, it may be vague, but you will have an answer.

This exercise puts you into a state of "now," drawing your power and will into the present moment while using that moment to access a purely qualitative state through your feelings. You have to be willing to trust your feelings and accept your inner truth or you'll have great difficulty with the exercise.

Third chakra individuals are not known for their patience, so you'll have a great opportunity to create some, as this exercise requires you to use all thirty seconds.

Self, Not Selfish

We live in an enigma. We are at once living in the Oneness of all things, but at the same time we see this universe of ours through individuated eyes. We say things like, "I think," or "I see" or "I am." And yet there is no separation between you and me. It is this enigmatic part of ourselves that we seek to resolve through the living of life, learning our specific lessons; that observer is not separate from observed but rather a part of the whole. This is the entire principle upon which all psychic and intuitive phenomena exist. Anyone practicing psychic abilities, remote healing, medical intuition and more, are operating within this paradigm.

The uniqueness of third chakra individuals can cause them to feel that whatever attention they draw to themselves, no matter how trivial, is selfish. Whether this is true or not does not matter if you take on the possible alienation and separation from your own goodness.

You doubt that what could be true, is true, and thus question your own authenticity and worthiness to hold truth. Not because you cannot. These issues are never because you cannot hold truth, but rather that you sense it only all too well and are up against the highest level of your own capacity to hold it. It is like your father giving you the keys to the car for the first time. Are you able to hold the responsibility given to you? Will you fail?

Certainly, all life is trial and error; the making of mistakes is the pavement that provides a firm ground for you to move forward. Your inner connection is so strong, that it impels you forward, through all manner of tribulation to learn the truth of life and self-empowerment.

You can suffer from taking everything personal. Believe it or not, I tell third chakra individuals to combat this by being a *little* more arrogant. Using the example of the king energy, no one disputes that the king is king. So, what matters is what kind of king do you want to be? By arrogance I mean you must accept that power is an *individual choice*. You see it all around you. Some people are in their power; some are not.

Since you cannot be effective from a position of weakness it makes sense to accept your power, but in doing so you must accept the accoutrements that go along with it, like the king must accept the trappings of his position. That kind of arrogance is not harmful, it is a simple, personal recognition of your power; a choice the third chakra individual must make for life.

The weaknesses of the third chakra personality include worthiness, self-esteem, comparison to others, and a lack of confidence in the power of your words. Taken in reverse, if you choose to become negative you could be an excellent manipulator.

As a third chakra personality, you can suffer from "Self, not selfish." Not able to perceive your Self as viable and valuable in the world, anything you accept is thought to be selfishly won. This creates a hollow space where you actually hold off receiving your own goodness.

Do you eat? Of course, you do. Eating is not a selfish consideration. Do you drive a car? These questions have to do with what it takes for you to go through everyday life and living. They are not acts of selfishness - they are just "Self." Thus, the third chakra individual must have a high regard for Self, just as the king must have for the office to which he was born. It is a responsibility imbued upon you at birth.

A swami came to visit me in 2001. He had come from his ashram in India to lecture around the United States and had heard about my work in light and sound.

While in discussion, he intimated that the government of India had declared him a saint in 1996. He did not want them to do it, but the government nonetheless proceeded with the conferral.

This is a man who can sit in a concrete box of fire for thirty minutes. Neither his person nor his clothes burn. Is it arrogant for him to accept his power, or is he demonstrating to others the power of human potential?

Should anyone be allowed to keep you from absolute truth and personal power? You must allow your Self to be powerful, to stand in the truth, and use the power of your will to manifest your personality as individuated.

The Law of Physical Manifestation – King Solomon's Temple

King Solomon was a powerful figure of Biblical origin, depicted as a man of great power to judge fairly. He commissioned a temple (King Solomon's Temple) to be built, and at the center was the "Sanctum Sanctorum" (holy of holies), the most holy place in the entire temple complex. This holy of holies had only one entry.

At the entrance, there were two giant stone columns on either side. Anyone entering the holy of holies through the single door would have to walk between these two stone columns. Doing so was symbolic of the Law of Manifestation.

Each stone column had a name. The one on the left was named "Boaz." The one on the right, "Jachin." The word Boaz meant "the word," meaning the spoken word of man. The word Jachin meant "The Law," with a capital "L," meaning God.

The word, spoken through the Law, creates the Manifestation. That is, when we speak our word through our higher Selves (God), the manifestation is set in motion by the universe, of which we exist in Oneness. This is the holy trinity of God. The two energies at the base of the triangle are the word and the Law; the apex is the manifestation.

This is the basis of manifestation for humanity. I tell people, "God has really good hearing; no need for us to repeat ourselves in prayer." We've only to state the desires of our hearts once, and the universe immediately sets in motion the mechanics to bring about their manifestation. To repeat ourselves to God is to imply that we have no faith in our word.

Higher and Lower Aspects of the Third Chakra

The higher aspects of the third chakra dominant individual represent the overcoming of the lower aspects. The seeds of the lower aspects remain, to serve your freewill should you choose to embrace, once again, an illusion.

Higher aspects of the third chakra:

1. Charismatic Leader
2. The Truth-Giver
3. Master Manifestor, Manipulator
4. Hierophant
5. Spiritual Leader
6. Person of Authority
7. Person of Authenticity
8. True Skeptic
9. Protector of the Innocents
10. Person of Ultimates

Lower aspects of the third chakra:

1. Power Struggles
2. Manipulator
3. Procrastinator
4. Narcissism
5. Powerlessness
6. Loss of Identity, Comparison to Others
7. Self-Worth, Self-Esteem, Confidence
8. Taking Things Personally

Higher Aspects of the Third Chakra Explained

1. Charismatic Leader

The charismatic leader is the bearer of truth and poise. Poise is grace and power together. Have you watched charismatic leaders speak? What is it about them that causes everyone to sit up and take notice? That 95% of communication that is nonverbal tells us when someone is accessing a higher level of truth, even if we do not agree with what they are saying.

It is not so much that you hold truth, as what you do with it in the moment. Yes, it is a huge responsibility to aspire to and hold great truths. It is larger still to administer them in the world.

Charismatic leaders hold the truth, power, and individuation that at once differentiates them from the group. The energy of uniqueness that could make you feel you've nothing to offer (because you do not see your power) is the same energy that is the basis for such powerful individuation in the charismatic leader.

The right use of power is a third chakra lesson. Being given power in a lifetime does not mean that you know how to administrate it.

2. The Truth-Giver

The truth-giver is one who draws, by reciprocity, the exact lessons to build the strength of their dominant third chakra. Such lessons are the liars and manipulators who purvey a lower level of truth for their own, linear ends.

Truth-givers, by definition of the third chakra, hold as much or more truth than most anyone around them. This is the beginning of the problem *and* the solution for the third chakra person.

Transcendent truth is owned by no one. The giver is liable to his current level of understanding - the truth *du jour*. When you are a truth-giver, there is much resistance, and sometimes doubt, about the veracity of why your own truth should be any more enlightened than anyone else's.

The soul-group calls in various individuals for the mutual evolution of group consciousness. The truth-giver is seldom popular, and you can often suffer the harmony through conflict of transcending relationships and friendships when you choose to have fidelity to your truth. Loyalty and fidelity are by-words of the third chakra dominance; they always come into question when the truth is offered. When it is offered in no uncertain terms it is also uncompromising in the sweeping changes that ensue in your personal relationships (loyalties) with others.

To avoid giving the truth is to procrastinate. However, you are not going to be so truthful that you stop strangers on the street to tell them what you think they really look like! There is a space, in between the extremes, where you can be in your truth (like the good king) and decide how to administer it.

3. Master Manifestor, Manipulator

Some third chakra personalities have the ability to manifest easily, for they are born with much power already. Most of these people seldom realize their natural power to manifest into physical reality. And, it seems that many do not believe that the process of manifestation is so very simple. That does not change the energy. The ability to manifest in some third chakra individuals is very powerful. It may come from the ability to see through the veils and perceive truth so powerfully.

That is not to say that the third chakra individual must go around and manifest continually, but for them it is very simple and natural. Manifestation includes physical things, such as money, but also can include spiritual (manipulative power), emotional (charisma), and mental (brilliance) forms. You usually do not suspect just how powerful your ability to manifest is, and often situations are created so you may acknowledge this power.

However, it is always best to start with the manifestation of simple things first, so as to build character and right action. As with many of life's lessons, you are given a small challenge and the outcome will determine the number and severity of other challenges. But weakness can lead to manipulative behavior.

Manipulation

If you go to a chiropractor or massage therapist, you've just been manipulated. Manipulation is neither good nor bad; it is what we do with it that defines character.

Some choose to manipulate for the good of humanity, some for the lower aspect of good for the Self. Those who choose the former represent the chiropractors, orators, politicians, musicians, and others who manipulate energy for beneficial purposes.

If, however, your truth is in the lower aspect, the manipulation can be for Self only, where the energy is used against others in order to maintain the lower level of truth.

To manipulate or to be manipulated. If you do choose to manipulate, it can be one of two types: positive or negative.

1. Negative manipulators use others from an egocentric position due to the low self-esteem and worthiness that is the lower aspect of the third chakra. Through the manipulation of others, you seek to build your confidence and to shield your own perceived shortcomings.

2. Positive manipulators would include, but definitely not be limited to, professions such as chiropractic and bodywork, where tissue, muscles, and bone are manipulated towards a higher goal of total health.

In either case, the manipulation is an extension of the power of the third chakra to manifest change, and to affect the external physical environment from your point of singularity.

There are also many situations in which others manipulated you from fear that if they ever let you become aware of your power *they* would have to change. Many such manipulative relationships exist until you become so angry that you either grasp your higher truth and make life-changing decisions, or procrastinate to the point of creating disease and illness.

Stanislav Grof, in his book <u>Spiritual Emergency</u>, discusses individuals (many with third chakra attributes) who have had several small epiphanies (spiritual openings). He discusses how one such third chakra person may be seated at the family dinner table in cosmic consciousness while everyone else is talking about the food. The third chakra person may feel he has nothing in common with many people around him, assume it is a detriment, and allow others to manipulate him because he does not yet perceive his personal power and truth.

The Magician card in the Tarot deck is a representative of the master alchemist; the male-energy manipulator who can blend the four archetypes (mental, physical, spiritual and emotional) into any combination. The third chakra person is capable of such manipulation, because they perceive the thing itself in its true essence and have the personal power to manifest (blend energies) to bring it forth.

4. The Hierophant

The hierophant is one of the major arcana cards of a Tarot deck. The major arcana represent major steps in the evolution of your consciousness through this and several lifetimes. The card is interesting to look at. In some decks, the hierophant is depicted as a man (male energy) looking out of the village and perceiving a great truth. Several village folk are gathered around the male energy, anxious to know what he sees. It is interesting to note that one of the villagers is the clergy (a local priest).

The truth transcends all religious and dogmatic attempts to frame it. I have had priests and associate pastors of churches come to me for private sessions because they had questions their religions could not answer.

If you are in Oneness, the answers of truth come from within and transcend another's ability to give it to you fully. But you can manifest people (hierophants) to come into your life who do hold great truth, and their representation through relationship to you will stimulate you to consider accepting a higher level of truth.

5. Spiritual Leader

Most third chakra individuals, by their nature, come to represent spiritual leaders, even if that is not their external path. Most are the leaders of their household when in a relationship.

It is because of the nature of the personification of truth, and power through truth, that you are perceived as a spiritual leader. By your very association, others tend to treat you as one.

That does not mean that you need to don robes and become a priest or nun. It means others will take a relationship to your dominant third chakra and treat you as though you should know the answers, the truth, and be able to articulate it back.

As you age in this lifetime you will take on (provided you don't procrastinate) more aspects of the spiritual leader. Holding the third chakra higher levels of truth makes it automatic.

6. Person of Authority

Other people will assume you know what you're talking about. At work, you can be promoted through no fault of your own. To be in authority is to hold truth with confidence and people will assume you have it, whether you do or not.

This is because their psychic relationship to you is built on your dominant chakra's basis in the individuation of truth: others assume your authority to be in place, because you are (unconsciously) showing them your dominant third chakra. Others will tend to want to do whatever you say because they assume you are consciously connected to the higher truth your third chakra emanates.

They will tend to treat you as though you should just know the answer, be able to handle the responsibility of authority, and have the command of personal power to carry it through.

7. Person of Authenticity

These third chakra individuals have no caveat: They are what they say they are.

In energetic interaction, the authentic person often attracts his reciprocal in people who wish to "try the authentic person on" to see if he is as authentic as his energy suggests. The contesting interaction is a power struggle to ascertain the pureness of the authentic state of the third chakra individual.

If pure in motivation, the potential exists to help improve the character of the soul-group by their right decision to capitulate to the higher level of truth the authentic person represents. It is not so much a personal capitulation, but to the essence of truth that emanates from the quality of the third chakra dominant individual.

All truth is personal as it pertains to humanity, but we all embody absolute truth by living in Oneness. This is precisely why we invite such third chakra individuals into our lives - for the experience of freeing our Selves from non-authentic externalization of our soul-quality.

Persons of authenticity may be quite unaware of their own qualities. We all are unaware of the beauties within us, dormant in our awareness, yet fully functioning as an emanation of our character through our given dominant chakras.

8. The True Skeptic

Sometimes during flower readings, I'll do a reading for what I call a true skeptic: someone who is willing to ask the questions that no one else is willing to ask. I am being complementary, as it takes courage to seek and demand the truth. Like the second chakra, accessing higher levels of your Self (success) is one thing; dealing with the success it represents is another.

Asking for truth as a skeptic is one thing, but you must be prepared for the truth you seek, because it *will* be revealed to you. It is you who must change to accept the higher level of truth; you who will be intimidated by it until you accept it. It is you who will be in anger holding a lower level of truth and knowing the difference. It is one thing to *seek* the truth; it is another to *live* it.

Skeptics, by their nature, are very much like scientists. Their life is a relentless pursuit of the truth. When finding it, they must adjust their perception of reality to fit the higher truth.

True skeptics eliminate the dross from what is essential; they rid the truth of the fluff that sometimes surrounds it. This is one reason why third chakra individuals make such fine spiritual leaders: they do not become lost in the very dogma they initially embraced as a form of the externalization of their spirituality. Eventually, the truth transcends all religion and dogma.

The price the true skeptic pays is differentiation from the consensus of reality that pervades mankind. The more skeptical, the more individuated into a higher truth, the more free you as a third chakra person become, unfettered by lower belief systems.

9. The Protector of Innocents

Some third chakra individuals take on an aspect that protects innocence. In other words, truth without caveat. If a five-year-old asks you whether he can play, do you say, "Define play?" The child will have no answer other than, "Just to play!" That is because he has no hidden agenda, no ulterior motive.

Innocence is purity without an agenda; it represents "the thing itself" with nothing hidden. Because the essence of the consciousness of the third chakra is rooted in reaching for the utmost absolute truth through personal endeavor, some third chakra people embrace that notion fully as to desire to defend those who cannot defend themselves, and to protect those who cannot protect themselves and have been preyed upon by others. And, by reciprocity, they invite people into their lives who are in need of refuge from the lies and divisiveness of the world.

As a third chakra individual, you have the ultimate sense of "right-ness," and by definition have the potential to stand in that higher truth among peers. The representation through relationship draws others near you who have suffered in a lack of innocence, for resolution in the energetic dynamics of personal interaction.

I've seen such individuals visit and support orphanages, work in triage centers, homeless shelters, shelters for unwed teenage mothers, etc. The third chakra, its power in the personification of truth, imbues a person to externalize that power by protecting others, hence protecting the philosophy of innocence in the world.

10. Person of Ultimates

Imagine you are driving your car and you notice a red button on the dashboard. You are puzzled at not having seen it before, and cannot find it listed in your owner's manual. Your urge is to push the button, but once pushed it cannot be undone. Not knowing what is going to happen has been overcome by the desire to push the unknown button.

Third chakra individuals set circumstances in their lives where they must choose between the unknown and the truth at hand. You must either hold a higher level of truth, or suffer from procrastination, confusion in emotional decisions, and the loss of your power. It is therefore an omnipresent force of energy that weighs upon you where you must make decisions of an ultimate nature, not knowing the results.

This differs from the second chakra individual in that the essence of the decision for you is rooted in the *motivation* for making decisions. For the second chakra individual, the essence of their choice is rooted in *faith*. The first is a quality of the individuation of truth and power (yang); the second is the quality of the will to be vulnerable to the truth of your feelings when there is no physical evidence of support for the decision (yin).

As a person of ultimates you will cast your Self in difficult positions of decision-making. Often, the decision is not uniformly popular if made successfully (in alignment with your inner truth). If you put off the decision, or do not stand in your power, suffering of some form will ensue because the lower level of truth was embraced.

Lower Aspects of the Third Chakra Explained

1. Power Struggles

The third chakra individual has a continual power struggle going on. That is not a bad thing. However, suffering comes from not making the connection between your struggles and your innate power to *overcome* them.

If you remember that the strength and weakness of the second chakra is the ability to continually create and reinvent, then it is easier to understand how the personal power of the third chakra individual can be seen as absent when it is not absent.

The lower aspect comes into play when you use the power struggle as an addiction in itself, a way of playing for power, manipulating the situation and others, the accumulation of material wealth, instead of using the beneficence of the higher aspect attributes.

There are many third chakra individuals, and many I know, who have turned the power struggle into its higher aspect by maturing and accepting their power when they achieve it, and by living in the higher truth as they know it.

You will have power struggles for life. The tests of personal power continue during your lifetime in order to learn the lessons of the third chakra. Look at it like going to a "chakra gym" — you increase muscle only when you work out.

Part of the lower aspect is rooted in your desire to be right even when you are not right. I notice that some individuals are not very patient and are very stubborn. In relationships, because of the lower aspect of their third chakra, they insist on being right all the time.

Manipulating a relationship in order to preserve a sense of personal power and being right only prolongs the power struggle, and continues to root third chakra individuals in their lower aspect.

2. Manipulator

As you can see, the manipulator is both a higher and a lower aspect of the third chakra individual.

I have counseled many people who are third chakra individuals. I asked one woman, around thirty-five years old, if she was dating men about ten years younger than she is. She was surprised, but said, "Yes," and asked me why. I told her it was because in choosing younger men, she could manipulate and control the relationship to her means.

The problem with doing this is that there is no real growth, because she is manipulating the emotions of the men, and in doing so avoids real challenge. This is a very safe place for her to be, but very unhealthy, as it guarantees she is living in a lower aspect of her dominant third chakra. Such lower actions always result in some form of suffering - from not manifesting what she desires, to physiological problems from anger due to procrastination of her personal truth.

We all manipulate. Withholding the truth while purposely manipulating is its worst, most unhealthy, form. Manipulating situations, from work to relationships, is based in the fear that you do not have the personal power to affect the changes you desire most: It is exhibited by comparing your Self to others, rather than standing out in your uniqueness. It is difficult to emphasize your uniqueness if you don't know what it is.

Many third chakra individuals manipulate for fear they will not be able to manifest through the truth itself, when by its nature imbued within them, they hold more truth than most others in their soul-group.

3. Procrastinator

Procrastinators put off action in order to avoid taking responsibility for their power. The power of the third chakra is as daunting to the mind as any other chakra. It is the power and truth that pours through the individuation of the third chakra that most people, upon incarnation, shy away from.

People follow charismatic leaders who are in the higher aspects of their third chakra. It is the energy of ultimates. These leaders make momentous decisions that change everything, once the truth is spoken and realized. Is it any wonder why some third chakra individuals have such difficulty with procrastination?

Procrastination can turn to addictions. *Addictions are just another form of deferral from your power.*

You can be addicted to anything - sex, drugs, rock'n'roll, alcohol, smoking, and numerous other substances and habits. There are addictions borne of emotional distress, the habit or substance becoming a substitute for soothing the emotional part of your nature in healthier ways. Even though there are numerous causes why you would embark on any addictive behavior, there is a strong attraction for the third chakra personality to head in such a direction.

From the point of view of the third chakra individual, the attraction towards addictive behavior is borne of "mentalisms" to deal with the energies representing its individuation into a single soul aspect incarnate. Mentalisms are the mind's way of dealing with the immense personal power of the third chakra. All mentalisms usually end because they are linear, mental attempts to deal with the consciousness that the third chakra represents.

Mental aspects cannot conceive of the qualitative aspects

alone; the desires of your heart, the emotional body, must reach through trust of Self beyond your mind's ability to conceive. Your heart must yield to what your mind cannot yet know.

Even so, I've seen many people smoke (dominant in the third chakra or not) as an addiction because they found it soothing. It is soothing to the emotional energy body. This may sound like heresy, but I really don't care so much that a person smokes, even though it's not the best of habits, because I know it is a way of calming anger, letting go of taking things personally, and dealing with emotional energy. I've even seen some of my clients exhale the smoke with a slight sound, like "haahhhhhh." That sound is a further expelling of the negative compressive emotional energy, which will be covered more fully in the chapter on the fourth chakra. Smoking is not a good habit, but without greater answers, it is a way of dealing with stress.

Any mental, attempt to deal with the consciousness of the third chakra can only succeed to the extent that you live in a third dimensional reality. This does not include the metaphysical part of your nature and hence creates separation. Your mind is continuing a behavior that either accepts a limited view of the truth, or is in denial of the truth and seeks to assuage the separation through diversion of the senses in limited mental form.

This is why all addictions end. It is because the mind is not enough to embrace the individuated truth that is constantly pouring through the third chakra. When you embrace the next higher level of truth, suffering is reduced and your soul moves on more optimally through its incarnation.

4. Narcissism

Narcissism grows out of a lack of confidence in your personality, but more importantly, it effectively removes you from your power in the present moment (where all your power is), makes you emotionally unavailable, and removes your participation greatly from the mutual evolution of the soul-group.

An emotional relationship with a narcissist involves three - you, the narcissist, and the narcissist's ego. The ego is based in the will to project a power that is absent from the heart. The narcissist becomes self-absorbed because it is also safer, in relationships, to do so without risk of emotional involvement.

Were they to give in to emotional involvement, it would mean to overcome the fear of the immense power and truth that the third chakra represents.

5. Powerlessness

"No one can help me" is the lamentation of lower aspect third chakra individuals who are rooted in powerlessness. You sense that you are beyond the assistance of others to obtain personal and professional goals because your task must be done by and for your Self. In fact, this can lead to not knowing how to ask for help, for you feel the press of your own personal power urging you to already know the answer.

Powerlessness is being cut off from the truth; it is feeling that your power is never sufficient to meet the tasks before you.

6. Loss of Identity, Comparison to Others

When the third chakra disposition is in its lower aspect, you will tend to compare your Self to others due to the internal feeling of deficiency in uniqueness. Again, your strength is your weakness - the power of Self through the uniqueness of being induces your mind to capitulate to that very same strength.

Instead of emphasizing your individuality, you spend time comparing your Self to the accomplishments and personalities of others. You are caught in the vicious place of desiring to emphasize personal identity and externalizing the power to do so. Taking the risk of accepting your power sets the course of individual distinction and "going against the herd" mentality.

Society has a way, through unwritten rules, to enforce like behavior. Those who operate outside the established norm are also considered to be outside the "consensus reality," and thus not part of it.

Many people throughout history have been ostracized, and more, because they were not only individualists, but also emphasized the power of a higher truth that flowed through them.

7. Self-Worth, Self-Esteem, Confidence

Worthiness and self-esteem issues are common for the third chakra individual, but certainly are not limited to that chakra. Many of us have felt confidence and self-esteem issues in life about a great many things.

Third chakra dominant individuals often have little confidence in their contributions to life and society because they live in great fear of their own power, even though they may live their lives by truth, be great detectors of deception in others, and even be great counselors. It is typical for third chakra dominant people to have little confidence in themselves, but to be astute givers of truth in helping others, and to channel their powers to help others attain optimal living.

It is at the maximum level of coping with the immense power of the third chakra that you begin to manipulate your environment and others to deal, on a mental level, with this incredible amount of energy. The sense of falling short is from the internal judgments that you makes when comparing your Self to others. With a low self-esteem, you will doubt your own veracity. You may even see the whole as a series of insurmountable barriers, due to the inner truth seen psychically through the third chakra and reported to your mind. And you may be constantly in a state of following the actions and decisions of others if you are in a weakened state.

8. Taking Things Personally

"Nothing is personal: only you can make it personal," writes Don Miguel Ruiz in his book, The Four Agreements. You as a the third chakra individual tend to believe that every criticism, every challenge is a personal affront. This is the higher possibility (consciousness) of the third chakra at work, but perceived through fear, creating a lower aspect.

It is the resistance to true power and authenticity that creates the moment when you will react in a negative, personal manner. The perception is that there is some deliberate manipulative conspiracy, either by other people or by spirit, against you when, in fact, none exists.

Even if it did exist, it does not serve you to respond from fear, as that instantly separates you from your higher aspect of truth, power, and individuation. The resulting anger may provoke a manipulative response, but more importantly, it separates you from being in a higher state of consciousness, and internalizes the anger itself in a destructive manner.

The power of the third chakra is to manipulate the third dimension through power and truth in a personal way. It is natural for the lower aspect to cause the negative reaction of taking things personally, and is exactly what third chakra people must rise above in order to live fully in their higher aspect. Give up the attachment to taking things personally. Let go of ego's desire to take on the world. Choose a motivation that is rooted in higher truth.

I would like to tell the story of Arjuna in the <u>Bhagavad-Gita</u> to emphasize a point about motivation: Arjuna is an army general in the days when opposing sides lined up facing each other, awaiting the order to charge. He rides out in the middle of the battlefield to assess the opposing army, deciding whether he should attack. At that moment, Shiva (God) appears to him and asks, "Arjuna, what are you doing?"

"I'm deciding whether to attack that army," he replies. "Do you think you should?" God asks. "Yes," replies Arjuna. "Why is that?" God asks. Arjuna gave God his reasons for attacking the opposing army. God then said: "Before you do, let me show you something first."

God opened up the gates of Heaven for Arjuna, and let him see the glory of it. After a short time, God closed the vision and asked Arjuna, "What do you think you should do now?" "I don't think I should attack," replied Arjuna. "Why is that?" God asks. Arjuna then gave his reasons for *not* attacking the opposing army.

The essence of this story is that it did not matter whether Arjuna attacked or not, but what his *motivation* was.

The soldier who falls on an exploding grenade to save his fellow soldiers is the same man who may commit suicide by cutting his wrists. What's the difference? He still dies.

The difference is in his *motivation* for dying; his *personal* decision. This is the definition of character that places you in higher or lower aspects of your consciousness. This is why it is so important that you think about what is personal and what is not. What is your motivation for taking something personally? What is your motivation for your actions?

Third Chakra Relationships

One of the most fundamental benefits that you as a third chakra individual offer to a relationship is to help individuate the power of the other person. Representation through relationship and inverse relationship dynamics bring you on the scene, sometimes to make another person angry enough to take their power back.

If you accept your power and truth, you offer to the relationship the power of an ultimate: "Do your best, and you can stay in relationship with me. Do it not, and I may exceed the truth that you hold and may also exceed our relationship."

You as a third chakra individual exceed most of your emotional relationships because you are constantly striving and exceeding your own understanding of the truths of the universe. Your own third chakra is forever provoking you to do so. As you externalize your understanding of greater truths, it sets the stage of conflict for the relationship to grow, or become eclipsed by the greater truth.

If you are not self-accepting, and instead embrace procrastination and manipulation, you become the ubiquitous "power figure" that dictates the terms of emotional exchange, keeps your Self well-insulated from any real growth, and extols a heavy, manipulative effect on your partner.

What a Third Chakra Individual Needs

As a third chakra individual you need to feel your own strength, truth, and uniqueness. You need to feel confident of your opinions and innate ability to hold and understand great truths of the universe.

You need to understand there are moments when you are the only one holding the truth; that the ability to do so inspires others to their own uniqueness so they can individuate and be in their power, too; and that holding the truth is sometimes lonely at the top, as it is for the king.

As a third chakra individual your word is power, your uniqueness separates you from the crowd, and in showing power, others assume there is nothing you need. You need to communicate the desires of your heart, and decide what kind of ultimate authority you are going to hold.

Emphasizing the Strengths of the Third Chakra

1. Anything that stimulates the acknowledgement of your Self, your uniqueness and individual character; promoting a sense of personal likes and dislikes; encouraging individual pursuits and interests. The emphasis is to promote the "I Am" presence through self-merit and individual contribution. What is it that makes you unique and viable as a human being?

2. Accept the availability of truth. An encouragement that truth is always available from within as in the recognition of no separation. You must realize, through personal effort, that the higher truths are borne within and any externalization through others is simply a mirror of the truths you hold.

3. Use the "Thirty Second Rule" exercise to make emotional decisions: For a *full* thirty seconds, ask your Self the following repeatedly, "What am I feeling now? What am I feeling in this moment?" At the end of thirty seconds, it may be vague, but you will have an answer.

4. Allow your Self to be powerful.

5. Don't repeat yourself. Value your words as powerful.

Healing Issues for the Third Chakra

The third chakra affects the hollow and solid organs in the mid-body, the biochemistry of the body, and some hormonal activity health effects. Mostly these effects are due to the retention of non-personal and personal anger, often towards the iniquities of the world or the sense of what is fair and just.

Other issues affected through the third chakra include:

- Thyroid (blood pressure, skin temperature, metabolic rate)
- The gastro-intestinal tract and the manner in which nutrients are assimilated through the tissues. Includes intolerance to artificial chemical derivatives in food and drink, dairy allergies, food allergies
- Biochemistry of the body includes PH and OH imbalances in the stomach, body and feminine organs. Biochemistry includes the skin, its sensitivity to metals, fabrics and plastics.
- Urinary system, including dehydration of organs and tissues, even if lots of water is being consumed (many third chakra women suffer from this). Also includes the adrenals.
- Sometimes shows up as problems in the nervous system, relative to muscle tension and can be anywhere in the body.
- For many third chakra persons, the issue is a matter of "getting the anger out". I tell them to get a punching bag, go yell at the ocean, go bowling and knock some pins down, but get the anger out. It is often an impersonal anger. Just as a room, any room, will collect dust, so also does the third chakra person collect anger.
- Anger has one positive quality; it motivates change. If Jesus could turn over tables in a temple and the Dalai Lama uses an air rifle (it's true) to scare away the crows when he's feeding the pigeons, perhaps it's OK for you to get your anger out.

Evolving the Soul-Group Consciousness

Because initial engagements between individuals and soul-groups always take place on the psychic level first, others who engage with you will tend to want to do what you say, because of the authenticity through truth that pours through the third chakra. It is because others tune in to this quality that sets the stage for you to define or run from his power. These are the very lessons set up by you to get you to step into your power.

Your authority comes from the psychic link through the emanations of the third chakras access to truth. As the quality comes through you, it is seen as authenticity: "What you see is what you get." The psychic impression given to others is that you would always speak with authority through a higher truth, and in many cases power is surrendered because of this psychic impression.

It does not always mean that you are aware of your power. Perhaps sometimes you may see it as a lower level ego attribute, the ability to manipulate others.

To evolve the soul-group consciousness, you as a third chakra individual must be living in your truth in a non-manipulative manner, and must have accepted your power as distinct. That represents the greatest possibility to the group of evolving their consciousness.

Chapter Ten

Fourth Chakra – The Empath

The fourth chakra is known as the *heart* chakra and the heart chakra individual is here to represent love. A fourth chakra dominant individual has two key features that differ them from the other dominant chakra individuals:

1. You would have had one or more sequential past lifetimes of right behavior and right action (dharma) to earn the merit to be in the fourth chakra.

2. You have physical issues that are systemic to the body, and localized, as well. This chakra affects whole systems - vascular, lymphatic, skeletal, muscular, etc. -where the other chakras do only to a limited extent.

With the evolution of consciousness in our world of today, there is a growing portion of the population who experience their own growing pains, and the growth of others as well.

In this instance, consider those who have incarnated with a heart chakra disposition. As one of these individuals, you must have had several lifetimes of dharma before qualifying or earning the right to incarnate in the heart chakra. It is through the accrual of merit, an individual accomplishment of character, that you carry with you from incarnation to incarnation. Thus you carry an inherent *experiential* goodness, different from an inherent spiritual goodness that we all have.

It also means that you come through in this lifetime, through that goodness, as psychically sensitive to all others around you. So not only are you faced with living your own life, you also are very sensitive to the energies of those around you. This can be to the extent you become a living sponge, soaking up emotional energies of other individuals.

Heart chakra individuals number about one in every twenty to twenty five people for a reason. Because the heart chakra is emotionally based, they are empaths. An empath is a person who psychically feels the feelings and emotions of others. Part of the difficulty of being a heart chakra individual is that you tend to "take on" energies from others. This is called "negative compressive emotional energy" and it is absorbed into your emotional energy field.

This can often create a problem because most empaths do not know that they are empaths. Not knowing you are taking on this energy in a non-physical way, you are unaware of the origin of your suffering. The negative compressive emotional energy can have deleterious effects on you because you also would not know how to clear the energy, or dispose of it.

Many heart chakra beings suffer continually, taking on the negative energies of humanity through having had many good past lives. They often do not see their own goodness, but rather take on suffering as a validation of their lives. They often sabotage their relationships because their minds are daunted by the purity of their hearts that they have *earned*. This is done through love, not as a purposeful self-destruction, but because of the intense self-realized goodness that the empath has lived in past reincarnations.

The Empath

We now know that as an empath you would psychically feel what others feel. You feel the feelings of others so well that you may not know those are not *your* feelings. There will be times when you ask someone, "What's wrong?" and you get the answer, "Nothing."

The truth is, you felt it empathically before the other person was even aware of the feeling. And, it's perfectly OK to do so. Most of us have no idea of this energy dynamic that goes on twenty-four hours a day. It is typical for us to completely underestimate who we really are

Empaths, as heart chakra individuals, are in a constant state of empathy, whether they are in the higher or lower aspect of their chakra. This is a central feature of the rest of this chapter, and it is the strength and weakness of the heart chakra individual.

Imagine growing up with these empathic abilities "on" all the time. It is easy to understand how there may be some emotional confusion! This is made even more poignant when parents are unaware or incapable of understanding the empathic child. Growing up in an emotionally overwhelming world, trying to communicate your feelings to many who have no capacity to understand you, you may hesitate to fully express what you're feeling.

Is it any wonder we spend many years, unfolding the petals of who we are, sometimes only very slowly?

The abilities of chakra dominant individuals in this and other chapters are not special; they are a part of who we really are. We try so hard to control our abilities, when the secret is learning to flow with them in concert with our higher selves from a position of trust, not beating them to death with our mind's incessant need to "know" how things work. As you have seen, the difficulty in understanding metaphysics is that you cannot get there with only your five senses and material mind. You have to reach out with your *feelings*.

You have an added disadvantage if you are born in the Western Hemisphere. You are not taught such subtle energies exist, that they are a part of you, or that you live in Oneness, not separate from what you seek. Though you see the blending of science and metaphysics becoming more and more understood and in natural relationship to each other, we as individuals must still make the personal and intimate choices to evolve our character through decisions of the vulnerability to accept our true Selves.

The empath is just a little like taking a drink of water from a fire hydrant. Sure, you get the drink, but you get so much more!!

Gullibility and Naïve-ness

Many heart chakra people, in the course of their lives (especially their love lives) will say, "How could I have been so gullible and naïve?" This comes from the empathic assumption that because you can accurately, intuitively see how someone could be emotionally whole and complete, you assume it is what that person wants as well.

In the real world, this is often disappointing as others do not live up to their possibilities, for it is in their freewill to accept or reject their greatness. And it is all too easy for you to blame your Self for being gullible, because you assume you were ignorant of the needs of a great relationship.

This is very puzzling for heart chakra individuals. You sense the Oneness, the emotional perfection in others. You do not see isolation, only integration.

Gullibility and naïve-ness do not come from ignorance, they come from *courage*. The empathic ability you have accurately sees another as he could be, but you assume it is your own ignorance, when you have it in complete reverse of the reality. You tend to think little of your true nature partly because in the West it has never been taught to us as children for the most part, and because it is easy to doubt and think the worst. It takes much more effort for you to be vulnerable to your Self, and for a heart chakra individual, that is saying a lot.

If your heart chakra really is dominant, imagine the immense courage it must take to be vulnerable to your own growth by staying emotionally open, at the risk of being devastated or overwhelmed by the very emotions you are trying to convey to others. Is it any wonder that heart chakra individuals have heart attacks, blood quality and pressure problems, myofacial, fibromyalgia, skin, cancer, depression, or just die early?

Being dominant in the heart chakra is no better or worse than any other chakra. It means the challenges are succinct for this disposition through your feelings and emotions.

Emotional Grounding

The heart chakra is in the middle of the seven chakras for a reason; it is the middle ground where mind and body meet. As throat chakra individuals must remind their metaphysical nature that they have a corporeal existence through grounding, so must heart chakra individuals ground *emotionally*.

Equanimity plays a large part in the emotional stability of the fourth chakra person, even more so than in the life of the second chakra person. That is because love is the central tenet, not creation. The more emotionally stable you are, the better equipped you are to deal with future challenges.

It is vital that you stay emotionally grounded, or much suffering will ensue. Once your emotions are stable, the qualities of stable mental, physical, and spiritual archetypes will follow.

Merit and The Law of Grace

Merit is an individual accomplishment of dharma, an accomplishment that creates purity in your heart. When an individual, especially a fourth (heart) chakra dominant person, has successive sequential lifetimes of right action and right behavior (dharma), merit is accrued. Merit is a highly individual attainment, like spiritual "frequent-flyer miles" and cannot be transferred to another person. It is the inherent goodness or purity of a life, or lifetimes, well-lived.

When enough merit is accrued in successive lifetimes, the Law of Grace is enacted through your higher spiritual contracts. It is similar to drawing a card in a board game and moving your playing piece ahead ten spaces without having to roll the dice.

The Law of Grace allows you to skip over certain aspects of a mission statement, assigned lessons and/or karma by erasing the requirement for linear experience associated with the lesson. Invoking the Law of Grace from lives well-lived sets a condition within your current life where there may lack a perception of worthiness for the blessings accrued. You may have no idea of personal inherent goodness, just an overriding feeling of emotional inadequacy born of great goodness and love.

It is a mystery how people can have such good past lives and be totally oblivious to their goodness. It is ironic that we, as humans, dwell more on the fear of being in our goodness than accepting that it is true, not only philosophically but also in accrual from lives lived.

Sometimes, karmic and mission statement events of suffering are removed through the Law of Grace from the life-path of fourth chakra individuals so that your life is freer to exhibit the qualities of your dominant chakra. This is one of the reasons why, when people ask me about what vocation a fourth chakra dominant person should pursue, I answer that it really does not matter, for you are more about holding the energy of love, rather than externalizing creative leadership or communicative abilities.

Sometimes, however, those events are enhanced to anchor you in the depths of your awareness of emotional strengths and weaknesses. In other words, how great the suffering and joy can be as a function of stimulating your empathy.

The subsequent comparison of the fourth chakra dominant person to others begins at an early stage. The compounding of strong empathy mixed with merit/grace can cause very mixed feelings, loss of identity, and emotional confusion. It is not that the fourth chakra dominant individuals don't feel well enough, it is that they feel only all *too* well.

The Law of Grace applies to your entire lifetime as a fourth chakra dominant individual. Whether you learn your life lessons through the development of character is up to you. It may be that along with purity, the hardest thing that you have to do is accept the grace with which you have been imbued.

Is it OK for one person not to have to suffer, when all around them is suffering? Is that a negative attribute of the fourth chakra dominant person? The pressure of this energetic condition can be severe early in life, sorely misunderstood and misdiagnosed.

There are many children in the world today, operating from their respective dominant chakras, who are heavily medicated due to a total misunderstanding of their energetic dispositions. When they come to me for a healing later in life, I have two healings to do, not one. The first healing is for the negative effects of the psychoactive drug that they have been taking, perhaps for years. The second healing is for the exhibited (physical, mental, emotional) weaknesses of their dominant chakra that precipitated the behavior in the first place.

Many fourth chakra individuals ask me what vocation they should pursue. I tell them it does not matter, and they begin reevaluating my skills as an intuitive.

As an aspiration to a vocation, it does not matter. As a fourth chakra individual you are not here to hold a vision, to give truth, to teach, etc. Your mere presence is healing in itself. I tell them that I don't care if they hang doors on cars for a living. Just do what you love and place a value on your labors. People will tend to heal just because you exist. It does not matter where you go or what you do, but to be more aware of your inherent strengths and weaknesses is to self-empower, and that is your greatest goal. By doing that, you help evolve the soul-group consciousness.

The Law of Symmetry

Because of the profundity of the heart chakra's love, there are no human words to express the depth of emotions that heart chakra individuals feel. Hence, your life's lesson as a heart chakra individual is to learn to communicate. It seems like a double-edged sword, because if you go further into accepting the love you represent, you tacitly accept that intensity in an ever-deepening relationship.

Therefore, many heart chakra individuals endeavor to demonstrate their communicative abilities through the Law of Symmetry. Put simply, if you walk into your friend's house and notice a picture hanging crooked on the wall, what is your first impulse? To straighten it, of course.

But think about it. How do you "know" what "straight" is? This is the root of the qualitative aspect of our multidimensional nature permeating every aspect of our corporeal, quantitative existence. That knowingness of symmetry, the orderliness of all things in their appropriate perspective, is *innate* to the heart chakra individual.

Because the heart chakra person comes to learn how to communicate the emotional profundity of love, many externalize the symmetry of love physically by becoming architects, designers, feng shui practitioners, etc. As love has been called the perfect symmetry, you are externalizing in that perfect symmetry what you cannot express verbally.

Therefore, as a heart chakra individual, you seek to place others in symmetry by communicating, on a profoundly emo-

tional energy level, that organizing principle that heals by association, or representation, through relationship. It is because of
this principle that others seem to heal, merely by being in your
presence. Chaotic people are drawn into your life because you
represent the perfect symmetry of love. Others are drawn to the
perfection it represents, through a relationship with you.

The Law of Symmetry is a way in which you can express the
desires of your life that cannot be expressed with any other form
of communication equally as satisfying.

Still, it is not enough for you to go around "healing" others,
because you must accept your Self fully in order to achieve your
goals of fulfillment in any given lifetime. It means that even
through the Law of Symmetry, you must employ healthy emotional boundaries, keep your emotional energy fields clear, and
use your discerning minds productively.

Healthy Emotional Boundaries

One of the key attributes the heart chakra individual must
hold is healthy emotional boundaries. I cannot stress this
enough. You must be willing to say "no" and mean it. You must
not equivocate about your emotional boundaries; it is all too
easy to have them transgressed by others, and most of the trans-
gression is subconscious.

Emotional boundaries accomplish two goals - one obvious
and one hidden. The first is that the boundaries give you a
fence to keep people on the other side. The hidden benefit is
that you now have a yard in which to be, room to live your life.

Without healthy emotional boundaries, you suffer terribly,
bobbing helplessly on any wave of emotion that comes along. By
that time it is too late, you are already in emotional overwhelm.
And from there you must work to be emotionally grounded.

It is easy to pour your Self into relationships, whether intimate or professional. You will tend to assume other people will
grow to how you have perceived them as emotionally whole and
complete. Healthy boundaries help to avert this most dangerous
of heart chakra issues

The Tibetan monks are very harmless people, praying and
meditating in their monasteries. They are very pure and sacred

beings, totally harmless to others. But they have great big doors on their monasteries because they realize that even though they are harmless, there are many people in the world who, by their freewill, are *not* harmless.

Heart chakra individuals have to be willing to exercise tough love. Any of you who are parents know what I am talking about. It is similar to when I am doing a flower reading and I say "I love you so much that I'm not going to let you off the hook." To let someone off the hook does not serve the other person, or your Self. You have to be willing to say "no." You have to be willing to allow others to suffer, if they must, to learn their lessons. You have to be willing to take responsibility for your Self, so much so that your "no" represents the highest state of love, even if others around you do not perceive it to be so.

Sometimes heart chakra people die early. They have absorbed so much negative compressive emotional energy from others that they manifest systemic and local issues. The compressiveness of the negative energy is what causes the manifestation in the physical, emotional, mental, and spiritual states.

As the throat chakra must be grounded in the physical plane and body, so the heart chakra individual must be emotionally grounded. That means, every moment is an opportunity to express your freewill. As the second chakra person must choose his ability to draw infinite possibilities from his dominant chakra, so must heart chakra people choose absolute love, as much love for your Self as you would give to anyone or anything. When those two energies become equal, you begin to live in your higher aspect, accruing dharma.

Emotional equanimity means choosing to be calm in the face of chaos. By your nature, you will tend to draw chaotic people and betrayers into your life because you represent the perfect symmetry of love.

You must consider your Self as precious. Some of the empowering techniques in this book may sound self-centered, but if you do not take care of your Self, who is going to? Remember, you are a magnificent being of light. You live in Oneness; there is no separation from you and what you seek.

The Feminine Principle

Most women and almost all men have no idea what the "feminine principle" means.

Imagine you are in a mountain meadow. Before you is the meadow, with flowers and ferns of every description, and beyond, a crystal blue lake framed by trees growing right down to the water. Beyond the lake are the mountains. The glow of the sun that has not yet risen has filled the sky with glorious predawn colors. A light mist floats over the meadow.

And there, at your feet, is a delicate spider web in one of the flowers of the meadow. It is filled with a thousand droplets of dew – each drop reflecting the entire scene of beauty just described.

The slightest touch by you would destroy the web forever. The fact that it can exist as that fragile and that beautiful in the same moment is the *essence of the feminine principle.* We are accustomed to use the power of the will to push. The feminine principle uses the power of the will to *allow*, to open a path inward whereby we are pulled forward through our heart's desire to be open and yielding.

You must enter through the feminine principle into the temple of your heart, embrace with your heart what your mind may not understand. You must be vulnerable to your greatness. It can be no other way. This is the life of the heart chakra individual.

Fourth Chakra Priorities

The heart chakra individual is here to represent what love is. You, by your mere existence represent that you've earned the purity and symmetry in your heart that emanates to everyone. It is that energy that the soul-group is relating to for its evolution.

It is very difficult for heart chakra individuals to perceive the purity that they've earned. Indeed, the key word is "earned." You represent the achievement of several lifetimes of dharma. It is not easy to place a value on what that love represents for you and for others in the world. As a result, many heart chakra people do not place a value on that endless love that flows through, and instead assume they must take on the dis-ease of the world.

While your path as a heart chakra individual is no greater or lesser than anyone else's, your disposition of love makes the path unique in quality and proportion to the number of other chakra dominant individuals. Your statistical prominence (about one in every twenty-five people is heart chakra dominant) makes your path one that requires as much, or more, attention to the specific weaknesses of the lower aspects of the heart chakra.

The life of a fourth chakra individual often centers on the "service with no service" soul's disposition. That is, many such individuals ask why they do not seem to have a particular task or specific job or career. It is because the qualities of the heart chakra place you in service, representing the vast majority of communication that is not physical, but is energy exchange.

It does not matter what type of work you do: All you have to do is show up and people will begin to heal from the perfect love and symmetry of love that you represent. Remember that while all your chakras are working, if your most dominant is the heart chakra, these will be the major life's experiences. Remember also that people will heal, just because you exist, so always place a value on what you do, whether it is a career or a marriage.

You, as an empath, are in total, direct immersion in the emotions of humanity, exercising compassion and evolving your soul by staying in your higher aspects. How is it possible, in this linear dimension, to adequately express the perfect symmetry of love? And, if your disposition is to represent what love is, how many times would you turn it around in your head, over and over, trying diligently to express it?

Fourth Chakra Communication

"In the same way, the Spirit helps us in our weakness. We do not know what we ought to pray for, but the Spirit himself intercedes for us with groans that words cannot express." (Romans 8:26, Bible, New International Version)

You are here to learn to communicate, but no human can express love in the purely physical realm. You can only represent it. The light is not the flashlight, the menu is not the meal, and the map is not the topography.

You constantly feel, even after a conversation, that your feelings were not fully expressed. This is a natural consequence because there is no physical, linear, quantitative way to fully communicate pure love and its symmetry of emotions that flow through your heart chakra. This is why so many heart chakra individuals communicate instead through intermediary devices that have perfect symmetry. They become interior designers, architects, Feng Shui practitioners, sculptors, healers, etc.

You, as a heart chakra person, are like the mountain lake of great depth. From a distance you cannot tell how deep it is. So many heart chakra people are not understood for that profundity of depth they represent, that their mere presence is healing. Only as you approach nearer can you tell the depth of the lake. Only as you attempt to see the depth of the heart chakra individual can you appreciate the amount of love they hold.

It is at once subtle and profound, and so easy for a profane world to overlook the great depth of beauty of the heart chakra individual.

Higher and Lower Aspects of the Fourth Chakra

Aspects of the heart chakra are determined by a sense of self-love. As with any of the chakras discussed in this book, the emanations of our higher consciousness coming through the chakras are most difficult to accept. Not because they are complicated or powerful in themselves, but because they are so very pure and simple.

Higher aspects reflect a life composed of the infusion of love, will, and wisdom. Lower aspects reflect fear, loss of Self, and fear of the lack of love, resulting in much suffering.

Higher aspects of the fourth chakra:

1. Love Itself
2. The Healer
3. Emotional Anchor

4. The Hub of the Many-Spoked Wheel
5. The Conserver and Preserver
6. The Person of Symmetry
7. Relationship with the Fairy Kingdom

Lower aspects of the fourth chakra:
1. The Human Emotional Pincushion
2. The Saboteur
3. Loss of Identity

Higher Aspects of the Fourth Chakra Explained

1. Love Itself

"To be what love is." Does that mean you walk around, your head in the clouds, feeling holy? No, it is holding the purity you've earned, the effortless movement of consciousness from one moment to the next, for you know in your heart that it is indeed true. It does not need to be true for anyone else but it does for you.

The essence of this higher aspect is doing everything to be in total trust of that love, that you are not separate from it. It emanates to you and through you with no separation. It is in this state that you offer the greatest possibility for others to aspire to their higher selves.

As second chakra individuals cause others to become inspired because they are inspired, so too will you cause others to aspire to their higher selves because you choose to hold your Self (moment to moment) in that purity. It is a freewill decision that requires your participation to allow your Self to hold that vastness of love the heart chakra represents.

Many heart chakra individuals run their lives by their heart, not their head, because they are meant to. If you emphasize the feelings of your heart, you sacrifice nothing of your mind and its ability to make rational and practical decisions.

You must decide if you are a heart chakra individual, and

whether you are retreating to your mind as a defense against the world Some heart chakra individuals retreat to their heads as a defense against emotional overwhelm: They become analytical and critical.

Do you want to know how to tell if you are a heart-based individual? If you are, whenever you become emotionally stressed or overwhelmed, you cannot think. It is because of the negative emotional compressive energies you've absorbed in the emotional energy body. The second chakra runs a very close second from emotional overwhelm, but is more associated with spreading oneself too thin, dispersing their energies into chaos.

Emotional numbness is a condition of the heart chakra when you have faced a tidal wave of emotions. It is so beneficial to imagine that you have a "volume control" so that you can regulate what you take on. In that way, you can prevent some of the emotional numbness that sometimes occurs. You'll not prevent all of it. Some lessons are necessary so that you learn from your life experiences.

2. The Healer

Communication that is non-verbal energy emanates from you at all times. If you are heart chakra dominant, others will think "healer" when they approach you. Although there are not many people who will actually think (though most entirely subconsciously) of that word, they will assume on some level that you possess skills to help with their infirmities. Many times it is the case that others take a psychic relationship to what you represent, giving you more accord for your skill than you may realize you have.

When you engage psychically with others, most of that interaction is when they are physically present, but they do not need to be. When you are on the phone, when you read a letter, watch TV, you are committing a psychic link, especially with your loved ones. These psychic relationships continue every day you are in your body, the interactions helping you to make decisions about the evolution of your soul.

When the energetic relationship is taken to the fourth chakra individual, the exchange is most often a healing to a certain degree. However, it is also most often unnoticed and unrecognized as such, because Western society is not trained or educated to understand energy in this way. The exchange occurs, nonetheless, and the result is healing through the absorption of negative compressive emotional energy by the fourth chakra individual.

For you as a heart chakra person, engaging with others psychically means two things happen: they take on a little healing energy from you, and you take on a little negativity from them. Remember, the reciprocity of your relationship to others is that you show them what love is, initially at great expense to your emotions, until you learn healthy emotional boundaries.

As you are healing others, consciously or not, you may notice how many people at the mall, grocery store, bank, etc., walk very near you and pause there for a moment. They are engaging close to your energy, to draw off a little healing energy. Most times this is not a negative encounter. These are people who aspire to their own higher aspects, who desire to heal their infirmities, and they are taking a psychic relationship to you for their healing. I grant you that for most people and most instances, this is on a purely subconscious level.

What would you do with this information if you knew it was happening in the moment? Would you be more careful with how you spend your energy, to whom you give it? This is not meant for you to erect huge emotional barriers to real interaction, but somewhere in the middle between extremes is found that person of equanimity.

What if you, like a sponge, were taking on all the illnesses, mental anguish, and emotional distress from those around you? What if you were taking those energies on for your soul-group? Would it explain how you're feeling, how it is sometimes difficult to cope with what you are experiencing? What if you were suffering but did not know from what, or how to heal it? Even a basic understanding of metaphysics and the dynamics of subtle energy helps to explain why some fourth chakra individuals have a difficult time staying emotionally even.

As others take relationship to what you represent they begin to heal, though there are those who are not interested in healing. Like the second chakra lower aspect, you may be constantly helping someone who has no intention of healing, in order to maintain an unhealthy, passive-aggressive and/or codependent relationship. This is where your healthy discernment and boundaries come in.

Something you may notice is that about every three to four weeks you may be completely down and out of energy, but not sick. For women, this is not part of the monthly cycle. This is a time of recapitulation, where your emotional energy field has become so saturated with negative compressive emotional energy that you must "recharge" your field by having a few down days. Rest, drink lots of water, pray/meditate, do the exercises in this book, and stay in equilibrium emotionally.

Although others tend to heal just because you exist, this does not mean you need to study energetic healing and become a formal healer. It means that your presence is healing as an individual who holds great purity from lifetimes well-lived. It means you cannot sabotage your emotions and live a healthy life at the same time. It also means you must take responsibility for your own greatness.

That means you hold your Self as sacred in that purity, knowing that everything you do to empower your Self also, in some way, has a healing effect on those in your soul-group, and humanity as a whole.

3. Emotional Anchor

The heart chakra individual can be the emotional anchor for a few people or for thousands of people. In the same way that you can represent healing through the purity of love, souls can take relationship to you to be the emotional anchor, or stability, for the group. I have seen this many times, where the individual is built to hold immense emotional energy, yet does not realize he is actively holding together the functional, energetic emotional dynamics for a group of people - sometimes a very large group.

It is so easy to miss the point that you as a heart chakra individual must be supported for your efforts. Most people have no idea the amount of energy it takes to hold this relationship, and if they did know, they should be doing everything to make you feel loved and comfortable. It is difficult because many of us do not even feel that we're psychic, much less taking energetic relationships to each other. Many of us have never been educated about how energy really flows and works, and thus we are limited to a less than optimal experience because we don't understand it.

You could move to another city, and the dynamics would be the same. People there would take psychic relationship to you, and you would mutually create the anchor for those who take relationship to what you represent as heart chakra dominant.

In holding this energetic disposition, the emotional anchor is like that pulsating hub of the many-spoked wheel, constantly interacting with souls on many levels of being, and requiring huge amounts of energy just to stay "even."

It is so imperative that you take very good care of your Self. Sometimes the biggest effort of all is just for you to realize who you are, and the tremendous responsibility of the position, the honor, you've earned to be able to help so many souls. It is easy to doubt that this is true, but this is how it works.

4. The Hub of the Many-Spoked Wheel

The fourth chakra individual often takes a position where many people in the soul-group relate to that individual as the spokes of a wagon wheel. The fourth chakra individual is the hub; always taking the "weight" on the axle of soul-group improvement from the many spokes (see Illustration #10-a).

Note here that no spoke touches any other spoke, but that they all attach to the hub. Also note that any given spoke never bears the whole weight, nor carries the weight of the other spokes. The hub stays in constant relationship to the spokes in the soul-group as the "wheel" (the entire soul-group interaction) travels forward through time.

This is also why fourth chakra individuals are found to be about one in every twenty five people, because they take a relationship to so many spokes (people), helping to anchor and heal the emotional conditions of others.

Thus the condition of some fourth chakra individuals can be very severe in that they are energetically allowing relationships to be taken to what they represent as purity and healing in this lifetime. By severe I mean that you can take on the infirmities, suffering, emotional, mental, and physical "issues" of another in a psychic relationship where you are the "hub" and another in-

Fourth Chakra Dominant Individual

WHEEL OF LIFE

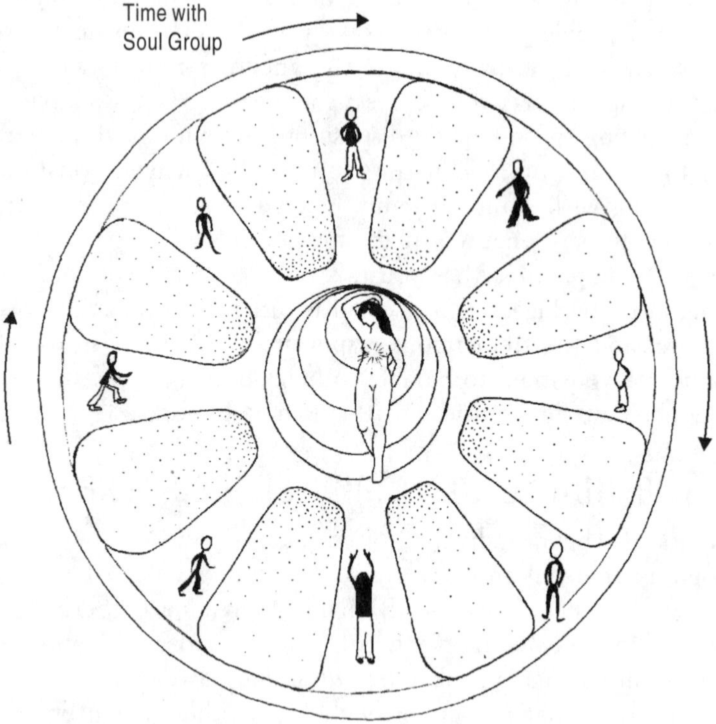

Time with
Soul Group

Hub of the many spoked wheel:
- Bears weight of axle of emotional relationships at all times.
- All spokes connect to hub.
- Can be a very large number of spokes
- No spoke touches any other spoke directly
- Wheel is in motion
- Each spoke bears weight of emotional relationship for only a moment, as the wheel is in motion.

Illustration #10-a: Empathic Relationships

dividual of the soul-group is the "spoke."

You can take on too much, often suffering some of the same issues as the spokes, or collectively amassing a tremendous amount of negative compressive emotional energy. The build-up of negative emotional energy in the human energy field can be compared to a water glass, where the glass is meant to only hold so much and no more. Add any more water to an already full glass and the glass "overflows" its threshold. In this case, the individual's energy field becomes denigrated because of emotional overflow.

This is why so many heart chakra individuals have illnesses that cannot be diagnosed or traced, because they initiate the healing effect through the hub and spoke energetic relationship to the whole of the given soul-group.

The Skip-Function of the Single Spoke in Relationship to the Hub

Viewed in Illustration #10-a, a single spoke (representing one person's energetic relationship to the heart chakra dominant individual) bears the full weight of the relationship only when located directly beneath the hub, as the entire wheel (soul-group) moves forward through time. The remainder of the time is spent in healing response and integration until the cycle repeats itself. Note that the spokes (individuals) may take different cyclic psychic energetic relationships to the person at the hub.

At the base cycle the individual takes the relationship through representation to the fourth chakra individual, obtaining some healing relief or exchange of negative emotional energy.

As time moves forward the individual cycles next into an integrative phase, where the effects of the healing and diffusion of negative emotional energy take place in the mental, physical, spiritual, and emotional aspects. These can vary according to time, karma, mission statement, relative health of the individual, and freewill choice.

At the peak of the cycle the relationship to the fourth chakra individual (hub) is the least energetic. Correspondingly, the energetic "pull" on the fourth chakra individual by the spoke (person) is also minimal.

The last phase begins the cycle once more, where the spoke begins to align energies, intent, and life-path into another direct contact at its maximum through time, at the base under the hub, where the exchange of energy is the most pronounced.

5. The Conserver and Preserver

The purity of the heart chakra individual, as you can see, externalizes to the physical, mental, and emotional levels of your life in several ways. It is the same with the other chakras: Souls will always externalize their personalities on the higher levels to the third dimensional personality.

There is a desire in the heart of the fourth chakra individual similar to that of the third chakra individual. It is the desire to maintain and preserve purity and to protect innocence. This often externalizes in the higher aspect through interest in ecology of the planet, preservation of what is pure in nature, culture, humanity, and conservation of things in life felt to be of a pure origin, or worth preserving.

These manifestations of the purity of the heart are a way of holding sacred, in trust, what that purity represents as the refinement of the innermost desires of our heart, beyond which there is no measure. That qualitative state cannot be quantified, but exists as a pure state of being, or Heaven on earth.

As a heart chakra individual, you bring Heaven on earth by grounding the purity you represent through the externalization of your custodianship of love, emanating to others through the symbolism of preservation and conservation. You will often champion causes that reflect a worldwide (system) effort in your desire to see humanity as whole and complete.

Those taking a relationship to you are ready to hold sacred their own inner vulnerability to aspire and surpass their understanding of love.

6. The Person of Symmetry

The higher aspect of symmetry brings the chaotic people into your life. They are your teachers of equanimity. They take psychic relationship to this special category of the heart chakra because the Divine organizing principle of love flows through you.

As stated in the Law of Symmetry, you just "know" what the

whole, organized system is, whether material, emotional, mental, or spiritual. That ability is very useful when applied directly to being a healer. But it also applies to seeing the complete connection between all the aspects of any activity, from the architecture of whole building systems, to understanding DNA sequences, to energetic practices in healing of individuals.

As the chakra gym example demonstrates, others are in your life to help you work out your lower aspect issues of wholly undervaluing the sublime ease with which you perceive the balance in all things.

Like the picture on the wall, a slight adjustment from you and everything is back in balance. This power is easy to abuse, but it is also easily abused by others. An example is the person who continually re-enters your life. You fix him, he's on his way, then he's back. It is when you finally say "no" that the cause changes and an improved effect occurs.

Always remember that this can be more effortless the more you allow it to be so. Effortless congruity is allowing the higher spiritual forces at work to be co-creators in your collaborative leadership through life.

7. The Relationship to the Fairy Kingdom

There are five kingdoms on the earth plane:

1. Humanity
2. Deva
3. Plant
4. Animal
5. Elemental (rocks, minerals, water, air, etc.)

The "deva" kingdom is the least understood of all the kingdoms. It can be the wind, the spirit that helps plants to grow in the way they do, the custodian of a mountain, a part of the breath of the earth. A subset of the deva kingdom includes the fairies, elves, gnomes, pixies, brownies, sprites, and so on.

Some heart chakra individuals, by way of their purity, have earned the right to associate with the fairy kingdom. How could you know if you do? There are two main ways to tell:

1. You constantly "lose" things but they show up later; car keys, bills, wallets, glasses, etc.
2. Things in your home are "rearranged" and no one you know has touched them.

One of my teachers, Dr. Hiroshi Motoyama, is the founder of the Institute for Parapsychology and Religion in Tokyo, Japan. His laboratory is on the second floor directly above his office. Dr. Motoyama has related how the fairies are constantly taking things from his office and transporting them into the laboratory.

Why would fairies be in the life of the fourth chakra individual? They represent a lightness and a purity, and they appear to ease your emotions, to help you find humor in the ironies of life, and to attend lovingly to you. I have found most fairies are fond of brushing most of you fourth chakra readers by the cheek, ear, or just under the ear, ever so lightly.

This quality of the fairies becomes a higher aspect when you are living in one or more of the other higher aspects of the heart chakra.

By the way, the number of fairies tend to *increase* in number as you go through life.

Lower Aspects of the Fourth Chakra

1. The Human Emotional Pincushion

Taking on everyone's negative energy is one way of getting attention, but it is devastating in the process. Many people suffer long and needlessly due to ignorance of the energetic dynamics involved. Healing from this lower aspect can take a tremendous act of the will to break emotional dependencies that are, at best, undefined.

Sometimes people heal only when the stakes are high enough and it has become "worth it" to heal. When it gets that bad, there is a long road of exerting the power of the will in healthy emotional boundaries.

One of the problems you have as a heart chakra personality is that you do not put enough value on your ability to receive emotionally, so you tend to compensate by giving too much of your Self. This results in a loss of identity that can go on for a long time. Many such people do not complain of their predicament or of the ensuing illnesses.

They stopped giving out medals a long time ago for how long you can hold on to pain. You must give it up and not value your Self by your ability to psychically take on other people's negative energies through your empathy.

We all desire love and affection but are not very good at communicating our desires to each other. Add to that a heart chakra dominance, and you have a recipe for disaster if you assume you can heal others by taking on their emotional issues. One of the first lessons I teach my students in healer's training workshops is not to take on the negative energies of the people they are healing. Some do anyway, as they must learn the lesson in their own way. Ultimately it degrades the emotional energy field and sets the stage for infirmities and illnesses to appear as a healing process of their own.

If you decided not to be the human emotional pincushion, what would you do instead? This is a valid and difficult question for some, as they have spent their life in service to others in the misguided notion that serving others is enough, but it is not. You cannot heal others from a position of weakness, and using your emotional energy field as a punching bag can only last so long.

To stop this lower aspect behavior you must first place a value on your emotions and ask your Self if it is worth the pain. You must give your Self as much love as you would anyone else, and you must love your Self fiercely, similar to the second chakra disposition. You must use the word "no" and mean it.

Emotional Neediness

Some heart chakra individuals become emotionally needy and become a different type of magnet that takes emotional energy from others. This is similar to the second chakra's vampiric lower aspect. The heart chakra individual in the lower aspect becomes the endless black hole, sucking energy.

This condition exists when heart chakra individuals feel they will never receive enough love, so they begin to pull the emotions of others. Have you ever felt drained when talking to someone? Chances are they were pulling on your emotional energy body. The problem is, until heart chakra personalities heal, they will continue to pull energy from anyone and everyone around them on a continual basis, with no end in sight.

Emotional Overwhelm

It is difficult to adequately convey just how sensitive the fourth chakra individual is to the feelings and emotions of others. Fourth chakra individuals are so empathic that for some it is a constant struggle just to stay evenly balanced. Even that much is sometimes too much emotionally.

Emotional overwhelm causes many a heart chakra individual to have fuzzy thinking when otherwise your mind works quite well. It is the saturation of negative compressive energies in your emotional energy body.

You can even feel an *emotional numbness*, a very strange feeling for a heart chakra individual. Again, this is because of emotional over-saturation, not because you cannot feel.

Perhaps this makes it a little easier to understand why fourth chakra individuals are here to learn to communicate. Imagine those whose feelings are "on" at all times, so sensitive to their emotional environment and to the feelings and emotions of others around them. Imagine being hit by the tidal wave of emotions that can come from one or more people, then imagine how this can be a blessing to the fourth chakra individual!

Actually, it is a tremendous blessing because there is, in reality, nothing to overwhelm. Once again, it is our linear and temporal mind doing its thing to try and bring Heaven on earth through the five senses only. It cannot be done. To bring Heaven on earth, you must unite your metaphysical nature with your physical senses through your feelings; feelings that transcend the thinking, into a qualitative state of "allowability."

Allowability is a term that means you cannot push on a door that opens inward. It means that only by being vulnerable to your feelings can you truly exceed your Self. This is that hard part of metaphysics that relies on absolute trust in your Self, and is not transferable from another. It is a choice, built and dependent upon your individual freewill to choose at all. This is what Joseph Campbell was referring to when he said that we all pick our own point of entry into the dark forest.

The more you are willing to allow through a fierce inner trust, the more growth in the evolution of your consciousness is possible.

Some fourth chakra individuals, however, experience a form of claustrophobia from having open emotional energy fields. When you are in a room full of people, your energy field can only absorb so much of the energy from others (and many times it is very chaotic energy) until you experience an urgency to leave. This is due to an instant and immediate contact with most everyone's energy field, and can be quite distracting.

It is also a sign that you have much to do to improve your self-empowerment and to create healthy emotional boundaries. There are always exceptions where you may require the lesson, have the mission statement, or karma, to experience such emotional overload. This phenomenon is much more common than you may think.

2. The Saboteur

Sabotage is validating the "I'm not worthy for love" lower aspect of the heart chakra. Recall that the chakra is multi-dimensional and the mind is not. Your mind has great difficulty coping with the higher dimensions conceptually, and you try to run your heart with your mind to make everything in this dimension fit into a nice, neat model.

Well, the universe is ironic, and it does not make sense to the physical mind; it is not supposed to. That is why you have feelings - to transcend the linear and embrace the higher level of existing.

Saboteurs often use negative self-reinforcing belief systems to validate the outcome: "See, nothing I do works. See, I'm not worthy of a great relationship." By casting enough doubt on it, saboteurs kill the relationship, validating their negative beliefs.

Again, it takes a tremendous act of courage, belief, and love in your Self, plus staying around healthy people, to change this self-destructive behavior. Since heart chakra people can be so sensitive, carefully choose whom you wish to be with, and choose those whom you would like to emulate. As you do so, the contrast between these friends and your old behavior will become apparent.

Emotionally Needy

The fear that "I won't get more love" is similar to what other chakra dispositions experience as the inverse to their true nature. Remember that we are suffering because we doubt our connection to Oneness. If you are a heart chakra individual, then you came here to represent what love is. It also means that you will doubt your purity and that you will never experience enough love until you begin to live in the higher aspect of the chakra.

This neediness is a dynamic that builds the saboteur's negative self-fulfilling belief system that ruins relationships to prove the negative point: "See? No matter what I do, I don't have emotionally-rewarding relationships." So many heart chakra individuals suffer quietly in desperation and resignation throughout their lives, assuming this to be true. It's not just an emotional malaise, but can eventually lead to other systemic problems of the mind and body as well (see *Health Issues*, later in this chapter).

To overcome emotional neediness requires a large act of courage to use the very same vulnerability that created the problem, though the act itself to change is gentle. Sometimes the greatest changes require the gentlest of gestures from the greatest heights of courage. It's strange how the gentlest gifts we give to ourselves sometimes require gargantuan acts of courage.

In The Prophet, Kahlil Gilbran expounds on the danger of love:

"When love beckons you, follow him,
Though his ways are hard and steep,
And when his wings enfold you yield to him,
Though the sword hidden among his pinions may wound you."

And yet, spread your wings you must. It is only by being vulnerable to love that you can love fully.

You must allow your Self to receive love, in the fierce recognition that there is no separation in the Oneness. That means you remain vulnerable and open to be loved, even though vulnerable to pain. It is your fierceness to be open to love that spirit (your higher Self) notices and acknowledges. It is the *effort* you make in the moment to be whole and complete, not the goal.

Sometimes the changes seem infinitesimal, but they are changes nonetheless. Be fierce in your desires. Never give up.

3. Loss of Identity

From my observations, most often fourth chakra individuals experience a loss of their personal identity early in life, from adolescence to their early twenties. If you are an empath, you feel what other people feel, only feel it so well that you do not discern the difference between your own feelings and the ones that are saturating your emotional energy body and fourth chakra.

If you have no real healthy emotional boundaries you would assume that what you are feeling are your own feelings. Eventually you begin to sense that when someone else expresses an emotion, you feel it but wonder why. This is where an identity crisis ensues, while you sort out your own authentic feelings from those around you.

Then begins a search for Self, and for healthy emotional boundaries, by creating circumstances and lessons that offer the opportunity for growth and discernment.

Fourth Chakra Relationships

One of the key errors that the heart chakra individual commits is very similar to the second chakra (both chakras are yin energy - receptive, emotional, nurturing). That is, heart chakra individuals are empaths (whereas second chakra individuals are mystics), and they psychically (empathically) see what their partner could be as emotionally whole and complete.

I have mentioned the difference between an accurate intuitive knowing of the other person's potential, and making the *assumption* that because you were correct intuitively, that is what your partner desires. Your partner may not be ready to embrace what you have so accurately intuited. And don't forget an empath's ability is always on, but your consciousness may be aware of your power to greatly differing degrees.

In order to have a great relationship you must exercise your healthy boundaries continually. Chakra dispositions are *life* issues, not today issues. It is all too easy to look for the quick fix, but consciousness is rooted in the effort, not the goal.

As a heart chakra individual you give of your Self through your most dominant connection to love on the highest level of consciousness. It is sometime difficult to perceive your own preciousness and sacredness as a being whose center is all about what love is.

Healing Issues for the Fourth Chakra

Physiological and psychological issues can develop from lower aspects of a heart chakra disposition. These issues can become systemic to your body, mind, and emotions, including problems with the heart itself, respiration, ribs, thymus (immune and endocrine system), skin, joints, fibromyalgia, blood flow and blood quality, and weight retention. Other issues include:

- Musculature, connective joint and tissue disorders, muscle tissue
- Vascular: veins, arteries, blood quality, blood pressure, blood sugar, enzymes, proteins. Blood: dissolved gasses
- Heart: rate, volume, beat. Heart function: arrhythmia, tachycardia, murmurs
- Nervous system: sympathetic and parasympathetic
- Meridian: all twelve meridian systems
- Skeletal: bones, bone marrow, bone structure
- Thoracic vertebrae, cartilaginous matter
- Skin: skin irritations, disorders, blemishes, rashes, etc.
- Allergies, arthritis
- Respiratory: lungs, bronchia, the act of breathing, asthma,

bronchial and thoracic issues. The inability of the lungs to exchange dissolved gasses with the blood.

Many such fourth chakra individuals suffer greatly without even knowing they are energetically taking on the negative compressive emotional energies of others. Unfortunately this can last a lifetime.

Marjorie Haynes has written an important book that discusses the amazing proliferation of fibromyalgia in the last fifteen years. Fibromyalgia has now been classified as its own disease: It is a condition where the individual suffers from pain in the musculature of the body. Many fourth chakra individuals take on the suffering of others, originating in the emotional energy body, and it takes time, sometimes years, to permeate the lower vibrational level of the physical body.

Psychological issues include a loss of personal identity, depression, loss of the ability to think clearly, personal sabotage, and a constant struggle to stay emotionally stable. Heart chakra individuals can instantly manifest issues of emotional depression, fatigue, and anxiety, because those are directly related to the functioning emotional energies.

It is important to understand the tremendous energy requirements you have as a fourth chakra individual. To maintain a healthy body and good stamina you must recognize that your body is like a factory, processing the emotional energies of others, especially in relationships. There are those who incarnate with very healthy and strong bodies and constitutions and who do not suffer from such emotional energy drain, but there are also many heart chakra individuals who do.

How to Emphasize the Strengths of the Heart Chakra

- Ground emotionally, just as the throat chakra person must ground his body
- Healthy emotional boundaries
- Love your Self as much as anyone or anything
- Never sabotage your feelings
- Being gullible and naïve is OK in innocence, but use discernment in relationships
- Accept the purity you represent; that you've *earned* through

past life dharma
- It's OK for others to heal, just because you exist
- You've no specific job vocation, though symmetry will always work
- Do what you love and place a value on it
- Communicate as well as you can, knowing no human tongue can express its fullness, and no human ear can hear its purity. Know it in your heart. Feel it in your heart
- Allow your Self to be emotionally correct when empathically observing others
- Do not take on suffering so that others may heal; transmute instantly any negativity you take on.

Evolving the Soul-Group Consciousness

When the soul-group takes a relationship to what the heart chakra individual represents, they are in many ways offering up their chaos for its own resolution. When you resolve the lens of a camera, you bring into focus all the elements for the scene you wish to capture. You as a heart chakra individual bring into emotional resolution the possibility of the evolution of the soul-group consciousness by:

1. Living in the higher aspect of your fourth chakra
2. Members of the soul-group make healthy choices for their lives from energetic encounters with you.

The symmetry of love attracts its inverse - chaos and neediness. By your nature you will attract the chaotic elements of your soul-group as the emotional anchor, healer, and hub of the many-spoked wheel. They take relationship to you to divest themselves of their suffering. They take relationship to you so they may aspire to the purity you represent from several lifetimes of merit through dharma.

The symmetry of love is the Divine level that balances the view of the picture of the world, the whole system of the mechanics of the universe, all intricately and sublimely working together as one. By your right actions you offer to the world their aspiration to hold the perfection of what love is.

The symmetry of love is perfect, and most daunting to the fourth chakra individual. If you can accept the limitless love that flows through you, you evolve your Self in the upward evolutionary spiral and everyone in your soul-group benefits from your vulnerability and courage.

Remember that sometimes the greatest acts of courage are enacted by the slightest and gentlest turn of your emotions toward love and truth, toward harmlessness, towards the courage to love your Self fiercely.

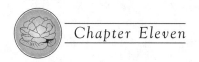

Chapter Eleven

Fifth Chakra – The Communicator

The fifth or throat chakra individual is the "step-down trans-former for God." You are to articulate what others cannot say by grounding information that others in your soul-group clamor for. In so doing, hopefully you hear the very message that you are bringing through, in order to raise the vibration of your own life. The difficulty is that you must be grounded, which renders you vulnerable to the feelings wrought through contact with the earth plane.

By definition of the chakra of communication, you as a fifth chakra individual are very psychic and well-tuned to the minds of others, and most times telepathic, even with animals and plants. I have known throat chakra individuals who prefer the company of plants and animals to humans because non-humans have no caveat, no hidden agenda. It does not work for very long as that behavior is ultimately unfulfilling for most human beings.

The vibration of the throat chakra, rooted in communication, daunts your physical mind into prescience (insight). That is, the higher, inter-dimensional communicative aspects of the throat chakra are an order of consciousness higher than that of the physical brain. Your mind capitulates to the strength of the throat chakra, especially if it is dominant, such that your mind attempts to do in the physical plane what the chakra does on higher vibratory planes. Your mind gets ahead of itself and you spend much time in the *future tense*.

Blending your natural impatience as a throat chakra indi-vidual with a high degree of psychic development, results in your tendency to finish people's sentences and to know where the next paragraph is going before you get to it. Because of the prescience of the linear mind, you are not the most patient person in the world. Your impatience is a real distraction from your spiritual power, if you sacrifice being present in the moment.

When your linear mind attempts to engage in nonlinear activity, the prescience leads to, at the very least, impatience and frustration. It can only enter the earth plane at a certain linear rate. Thus your frustration in communication. The prescience can be unrelenting. But this impatience is not helpful, nor is it temporary.

Your frustration can lead to a racing and frenetic mind. When this occurs, you may go "out-of-body" easily and soul-travel or spend a lot of time in the astral plane. Examples that are similar to being out-of-body are daydreaming, watching television in a hypnotic manner, or finding you've driven your car miles down the highway without consciously paying attention to the road.

And yes, it is true that you may be talkative, sometimes without really saying anything, because of the strong and misunderstood energies that are coming through your throat chakra as the teacher and communicator. Such unchecked verbosity is fairly common and often a mark of being out-of-body.

Why is this important? Because if you are in your body, you can feel, and if you can feel, you can feel pain. So, most throat chakra people are pretty smart. They stay out-of-body through various pursuits and pastimes, though you cannot register those "spiritual frequent flyer miles" for having been here on the earth plane experientially by being out-of-body. Even so, many fifth chakra personalities spend a lot of time on the astral plane. Look around in a supermarket or department store and you can observe over half the people there are not fully present.

Shallow breathing, loose focus of eyes, loose mind concentration, thoughts running rampant, speech rapid and unconnected; these are all signs of an ungrounded person. In time, it becomes very easy to spot the throat chakra dominant person, even without using psychic abilities.

Hidden side effects of being out-of-body too long are lack of productivity, feeling as though your life is not effective, feeling alone, aloof, detached and separate from your Self, loved ones, and community.

Being out-of-body produces these negative effects (lower aspects) of the throat chakra when it has become excessive. If it continues to worsen, this is where disease and illness begin in the mental, physical, spiritual, and emotional states of your being.

Grounding is the principle of uniting as above, so below. It takes your will power to accomplish this because the communicative aspects to the higher realms yield to a condition of not listening to earthly advice or counsel. So many times I have counseled fifth chakra personalities, only to have them return quickly to lower aspect states of behavior and continual out-of-body preference.

The out-of-body experience is a life-issue for fifth chakra individuals. It means you can work on the issue of "groundedness" and presence as much as you want, but you will have to do it for your lifetime. This is because you are here to teach and communicate, and you are also here to learn to feel. I have clients who reveal they've been working on certain issues for years: How come they have not overcome them yet? Some of these issues are yours for life.

In a way it is like going to the chakra gym to work out. We create the resistance in our lives so that we will grow from our lessons. You cannot grow by just looking at the weights; you have to lift (power of the will in action) them. By working out, you become strong. The next time you have a challenge, because you have worked out in the throat chakra gym, you'll be less likely to fall. And if you do fall, you'll be less likely to be injured.

With suffering and effort come due reward of the evolution of your own consciousness through the evolutionary spiral. Through those endeavors to improve your Self, you offer the greatest gift to humanity - that of the evolved soul. When others take a relationship to what you represent, they have a greater opportunity to heal and grow because of your own personal choices to hold your Self in the higher aspect of your given chakra dominance.

The fifth chakra is the jumping off point to much higher realms of existence. If you imagine the steps (I must admit to looking at it quantitatively) between chakras one through five as single progressive notes on a piano, then imagine the distance between chakra five and six as a whole octave, and you begin to understand the precipice of consciousness upon which you stand if your fifth (throat) chakra is dominant.

The sixth chakra is an octave of energy above the fifth; the seventh is another octave above the sixth. Be aware that having one chakra dominant over the others is not better or worse; it is an experiential perspective of life in this dimension.

When viewing consciousness in terms that you can grasp, you as a fifth chakra dominant person are at that place where Heaven and earth, the non-physical and the physical, truly meet. Hence, your lesson is to "feel" by grounding your tremendous energetic communicative abilities with the earth plane.

Remember the Hermetic principle "as above, so below"? Your purpose as a fifth chakra individual is to unite above and below, Heaven and earth, by articulating what cannot be said to humanity. As you will see later in this chapter, the collaborative workings of your soul-group actually create the mild vacuum for you to appear.

Here we have a problem. If you are a step-down transformer for God, and God is all possible expression, what and how are you to communicate?

God is known as the "ineffable," whose existence cannot be explained because his/her existence is all-encompassing. Western philosophers have a difficult time with two things:

1. Describing the existence of God
2. The problem of language

Describing God is impossible, the philosophers argued, for in order to describe something you must first stand outside the experience of it. If God is the all-encompassing All That Is, there is no way that you can stand outside of that experience to describe it; "over and against itself, thus constituted," as some Western philosophers would say.

As a fifth chakra individual, you have the ability to "step down" the energies through your soul and monad to give to humanity an explanation and articulation of why things work the way they do. You have the ability to telepathically engage with other people, plants and animals, and can engage in prophecy. Although I do not recommend it without adequate teaching, you make great channels for ascended beings. It is the teacher within that externalizes through you. But what language to use to communicate effectively?

Language as Western society knows it, is composed of symbols to help us communicate. For example, let's say I just bought a beautiful wood table for my dining room, and I call you on the phone to tell you. You ask, "Rick, what does it look like?"

How long do you think it would take for me to fully describe everything there is to know about my new table to you, so that you would know as much about it as if you were standing in the dining room right next to it? Now imagine the fifth chakra individual, psychically seeing all of what the table is, and attempting to communicate to humanity what he sees. It's like blowing your breath out through a soda straw. It can only come through so fast in this dimension, limited by time and space.

We use language as a convenience for communication, but the symbology of language has cost us a great deal in the supposed benefit of expediency of using a single word to describe the vast character of the "thing itself." Throat chakra personalities are in direct psychic contact with all of this information; it is one of the primary reasons why they are so impatient. The press of psychic information coming through your mind and expressing through the limited linear communicative abilities can be exceedingly frustrating.

You as a fifth chakra individual will get information first, before those in your soul-group, for the purpose of disseminating the information to that group. You must illuminate, elucidate, and make information palatable for others in the world, helping them to understand what they cannot know. That sounds very cryptic. It means that you are the holder of great knowledge, but must also dispense it to humanity. Humanity will help set the circumstances where the most exact setting and application are possible for you to articulate. It does not have to be the spoken word: It can be anything that is communicative.

You must continually remind your metaphysical nature of your corporeal presence. This is a life issue. In my experience, it is very difficult for the throat chakra individual to remember to stay grounded.

I remember doing healing work on a fifth chakra dominant woman in Calgary, Canada. She made her living as a psychic, but was house-ridden, in recovery from an ongoing battle with cancer. After the energy healing session, she immediately went back out-of-body and started babbling a mile a minute. She went right back to her old habits.

Everyone goes out-of-body occasionally. When you are out-of-body (ungrounded) you are less than fully conscious of your surroundings and of the present moment.

The reason grounding is so fundamental for you is that you are *so often ungrounded*. This is due to the strength of your dominant fifth chakra. It easily assists you to go out-of-body, reaching higher dimensional levels of awareness, and drawing in higher intuitive abilities. It is a wonderful place to be, but you cannot be there all the time because the earth plane is where you must be to work, in order to achieve those "spiritual frequent flier miles" from having been here.

There is the example of a lovely jazz singer from Manhattan who sent me a CD for evaluation. She is throat chakra dominant. I told her that her singing would sound much better if she were grounded when she sang. She was puzzled and took offense. I explained that when you are in your body (grounded) you are in direct energetic contact with others, which they can tell on some level of their being. If you are *not* in your body as a singer, listening to you would be like listening to a tape recorder on the stage instead of a live performance. It is just not the same, and real communication contact is not effective. It is like talking to your friends on earth from a tin can phone out in space. They don't "see" you, as you are out-of-body and unavailable; they only hear the sound, but not the real content.

If it were a loving relationship, you would be perceived as emotionally unavailable to your partner. This concept is discussed more in the relationship section at the end of this chapter.

It is so difficult to break the attachments to methods that seem to reduce your suffering, but don't last, because the methods do not incorporate a spiritual (metaphysical) knowledge and practice. If you continue ungrounded, you will pay the consequences through your relationships, health, and spiritual evolution.

You can find some humor in the specificity of the fifth chakra. You, as a fifth chakra dominant individual, could be at a party the night before and the next day your friends could ask why you weren't there. You protest that you were indeed at the party. This happens often to fifth chakra individuals. Your specificity can be so fine that others cannot perceive your communicative abilities, or worse, your physical presence.

Why is this so? Because the vibratory rate of your fifth chakra is very high and very fine. It is the cause of the most major of your problems as a fifth chakra personality, that of communication. Something was mis-communicated, misconstrued, there was a misconception, or communication was misinterpreted.

Sometimes you will assume that others have heard you, or understood in the manner you communicated, but often it is not the case. Other times you will be mystified why no one understands you.

Since your vibration is very fine, individuals may hear but not understand you. You must use phrases such as "Repeat back to me what you think you heard,' and you will be amazed to find that your communication was not perceived accurately.

Sometimes people will ask you "What did you say?" It is not that they could not hear you; they are struggling on the metaphysical level to tune in to the high vibration of your high-frequency throat chakra energy.

Communication is a two-way street, and it has many forms.

It is Yin (receptive, incoming)
- I hear
- I see
- I smell
- I sense by touch
- I taste

It is Yang (outgoing, manifestative, assertive)
- I speak, I sing, I act on a stage

- I write, I compose E-mail
- I play music

The nature of the intuitive communicative abilities is so strong coming through throat chakra individuals that often they will not perceive their own talent, but will tend to become frustrated and alienated because of that talent. And so it is with each chakra we've looked at. The great inherent strength of each chakra is the weakness at the same time.

Letting Go of Information

One of the hardest things for throat chakra individuals to do is to let go of the information they give to others. The reason for this is the psychic connection through the well-developed throat chakra. You will feel (and depending on the level of awareness, not always know) the trueness of the information you receive. Thus, when you give such connected information to another, there is an investment in the other person following through. Often it is not the case, as freewill predominates, and anyone has the ability to refuse good information, and even healing, should they choose.

So, there is an attachment to the information you give because you have difficulty letting go in terms of what the other person does with that information. The objective is to allow the individual receiving the information the ability to choose whether to follow it, and to allow them to take the responsibility for the information, regardless of the outcome. This can be a very large stumbling block if you have a strong throat chakra presence, as you may be very invested in the goodness of the outcome. The more investment, the more limiting it is for you, because you cannot *make* another person understand or follow you.

Channeling

One who "channels" acts as a conduit for sentient beings that exist on higher levels of awareness in higher dimensions. As a conduit, the channel ostensibly also brings through higher wisdom, with the proviso that the ego is completely out of the way, in order to bring forth the purity of the message. As a throat chakra individual, you are particularly well-suited for this task, as you have the proper "plumbing" already in place.

It takes much preparation and training to be a good channel, plus a solid understanding of your Self as a functional and Divine part of all that is. There are many so-called channels in the world who channel nothing but their own egos. This makes it very difficult for authentic channels to be viewed as authentic. This difficulty relates to our fundamental problem with metaphysics: How do you know the information you're getting is true and correct, especially if you are not getting it directly from Source?

I'm writing a book called <u>Speak for Your Self</u> that takes a stand against channeling without adequate training and preparation. For a throat chakra person to try channeling without serious training is to throw gasoline on a fire. I cannot emphasize enough how important it is to develop your own inner trust and Divine connection first, before you decide to channel someone else.

No One Knows Me For Who I Really Am

The greatest fear of the fifth chakra individual is that no one knows you for who you really are. Because your vibration is such a high frequency, it can be difficult for others to tune in to what you are attempting to communicate. It is not because you cannot communicate; it is because you perceive higher levels of communication without consciously understanding their level of vibration. Often, when others are squinting their eyes to understand, they are attempting to tune into that communication that is energetic, not physical.

Because it is sometimes difficult for others to tune in, the ensuing problem for fifth chakra dominant people is that they can feel no one knows them. The alienation and detachment the fifth chakra dominant person feels can lead to a resignation from humanity (See the Hermit lower aspect), and even a rejection of humanity.

Many *will not* know a fifth chakra dominant person for who you really are. This emphasizes the point that you must be grounded and aware of your physical presence. In being grounded, you offer the opportunity to others to "see" you energetically, at least according to their spiritual and intuitive development. Some people will not be capable of seeing the real you no matter what you do, for the problem is theirs, not yours.

The Gross Earth Vibration

When your fine throat chakra vibration meets the gross (rough and uneven) vibration of the earth plane there can be much resistance to growth. Many throat chakra people have a difficult time being here and relating to the exigencies (little emergencies) that are a part of everyday life. You must be grounded into this vibration to be efficacious, but by grounding, you may feel even more. Even though grounding leads you to the possibility of feeling more, and not all feelings are pleasant, it is a necessary element of a healthy fifth chakra.

One of my teachers is throat chakra dominant. When he was born, his feet and legs were turned up into his body. The symbolism was that the earth plane of vibration was so "gross" that it was difficult for the lower part his physical body (feet) to even touch the ground. That is classically the part of our body that makes contact with the earth. It is why so many throat chakra individuals have problems from the knees down.

My teacher had to have multiple surgeries so that by the time he was five he could walk with braces. By the time he was ten he could walk unaided. I have counseled several throat chakra individuals to find they have had leg, body architecture, and blood circulation problems as children.

Can you imagine spending the first ten years of your life with such great difficulty even touching the earth plane? But so it is with many throat chakra individuals who quite naturally spend a lot of time distracting themselves from the heaviness of this dimension and avoiding being fully in body. Many are daydreamers, smokers, and escapees from the rougher parts of this dimension.

The earth vibration can be very difficult for you to navigate due to your highly sensitive communicative (energetic) abilities. Walking through such a gross vibration is a natural inducement for you to go right out-of-body. And yes, smoking and drinking do soothe the emotional nature and the out-of-body experience, but since those habits are not a holistic approach, the behaviors may only last a while before ending.

Fifth Chakra Reciprocity

Although certainly not exclusive, you as a throat chakra individual will attract those who can feel emotionally (fourth chakra empath and second chakra visceral) in order to allow you to feel the earth plane.

When you understand that 95% of all communication is non-verbal and non-physical, that it is energy on many other levels, then an understanding of the true dynamics of communication is possible. We all take psychic relationships to each other. When two people meet, there is a dialogue on a very high level, seldom conscious, where the true communication is held, agreements are made, and karmic implications and/or freewill choice decisions are put into effect by both parties. The higher dialogue includes a precise recognition of the chakric attributes of the other person, any karmic ties, and reciprocal possibilities, in order to work out a life's mission.

Through that same 95% that is energy, the throat chakra person heals, in others, the ability to comprehend and understand. It is because the fifth chakra person represents, as dominant, the character of higher levels of communication that draws people who wish to engage a higher level of understanding.

When you engage with a fifth chakra personality, you will think "teacher" or "communicator" or "expediter of information," although almost never consciously. There is a position into which the fifth chakra personality is placed where a person or soul-group of people will engage him to bring in psychically to the earth plane pertinent information relative to the evolutionary spiral of the soul-group.

The majority of communication that is not physical ensures

that the dynamics of the possible relationship are functioning in *both directions*; that each individual in the relationship has the possibility of receiving the lessons to which he aspires.

As an individual with a strong throat chakra presence, you will tend to draw individuals to you who have difficulty framing or articulating their desires. If you are in your higher aspect, you will know how to put into words, music, etc., the expression through communication that others cannot say. The lower aspect throat chakra individual spends a lot of time in inefficiency, and thus suffers.

The Pyramid on the Dollar Bill

Have you ever examined the back of a one-dollar bill? The pyramid depicted is not an American idea - it is Egyptian. It comes from the Egyptian saying, "God sees you, you don't see God."

If you look at it closely you see several stone courses leading up to a plateau. Above that is a small empty space, and above that, the "all-seeing eye of God" in the capstone.

The fifth chakra individual fills in the space in the middle, between the courses of grounded humanity, and the all-seeing eye of God. You are here to translate that all-seeing Presence into language that is palatable for humanity. It is not just the language of semantics and understanding, it is your presence that induces the activation of higher levels of communicative awareness: that one is psychically connected to everyone and everything in Oneness. Your innate ability is one of the reasons your mind works so well, but also at times believes you are just not communicating with the world. The world sometimes cannot "hear" you. There are ears to hear but sometimes no real hearing takes place.

If the space above the courses of stone (who are humanity) is transparent, who could see you or what you are trying to accomplish? Who could understand you to acknowledge you? Yet *you* perceive the all-seeing eye of God; you are sensitive to higher teachings, and the qualities of the fifth chakra dominance flow through you whether you are aware of it or not.

Grounding

Think of the grounding experience like a lightening rod. If it is suspended in air and lightening strikes it, the lightening has nowhere to go. However, if the rod is grounded, the lightening is grounded on the earth plane. To extend the metaphor, if the lightning grounds, the fifth chakra personality can now connect and communicate with the earth plane and get his message for humanity across. When grounded, not only are you in the here and now, but you are able to fully express your abilities onto the earth plane. In a way the throat chakra individual helps to accelerate the learning of others.

Grounding in its essence and all its forms is always reminding your metaphysical nature that you have a corporeal presence. It is uniting Heaven and earth in one moment, in every moment, through the power of your will. It is one of the hardest things you will ever do, because the tendency is to be out-of-body, as the fifth chakra pulls you up and out of this plane.

What is grounding?

• Breathing techniques, including yoga, Pranayama (the science of breathing) Yoga, Tai Chi, and Qi Gong are excellent forms of being grounded. The breath is central to our existence.

• Grounding stones: Smoky quartz, obsidian, malachite, hematite, and black tourmaline are all grounding stones. You can use them to stay grounded by just having one in your pocket or on your person within an inch of the body. The stones themselves do no grounding, but have properties that act as a mnemonic device to assist the wearer in being grounded. Size is not important: a stone the size of a dime is sufficient. At the end of every day, hold the stone under running water and think the word "clear."

• Walking by the ocean, water, rocks, trees, mountains, is grounding. Getting your hands in the dirt, planting flowers, etc., is grounding.

• Anything in, on, and around water, including water fountains in the home and aquariums, is grounding.

• Eating can be very grounding. Some people say eating chocolate may be grounding. It may not be true, but it's fun to think so.

- Air ionizers are grounding. (Smoking can be, too, though not healthy.)

Grounding is placing your intention to be in the here and now, to be totally focused in the moment. Grounding is the awareness of your physical presence, in the body. Being grounded prevents psychic manipulation.

What is <u>not</u> grounding?

- Excessive talking
- Talking on the phone
- Watching TV
- Driving a car
- Using a computer

These are things we all do regardless of our chakra dominance, and so we are not going to be in our bodies at all times, nor should we be. Just be aware of what is not grounding and bring your Self back into focus.

If you are driving and feel ungrounded, pull off the road, stop, and do the breathing and meditation exercises in Appendix A, or do some yoga, Tai Chi, or Qi Gong. A grounding exercise can be done at any time, but it only works if you apply it. If you think of grounding without the will behind your intention, it won't work.

Grounding is a state of being, not a location. It is a *choice*.

It is also a two-way street, energetically. If you ground, you are the lightning rod that contacts the earth, creating the possibility of Heaven on earth by articulating higher knowledge through communication that is not verbal or physical. At the same time, though, being grounded yields you to your own vulnerability to grow and gain soul's experience through the feeling sense of the third dimension. For some, it is all they can do to be grounded, moment to moment.

But grounding is what you must do to learn the feeling state of consciousness in your corporeal body, while maintaining the conscious connection through your throat chakra to higher realms of existence.

For the everyday person with no knowledge of metaphysics, the application of this information can be quite a stretch. It would be a start for such an individual to practice the grounding techniques, especially the breathing exercises. And, they must be practiced often and with presence of mind through the will. Only by applying these principles can you have success in being grounded.

There are many hidden benefits to the application of grounding techniques. Feelings of greater productivity, increase in perception of communication, and feeling more "present" are all the benefits of grounding the throat chakra activity.

Golden Mean Spiral

A component of the energy through the throat chakra, as seen from a side view, shows this winding energy emanating from the throat chakra and ending in the pineal gland, located in the center of the brain *(see Illustration #11-a)*. This is a phenomenon I've noticed after years of spiritual counseling. The spiral is present in *all* individuals, regardless of their chakra dominance. It is energetically linked to the function of the throat chakra. If there is a problem in the chakra, there is usually a problem in the spiral of energy as well.

The spiral of energy begins in the throat, affecting the thyroid gland (skin temperature, blood pressure, metabolic rate), then passes through the occipital area of the brain (short-term memory, ocular/visual center), through the frontal lobes of the brain and eyes, through the corpus calossum and affecting the small bundle of nerves that connect both hemispheres of the brain, and ends in the pineal gland. It is shaped like the golden mean spiral and is created and affected by the functioning of the throat chakra *(see Illustration #11-a)*.

The function of this spiral of energy is to interface directly with the biochemical, electromagnetic, and neurological aspects of the brain, eyes, ears, cochlea, and all matter in the skull, including thought processes, psychic perceptions, telepathy, emotions, etc.

So often when there is a difficulty with the throat chakra, there are associated difficulties along the line of the spiral of

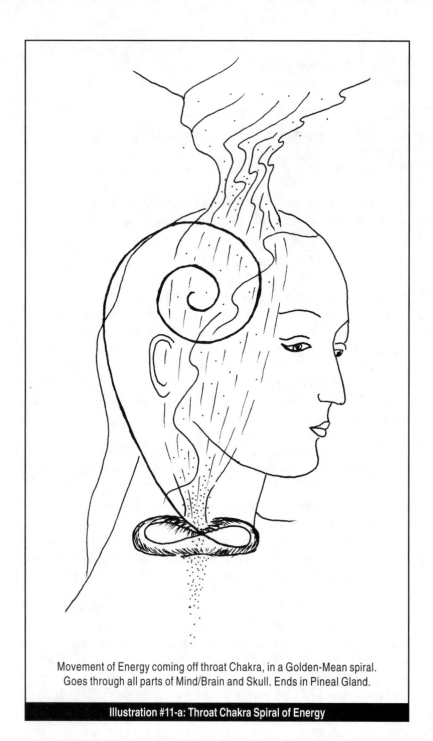

Movement of Energy coming off throat Chakra, in a Golden-Mean spiral.
Goes through all parts of Mind/Brain and Skull. Ends in Pineal Gland.

Illustration #11-a: Throat Chakra Spiral of Energy

energy. Hearing loss, imbalance, short-term memory, dyslexia, and interrupted sleep patterns, are all related to this spiral of energy, and thus to the throat chakra disposition.

When the throat chakra individual practices grounding techniques it helps to heal and improve the flow of energy in the spiral as well.

Fifth Chakra Priorities

As I've emphasized, the fifth chakra individual is here to articulate what cannot be said, by bringing higher communicative information through to this earth plane. Communication does not only mean the spoken word, but any type of communication: E-mail, poetry, sculpture, teaching, singing, etc.

It is a tall order when you consider there are so many problems in communication today. Even those of us who are on the same page on certain issues find difficulty coming to a consensus of opinion.

Society likes to enforce a consensus of reality through unwritten rules and accepted patterns of behavior. Those who strive to be in the higher aspects of their dominant chakra must face the smothering embrace of the group fears, the lower levels of truth, and the resistance to growth that seems to be the pattern of human behavior we call the status quo.

The fifth chakra person comes, most often, to destroy illusion. Coming onto the earth plane as a destroyer does not sound like a peaceful mission. But, as Buddha was fifth chakra dominant and quite the teacher of harmlessness, he also had to help his monks overcome much of their lower level understandings of "teachers."

You know the saying, "When the students are ready, the teacher will appear." With the throat chakra individual, when the teacher is ready, *the students will appear.* When you, the throat chakra individual, accept the power of your immense psychic ability to see great teachings and to make clear what the rest of humanity has created the mild vacuum to understand, you accomplish what you came here to do.

When you impart great teachings through whatever medium

you choose and are willing to let go and allow others to become responsible for the information you give, you are avoiding living in the lower aspect of the throat chakra; the attachment to the outcome.

Similar to the second chakra, you can see what is coming. Not as a vision, but rather as an explanation. You are not here to impart a vision on humanity like the second chakra, but to help humanity understand a higher, more efficient interaction with its own higher Self.

Like the third chakra individual, you are not the most patient person who ever walked the earth, but you must be grounded and focused to be effective and avoid the pitfalls of the throat chakra lower aspects. You must always work to be focused, to understand what it is to feel, and to not be distant from those feelings.

You represent communication and teaching, the imparting of higher levels of understanding that humanity has difficulty grasping. The elegant collaborative leadership of ourselves as spiritual beings has your higher Self orchestrating the many opportunities for you to grasp the higher teachings and communication that would otherwise effortlessly flow through you. As with any chakra, presenting the opportunity to others and receiving it are two different actions.

You should avoid being only the teacher if it means you are teaching so well that you are not allowing your Self to feel, rendering you emotionally unavailable. This is one of the biggest challenges for those in a relationship with you. If you are not grounded, there is a potential for many problems, due to a lack of true, grounded communication.

You can feel very distant from the ones you love, even if they are standing in the same room. The very same psychic abilities that make you so strong also create difficulty for your mind to ground this power onto the earth plane. The strength is the weakness. Until you are using that grounding in a focused manner, emphasizing your existence in the moment, you will tend to be ungrounded. That ungroundedness has negative effects of feeling alone, aloof, detached, separate, and having nothing in common with others.

To feel is to be fully in-body and that can be quite overwhelming to throat chakra individuals, to the point they feel their intellectual abilities are impugned.

If you knew the contents of a dictionary, would it make you wise? Knowing the vastness of what to communicate to the earth plane is not the same as grounding it through you. Feeling the import of what you impart is something else again. To attach value, wisdom, and appropriateness includes a due regard for the feelings of others. You cannot just impart information to the people on this planet, be distant from it, and avoid suffering. To do so assures you are in the lower aspect of your chakra.

The resistance to ground is natural for the fifth chakra individual just as the resistance to do only one thing at a time is natural for the second chakra individual. By not grounding, you do not have to feel, and by not feeling, you do not have to feel pain because you are not in your body.

To learn to feel is to accept your Oneness; the "as above, so below" that unites your metaphysical and corporeal natures. It means you are emotionally available and able to connect to the very communication you give to others. It means you cannot hold the physical world at bay while you teach and communicate to it. You cannot be separate from what you do, or you will suffer.

To feel does not only mean to intuit. It means your emotions are reacting to the experience of fully feeling your physical presence here in the third dimension, something that is very hard for some throat chakra individuals. You know how it is. We get used to what works in our lives, only to have some challenge set before us. We were in our ignorant bliss before the challenge appeared. Why should it change now? Remember, you are setting these lessons for your Self, and the Law of Reciprocity brings the people into your life who will represent your visit to the chakra gym to work out with your lower level aspects, until you overcome them.

The lessons keep coming until you are not attached to the lower aspect. You begin to really feel from having accepted your heart's reaction to being in-body, and you begin to feel that our life is more productive; that you are really getting done the things you came here to do.

There is no other way for the throat chakra individual. You must ground and be fully present in the moment, pulling in all aspects of your nature. It does not guarantee that your communication and teachings will be heard and absorbed by others, but you will have achieved what you came here to learn.

Higher and Lower Aspects of the Fifth Chakra

Aspects of the throat chakra are determined by the grounding of communicative and psychic abilities. As with any of the chakras discussed in this book, the emanations of our higher consciousness coming through the chakras are most difficult to accept. Not because they are complicated or powerful in themselves, but because they are so very pure and simple.

Higher aspects reflect a life composed of the infusion of love, will, and wisdom. Lower aspects reflect fear, loss of "feeling known," and fear of the lack of communication.

Higher aspects of the fifth chakra:

1. The Communicator
2. The Teacher
3. The Ambassador
4. The Networker

The lower aspects result in much suffering, including physical, mental, emotional, and spiritual issues.

Lower aspects of the fifth chakra:

1. The Mentalist
2. The Know it All
3. The Emotionally Distant Individual
4. The Hermit

Higher Aspects of the Fifth Chakra Explained

1. The Communicator

The communicator is the coordinator and expediter. You would be the one who is like the freeway interchange or nexus. Imagine cars approaching the interchange and taking the ramp to go from north to west. What if a single car is parked on the ramp? What would happen to all the oncoming traffic taking that ramp to go west? It would stop.

The energy of communication is dynamic; it is in ceaseless motion. In physics, the term "flux" relates to an energy that can be measured only when something else (another energy) is in motion. Moving a magnet through a coil of wire creates a magnetic flux that can then be measured. If the magnet is not moving, there is no flux.

These two examples are meant to illustrate that the throat chakra individual helps with the movement and propagation of the articulation of energy that is known as communication. If the flow stops, the communication stops. In a way, by your mere presence, you help to accelerate the learning of others by the fluidity of relationship.

When someone speaks, your ears hear the sounds and the nerves in your cochlea convert them into *time-code sequences*, pulsed electrical signals based on frequency and amplitude over time. That means that your brain takes in information over time and makes intelligence out of the sentence after it is spoken. What if you are a throat chakra person, who by your great psychic abilities, does not have to wait until the words are spoken to complete the sentence? What if you can tune in to the mind and thoughts of others, as well as your own intuition, to know something before it happens (precognition)?

As the communicator you are here to provoke a response from others by establishing a method, a nexus point, by which communication can take place. This higher aspect of the throat chakra speeds up and makes more efficient the manner in which others assimilate and articulate their own information.

When others take a psychic relationship to what the throat chakra person represents through their higher aspect of communication, they increase their ability to communicate in higher psychic levels, also helping to elevate the soul-group.

Martin Buber, in his book I and Thou, speaks of a "betweenness" that occurs between two individuals having a conversation. That betweenness represents the possibility of all understanding that could take place in the communication, but it does not mean that it will. You cannot force anyone to understand anything. You must *allow* your Self to understand, to create the space where understanding is possible.

Because of the fine vibrations of the throat chakra, and because of the tentative nature of existing here in earth's vibration, once again there is the possibility of feeling if you are grounded. To be grounded implies a vulnerability to those feelings.

2. The Teacher

Being born as a "teacher" does not mean you must teach from a pulpit or podium: It is an energetic disposition of the fifth chakra by which others take relationship to what you represent. It is your orientation towards life by an active association (whether you are conscious of it or not) with communication from higher levels of being.

You'll notice that others often will assume you should just know the answer. Remember, we are psychically connected to each other, long before the mind thinks a single thought. Others will tune in to your dominant fifth chakra, and assume you are composed of knowledge sufficient to give the answer, explain the problem, etc. It is their energetic reciprocity to your dominant chakra that collaboratively creates the situations to interact, the urge to grow and understand who you are.

Teachers who have come to the higher aspect of the fifth chakra have mastered their frenetic thoughts, or at least come to terms with the fear that drives them. There was an orator who said: "When I give speeches, I've never gotten completely rid of my butterflies (fears), but I have made them fly in formation." You may always have the tendency to be impatient, have a racing mind, and be ungrounded, but the effort to overcome is what defines your character.

The more you as a teacher ascend to your higher aspect, the more you ground esoteric teachings (ways of understanding, including telepathic awareness) and the articulation of communication, so that higher levels of understanding are not only possible, they are now viable. When there is a soul-group desire to attain a more viable way of interconnecting and assimilating knowledge, the vacuum is created to draw in the teacher with the most exact skill sets for that group. When the higher aspect teacher perfects his life, he becomes available to the students, who appear when the teacher is ready.

Frequency Matching

One of the skill sets that accompany your throat chakra higher aspect of teacher is "frequency matching." This is an intuitive ability to match the thought-stream of others, such that real communication may take place. You see a lot of emphasis on communication in company sales techniques. The essence of it is rooted in the energy of the throat chakra. When it is developed as a higher aspect, you and those with whom you communicate have the greatest opportunity to grasp yet higher aspects of the consciousness that flows through your chakras, or the best possible infusion of your soul qualities.

Frequency matching is similar to tuning a radio. Moving the dial slightly makes the difference between hearing the station clearly and hearing nothing but static. Throat chakra individuals already have psychic abilities fully functional in the communicative aspect: Tuning is using the power of the will to *allow* your Self to receive what another person is emanating psychically. It is matching the other person's frequency and then relating your message back to him in the same manner.

In the mundane sense, if they laugh – you laugh, if they are all business – so are you, and so on. In the metaphysical sense, which is much more important, you are tuned to the way in which they perceive their reality, the way their cognitive abilities focus and process the communication into meaning.

I tell my students, "What I say does not mean anything. What you *do* with what I say; that means something." Once you've tuned to their "frequency" you relate back to them in terms they can understand, but it is more than a choice of words, it is the power of the will to see someone for who they really are.

This subset of the teacher works very well for the ambassador higher aspect, below.

Transcendent Thinking

Incorporating the "as above, so below," Heaven on earth that the throat chakra individual must do (as any dominant chakra must) is melding the physical, thinking mind with the transcendence of higher awareness. A mark of your evolution would be the degree to which these two states are seamless with one another. If it were truly seamless, would you know it? Remember, you cannot *make* it seamless, you must *allow* it to be so.

To think in such terms, you must be open and receptive to your own abilities. To have strong psychic and telepathic abilities and to use them functionally in the third dimension is to challenge your linear mind with non-linear states of awareness. The more you allow your Self to use the awareness, "the space in between your thoughts" (as Deepak Chopra would say), the more you bring your prescience into a grounded focus, and the more you live your life on purpose rather than merely reacting with thoughts alone.

Transcendent thinking works only in the moment: You cannot plan it, you must be it.

The Destroyer

Many of the higher aspect teachers are destroyers. Of course, when we hear this word we often do not think of it in positive terms. However, in this context, it means to *destroy illusions*. Many times teachers will show up in the soul-group only for a short space of time. Their energetic presence causes the old teachings and belief systems to come up for review, and if the soul-group is progressive, the better understandings and higher awareness are grasped as the illusions are destroyed.

It is interesting that in some of these cases the teacher shows up, remains in the soul-group for a short time, then leaves. The effect is that the core energetics of the way the soul-group members relate to each other is affected by the destruction of illusion, and as the teacher leaves, the soul-group re-attaches energetically to each other, establishing better, more aware relationships that continue and deepen long after the teacher is gone.

Often the teacher will be pulled into many diverse soul-groups. The groups will not get along with each other, but the teacher/communicator will have free passage into all of them. The teacher helps to destroy any illusion as to why one group should be separate from another (destroying the fears that separate them). The result is that the groups will tend to lose their disdain for each other and meld energetically along common, higher aspect and awareness goals.

3. The Ambassador

The ambassador must use tact, finesse, and diplomacy to get his point across. One of the more difficult tasks for the higher aspect of the fifth chakra individual is how to use that communicative ability to reach others.

If you were to walk into a third grade classroom to teach the students about quantum physics, how would you do it? What words would you use? The subject matter is not the difficulty; speaking in a way the third grade mind can understand is the difficulty. But you as a fifth chakra individual are equipped to do this because of the psychic nature of the fifth chakra, rooted in communication. What words would you choose? The ambassador knows the protocols of communication, and is well-suited to create the perfect match where true communication can occur.

Imagine you are an American in France. You are in a restaurant in Paris, and you say in English to the French waiter, "I would like to have some eggs." He does not understand you. What do you do? You say it louder, "I would like to have some eggs!" with authority in your voice. Is that going to make him understand you? Of course not.

You must use psychic abilities and telepathy to make your communication palatable to the listener. You must be the artful sculptor of communication, the creative knowledge flowing effortlessly through you in a manner all can grasp and internalize.

4. The Networker

The fifth chakra person is a living nexus point. That is, think of a nexus as a freeway interchange, where the cars are facilitated to get where they wish to go by a series of ramps that speed the efficient flow of traffic. Any car that stops on an onramp would impede the entire flow of traffic wishing to go in that direction.

So by definition, the energy (cars) must be allowed to keep moving in the most optimal manner. The fifth chakra person acts as an "energy interchange"; networking, optimizing and enhancing the flow of communication and meaning between and among people. The throat chakra enhances and even heals the possibility and ability to comprehend, if grounded, for oneself and for others.

Of course, the more grounded the fifth chakra person is, the more efficacious their life and the possibility of those **around them to** increase, by reciprocity, their awareness of meaning, understanding and communication by representation through relationship. In this case, the fifth chakra person is optimizing the connections and flow of consciousness for others around him. This also means that the fifth chakra person may often find themselves in the position where they are acting in the capacity of networker (consciously or not) for a few people at a time, to various groups simultaneously, to large groups.

Lower Aspects of the Fifth Chakra Explained

1. The Mentalist

Mentalisms are pure distraction for the throat chakra individual. As you will see here and in the next chapter on the sixth chakra, mentalisms are ways of dealing (quantitatively) with the higher awareness coming through you. Mentalisms stunt the higher awareness by forcing it to "fit" in practical and pragmatic patterns of linear and temporal thought. Being rational and pragmatic is a wonderful tool for the third dimensional mind, until the interface between this and higher realities is considered. It is in the resolution of the two that we get into trouble. The mind wants to make sense of what it is receiving inter-dimensionally.

When the throat chakra is dominant, your mind fears it will never assimilate such knowledge, so it reacts by creating strong mental barriers that use words like practical and reasonable as foils for true, higher understanding and awareness.

Mentalisms are fear-based defense mechanisms that use the power of your mind to force higher-level awareness to fit neatly into this dimension. It doesn't and it won't work for long, though some individuals take these mentalisms all the way to the end of a lifetime. In some future life perhaps their mentalisms give way to transcendent thinking.

2. The Know it All

Knowing everything is like being a fluorescent light bulb. It is bright, but there is no warmth. It is not enough to know: you must *apply*. And for the throat chakra individual that means you must be grounded in your knowledge.

Many throat chakra individuals (and some second chakra analytical types and heart chakra individuals who hide in their minds) assume that if they accrue great knowledge it is the same as an evolved consciousness. This is a fundamental misunderstanding of quantitative vs. qualitative reality. It does not matter how much you know, though knowing things is neither good nor bad. It is the awareness (wisdom and will) with which you apply what you know that allows the definition of your character to evolve so you may infuse your soul-quality into your personality.

You may be brilliant, and many throat chakra people are. *But a high intellect is sometimes a real impediment to spiritual growth.* You can assume because you know a lot, that you know a lot. You must be careful what you put into your head as "knowledge." If it is only of the third dimension, it is limited, quantitative thinking and does nothing to help ground you. There are many individuals who are like walking libraries of information - but that is not enough.

You could know every esoteric teaching, every metaphysical technique, and that in itself does not make you higher in consciousness. You must use your will and vulnerability, face your lower aspects, and overcome illusion in order to grow. Does going to church make you holy?

Do not let "knowing everything" take the place of your own enlightenment. It is a trap, a very elegant one, but a trap just the same.

3. The Emotionally Distant Individual

When throat chakra individuals are ungrounded, giving and receiving love is like talking to them from the next room. There is no real contact through the 95% of communication that is energy. Being ungrounded and having a racing mind together ensure the fifth chakra individual is emotionally unavailable. You may be impressed with his mental prowess, but there is no real emotional connection. No real progress is made towards what the throat chakra individual came here to learn, to feel.

You can imagine that just like with any other chakra, these lessons are difficult and demanding. So many times we ask the universe to help us as long as we don't have to face our strongest test. And what do you suppose the universe answers us with? *The strongest test.*

Worse, if you as a throat chakra individual are unaware that you are engaged in such behavior, the condition can go on for some time before the lesson is created for you to learn from the experience. The only way to break an illusion is to recognize there is one. This Catch-22 seems insurmountable, but if you recall that we are eloquently constructing our own lessons from our higher Selves, then the lessons that follow are the exact match for our fears and resistance.

It is not too hard to look around you and make assessments as to who is emotionally open and who is not. You may wish for them to have progressed further than they may be, but the evolution of a soul is a highly personal endeavor. *The best thing you can do for others is to be an example of perfection your Self.* From that position, they may take a relationship to what you represent and improve their lives. It doesn't mean they will, but by your actions you offer the world a better choice.

If you are a throat chakra individual, you must not mentalize and rationalize at the expense of your emotional availability to others. This is really asking a lot because it makes your fine vibration available to feel the pain that is sometimes associated with emotional closeness and intimacy to others. Never would you sacrifice one ounce of your integrity, only sacrifice your fear. You'll find that when you ground your Self you also ground the strength to meet any challenge.

It is all too easy to forget who you really are. Grounding your metaphysical presence into your corporeal nature also makes all of that transcendent awareness instantly available to you, so you do not have to attach the fear to the emotion, or the resistance to your physical mobility (the ability to move freely through the seas of emotions in this dimension).

4. The Hermit

Hermits are those who go away from society into the cave of their own desires, only to once again emerge and rejoin society. Jesus Christ went into the desert, Buddha sat under the bodhi tree.

The fifth chakra individual, similar to the second chakra, will at times withdraw from society into a private astral world for a time. The price you pay is that of the alienation and aloofness you feel from society. Having nothing in common, retreating to the daydreams and non-grounded out-of-body experiences, you can spend a great deal of time as the hermit, perceiving it as an emotionally safe place to be.

The safety is real and illusion at the same time. You may feel the security of non-engagement (the fifth chakra individual can be in the lower aspect role as hermit, even when in a relationship), but suffer from not being integrated. Separation creates suffering, and so the hermit will often re-emerge tentatively, if he sees the value in doing so.

The hermit can have a very dark side. The throat chakra individual can feel so emotionally cut off from society that he becomes suicidal. "Why bother, no one hears me," he may say. He can feel that no matter how hard he tries no real communication is taking place. It can sometimes take a very long time for the lower aspect hermit to rejoin society: He can become an isolate.

Release the Attachment to Outcome

One of the hardest things for throat chakra individuals to do is to let go of the information they give to others. It is because the throat chakra individual is "dialed in" psychically and knows information before most others do.

"Am I the only one in the room who knows what's going on?" the throat chakra individual may ask. Yes, you have to be, because you are there to hold and impart the communication and teachings from higher levels of being. You are put in situations to just that end.

It also means that once you have the information and give it, let go. It will be very difficult because, like the second chakra individual, you'll know that what you're saying is correct, but others may not be ready, willing, or able to understand what you've given them. Frustration aside, you must let go of the information and allow others to become responsible for what you've communicated.

The fact that you may be throat chakra dominant means that you would fear that you do not know enough and will not get enough information and communication. This is the illusion - a very powerful one. When you let go of your fear, you'll find your psychic abilities work as well as they ever have. When you ground you'll feel the efficacy of your communications, especially when you let others become responsible for the information.

Imagine being a prophet telling humanity what is to come and no one listens to you. Imagine having psychic abilities so good that you do know what is coming, can tell what people are thinking, and are in telepathic relationship to others as well as with plants and animals. That is the throat chakra individual. Is it any wonder you might feel so daunted by your given dominant chakra?

Allow your Self to be right. Let go of the information when you give it.

Fifth Chakra Relationships

Being in relationship with throat chakra personalities can be a great experience. It depends on how much time they spent getting grounded before they met you. If they are working on it while in relationship to you, it means you too are working on some issues. The Law of Reciprocity will ensure you both have a lot to do.

If the throat chakra individual is in his higher aspect it means he is grounded and focused. That especially means he is emotionally available to you. If he is in his lower aspect you will have to deal with his daydreamer disposition and some emotional aloofness through his mentalisms and intellectual prowess. The lower disposition also means that his mind never really lights in one place for very long, so the conversation and the goals of the relationship may skip around a little and suffer from lack of a strong foundation.

If you are in a relationship with a throat chakra individual, think of the words "ground" and "clear" when you are communicating with him. It may not make him ground, but it will represent a healthy opportunity for him to do so. If anything, your steadfastness will amplify your perception of his ungroundedness because you will see it much clearer if *you* are grounded.

Can two throat chakra people be in relationship to each other? Briefly, of course they can. It can be a great relationship if each is working on staying grounded and focused.

To keep throat chakra individuals in a relationship you must understand that sometimes their communication is like the wind. If you'll stand there long enough and allow the wind to blow past you, the real message is not far behind. It will take some patience and fierce trust of your true perceptions beyond the strong mentalisms the throat chakra person can project as his protection mechanism. To improve the relationship, *you* can do the grounding exercises. At least one of you will be grounded.

Being in a higher aspect, throat chakra individuals may have many endeavors and interests to keep their brilliant minds busy. Don't make the mistake of assuming brilliance means intelligence. There are many throat chakra individuals who have normal intelligence with brilliant telepathic energy flowing through them. They are very well telepathically linked to their environment. Becoming aware of their strengths is best and most holistically served by becoming aware of their weaknesses.

If you are more aware of your partner's fifth chakra dominance than he is, the choice will always be his as to the development of his character. You must decide when it is appropriate to help and when it is appropriate to allow him to learn the lesson for himself.

Healing Issues for the Fifth Chakra

We all have healing issues, though I've noted specific illnesses related to each chakra. The fifth chakra, because it is located in the neck, is certainly related to that area (all bones, tissues, glands, etc.), but also relates to the head and mind, and the affects of its concomitant golden mean spiral of energy that ends in the pineal gland.

The affects include neurological, emotional, intellectual, and spiritual issues. However, parts of the rest of the body are also directly affected by throat chakra function, such as capillary action in the fingers and toes, the architecture of the lower legs and extremities, and certain skin and sensory sensitivities.

Other issues include:

- Musculature
- Knees, shin splints, cramps in calves
- Problems with the architecture of the body, arches, ankles, shins, calves, heels, pronation (the way you walk, heel-to-toe)
- Cervical vertebrae, thyroid, cochlea, headaches, etc.
- Tumor in the brain, sinus, teeth, jaw misalignments, cervical vertebrae, anything around the head
- Golden mean spiral: memory, dyslexia (aural, visual, conceptual), sleep cycles (pineal gland; serotonin/melatonin)
- Emotionally distant, the "know it all," the mentalist, the frenetic mind
- ADD (attention deficit disorder)
- Alzheimer's disease, confusion, altered personality states
- ALS (Lou Gherig's disease), neuromuscular degeneration,

loss of physical mobility.

How to Emphasize the Strengths of the Throat Chakra

- Ground: Stay in your body as much as you can
- Improve your patience
- Make eye contact with others, and feel your physical presence
- Breathe
- Be careful what you "think" you have to know. Watch what you put into your mind. Watch out for "too complete an understanding."
- Hug and embrace in your relationships. Make physical contact

The Daisy Pattern of the Fifth Chakra

Many fifth chakra individuals will find themselves on a looping path that is very similar to the daisy-like illustration (*see Illustration #11-b*).

You begin outward bound along your path, mutually pulled by an externalization of your soul's purpose, and by the desire of the soul-group to invite the teacher to destroy their illusions as to why they should suffer elitism from other soul-groups.

As you "head out on the daisy petal," you are externalizing your soul's purpose, but also are continually confronted with the decisions that are part of your character development:

1. Are you communicating outwardly: speaking, writing, E-mailing, etc.?
2. Are you communicating inwardly: listening, hearing, perceiving, etc.?
3. Are you grounded?

As you progresses outward, the energetics are set in place for the development of your personal character. When you reach the end of the petal, you are in the dynamics of that soul-group entirely. At the appropriate moment there is a disengaging (on many levels) where the soul-interactions have reached a completeness, whether successful or not, depending on the individual freewill decisions of all.

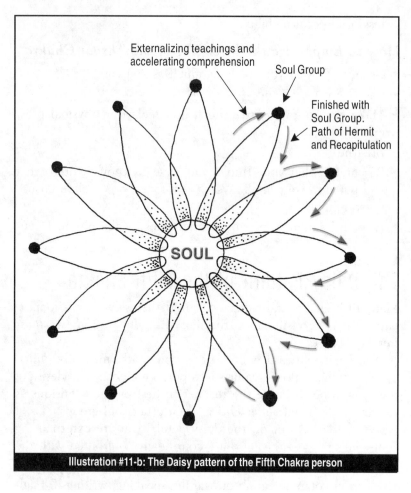

Externalizing teachings and
accelerating comprehension

Soul Group

Finished with
Soul Group.
Path of Hermit
and Recapitulation

SOUL

Illustration #11-b: The Daisy pattern of the Fifth Chakra person

As you leave the dynamics behind, you engage in the energy of the hermit. You pull in your energies of communication and affiliation for the recapitulation of your own inner resolve, and coherence to your soul's purpose. The time it takes can be a few hours to many years.

As you reach the center (core essence) you begin to gather the internal resources of your consciousness to make another sojourn out on another petal, to another soul-group that has a different energetic than the one experienced before.

The variety of soul-groups in mutual attraction to the throat chakra person also helps develop the consciousness in the second chakra - the need for variety and for the visceral, experiential interactions that help ground the throat chakra individual.

Some petals may overlap slightly, as the throat chakra individual may be involved in varying degrees with more than one soul-group at a time.

Evolving the Soul-Group Consciousness

Soul-groups will exert a mild vacuum on the fifth chakra personality to draw him in as teacher, for the purpose of the articulation of energies, through communication, for what they cannot yet express. Through this mild vacuum of energy he approaches various soul-groups and disseminates, illuminates, and articulates communication, 95% of which is energetic exchange. If he dwells in the higher aspect of his throat chakra, it represents the highest energetic advantage for the evolution of the soul-group that brought him in.

Often the fifth chakra personality will be allowed in several diverse groups of individuals, where those groups would have nothing to do with each other. This is a necessary part of helping to destroy illusion within those soul-groups, especially the illusions that separate the groups from each other. As the groups pull the fifth chakra personality in, he defines the nature of his character through right action (dharma) or capitulates and extends the cycle of interaction between himself and the soul-group, and also between the groups.

Soul-group individuals have a great opportunity to destroy their illusions when they take a relationship to what a throat chakra individual represents. It is they who create the space for the teacher to show up or come into the group. The soul-group is offering to the throat chakra individual the opportunity to teach and to communicate. After all, if there are no students what can the teacher teach?

The decision to evolve for members of the soul-group (and the throat chakra individual), as always, is of freewill. The greatest of teachers can show up on the earth plane but they can be rejected, ignored, or even killed for what they teach.

When others take a psychic relationship to what the throat chakra person represents, they increase their ability to communicate in higher psychic levels, also helping to elevate the soul-group, because the throat chakra individual offers the possibility of activation and acceleration of the group consciousness (more so if grounded!).

The communicator will induce the soul-group to enter the nexus, if they are willing, for that activation and acceleration. It depends on the evolution of the throat chakra individual. There are many such individuals in the world who may be only dimly aware of their tremendous abilities.

Sometimes your higher Self will induce you to move around the planet like a chess-piece. This is to give both you and your soul-group the maximum exposure to the emanations of your dominant fifth chakra. Many throat chakra individuals have the desire to travel, but it is also because their various soul-groups (who may be geographically diverse) are also exerting that mild vacuum for them to show up.

It could be that if you were disposed to communicate in an electronic manner (E-mail), there may not be so much physical travel, but the effect and diversity would be the same, perhaps even more so as others tune into your communicative and teaching gifts.

The more aware you are of your abilities to communicate and emanate higher teachings, the more the people of this planet may accelerate their evolution.

Paramahansa Yogananda used to say, "God loves to have His skirt tugged on by us." I take that to mean we are best served if we are eager for our evolution. Why wait until the next seminar to be enlightened? Why not now? Accept your teachings. Accelerate your evolution. Use your will power. Now.

Chapter Twelve

Sixth Chakra – The Prophet

The sixth chakra (brow center) is at the edge of the human potential and possibility of achieving a plausible explanation as to its influence in a person's life. Picture the vibrations of chakras one through five as you would the notes on a piano, one following the next. The vibration of the sixth chakra, however, is a full octave above the fifth (throat).

The number of people I've encountered with their sixth chakra as dominant would be about one in every two to three thousand. Over the years I have found only a few individuals who have a sixth chakra dominance because it is so rare to have one's influence focused there. In fact, it is so very difficult to describe that the consideration in this chapter of the sixth chakra's influence is cursory at best.

If the fifth chakra represents the communicator and one who is psychic by default, then the sixth chakra individual would represent the "clairsentient." The definition of clairsentience is literally "to know that which cannot be known." Clairsentience is the highest of all psychic abilities wherein one simply "knows" rather than sees, hears, etc., a particular phenomenon. This state of knowing is pervasive to the individual's awareness. So much so that the individual is often unaware that the advanced state of clairsentience exists.

In some cases, individuals with a different dominant chakra may also benefit from a reference to the influence of the sixth chakra. This often adds prominence to the given dominant chakra, enhancing its native strengths (and weaknesses).

If the sixth chakra is dominant, the effect on one's life includes the prescience of the fifth chakra to a higher degree. Its influence causes one to be absorbed in the future, to the effect that the mind is always considering the next move, the next sentence, and is exceptionally busy at most times with many concurrent thought patterns. The sixth chakra conscious person will often slow down within the body of an endeavor or conversation with another in order to keep the event or the conversation flowing and not stilted. The prescience assures that there will be some suffering from being able to think of far more than that which can be accomplished in the moment. The sixth chakra individual's mind can zip out to lateral thoughts and streams of consciousness, often simultaneously.

The mind thus capitulates to the power of the sixth chakra, in most cases, by succumbing to the state of prescience due to the lack of any physical evidence or information that this is leading the individual to imbalance.

One tends to live in the future, not focusing on the present moment. The consciousness that comes through the sixth chakra affects the four archetypes of being human: mental, physical, spiritual, and emotional in terms of paradigm shift. That is, *the sixth chakra individual grounds new paradigms for humanity.*

Usually when one learns of the imbalance of too great an influence of the mind, this is brought on by emotional suffering, which brings on the contemplative moments to reflect that the mind suffers from mentalisms.

Many sixth chakra dominant individuals have the sense that they are ahead of their time; that they may have been born a few years too early. Indeed, this is very close to accurate, for the clairsentience literally makes the individual prophetic. This is at once wonderful and ponderous.

It is so easy to underestimate the amount of energy that pours through our chakras. It is so easy to misunderstand, because of our illusions, the higher noble aspects of who we are and what we represent as magnificent beings of light. Perhaps, after an understanding of the presentation of chakras two through six you may understand how no one is in the seventh chakra.

Sixth Chakra Priorities

The sixth chakra person is here to ground and incept onto the earth plane a new paradigm that is being seen for the first time by all humanity. Like the fifth chakra teacher, when the sixth chakra prophet is ready, the people will appear to take relationship to what the sixth chakra person represents.

The paradigm is the new way laid at the feet of humanity, brought by the prophet who sees it clearly. And so many times, instead of gently stepping up to its higher truth, we walk on it as it were a carpet. Sixth chakra individuals are misunderstood much more severely than even fifth chakra individuals.

Their mere presence is an acceleration of thought to the threshold of tentative acceptance of a paradigm not yet experienced, which threatens the very thoughts that brought one to this precipice of the concept of "Self." As the heart chakra individual heals by his presence, as the fifth chakra individual can accelerate communication and articulation, the sixth chakra individual incepts the known from the unknown and offers it to humanity. Many times it is through the children: those with autism and Down syndrome, and the savants. Sometimes it is through what we call the "indigo children," a euphemism that barely describes their true nature as bringers of the tender branches of our own evolutionary upward spiral.

Please recall the statistical relevance of the sixth chakra individual. They are usually about one in every two to three thousand people, and quite rare. And yet so many times sixth chakra individuals have so little grasp of what they are grounding onto the earth plane. It has nothing to do with intelligence, and sometimes not even so much awareness as the confidence it takes to grasp with the heart and feelings what the mind itself cannot yet know. This is why it is imperative for sixth chakra individuals to constantly endeavor to be in their hearts.

The sixth chakra individual is here to learn to be in their hearts, to ground that tremendous consciousness that flows through the mind into the heart. As heart chakra individuals must ground themselves emotionally, and as fifth chakra individuals must ground their metaphysical nature into their physical body, sixth chakra individuals must focus on being in their heart in the state of lovingness. This is the Heaven on earth, where the dawning of the new paradigm rises in the east through the mists of our yearning to be conscious beings.

If the sixth chakra cannot ground, they also cannot live fully in the higher aspect of their being, and the full impact of their presence, rare though it is on this plane, cannot be grasped by those of us who helped collaboratively create the possibility to take relationship to what they represent.

The sixth chakra individual can suffer greatly, often early in age. Many can stay in the lower aspect of their sixth chakra for an entire lifetime. And there are many people with neurological disorders, many autists, who are completely in their hearts but not able to externalize their gifts in a manner we can understand.

They may also suffer because the lightning that flows through the throat chakra individual is magnified through the sixth chakra individual, and thus represents the perception of an insurmountable challenge to ground. His mind capitulates, even though the individual is in his heart, and the true externalization of his soul-quality is not yet realized.

Nothing of his exceptional mind is sacrificed by choosing to be in that qualitative state of the heart. The paradigm becomes grounded into reality if the sixth chakra person is able to ground himself through heart-centered focus of activity. As he successfully grounds through heart-centered awareness, the consciousness grid of this planet is affected with the new paradigm of human consciousness. That level of consciousness, through the soul-group activity, is available to all through our collaborative efforts, but remains in the freewill of all to accept or reject.

Higher and Lower Aspects of the Sixth Chakra

Higher aspects of the sixth chakra individual allow humanity a glimpse of an accelerated, evolved humanity. Lower aspects reflect an abstraction of the true reality due to fear, and loss of contact with grounded reality.

Higher aspects of the sixth chakra:
1. The Prophet
2. The Clairsentient
3. The Person out of Time

The Lower aspects result in much suffering, many times early in life.

Lower aspects of the sixth chakra:
1. The Abstract Mentalist
2. Emotional Imbalance

Higher Aspects of the Sixth Chakra Explained

1. The Prophet

The positive aspect is that these individuals ground energies and information that are previously unavailable to others, either in the soul-group or on the planet. These individuals would be the first, the prophets, to bring in the new information, the first to ground it onto the earth plane. Their life's purpose is to stand at the edge of what humanity understands and offer the fruit of high truths.

Several Tulkus (a former Lama or Rinpoche with full memory of a past life) represent sixth chakra dominance. Unfortunately, the first thing to get stomped out in the history of our human evolution has always been the truth. Many sixth chakra individuals are martyred, one way or the other, either outright or by being swept under the rug of consensus reality.

Prophets usually suffer in their "home town." Many people are so inured in their daily affairs that prophets at the least go unnoticed and ignored, or at most are scathed in ridicule and obscuration. Many sixth chakra prophets are induced to leave their homes either literally or figuratively in order to find themselves and to find people who will listen to their prophecy.

Many sixth chakra people have no idea they are the paradigm-bringing prophets, the souls who externalize because they and humanity are at a nexus point to make the decision to advance upwards on the evolutionary spiral.

Humanity only dimly awakens to such individuals. It takes great effort on the part of those of us whose sixth chakra is not dominant to truly see those sixth chakra individuals. We must see them with our hearts, not our minds.

2. The Clairsentient

If you knew what could not be known, how would you share it with others? If you did share it, how would they understand what so often only you can see? Is it as simple as the fifth chakra individual making the information palatable to others?

It is not so easy. The clairsentient higher aspect of the sixth chakra means you see, feel, taste, touch, hear, and smell what cannot be sensed or known. It is the transcendence of the senses to a higher state of being that cannot then be explained through those same third-dimensional senses. The difficulty of the fifth chakra individual is amplified by an order of magnitude, though the intuitive information of the clairsentient is exceptional.

Any higher aspect of the sixth chakra is especially well achieved if the individual can be in his heart. The heart-centered exercise, which came to me in meditation, is something I've been teaching for over ten years. It is an essential tool for all of us seeking to allow ourselves to be more intuitive. It is a lifesaver for the sixth chakra individual.

3. The Person out of Time

How would people react to you if they felt you were born years ahead of your time? Are all your friends older than you? How would *you* react to people in the world if you felt you were born years ahead of your time? If you are sixth chakra dominant and a prophet - who would have the ears to hear what you have to say?

Just as the fifth chakra individual, you must live up to your higher aspect and give the communication, but you must also let go of it once it is given. It is hard enough to attempt to relate to those you feel you've nothing in common. It is even more difficult to let go of the information you give. Several geniuses have given gifts to humanity that lay dormant for fifty years until humanity can appreciate them.

Alice Bailey channeled the Tibetan "Djwal Kuhl" in her writings in the 1920's, but a lot of that information could not be understood until now. Even so, many who read her works are confounded by the message.

It is best for sixth chakra personalities to be absolutely confident of who they are, but to also be absolutely humble in the moment and let go of what they teach after they have made the effort. They must allow humanity to catch up as best they can, if and when they can. Far better it is for sixth chakra personalities to live in their higher aspect and instill the paradigm to humanity through the 95% of communication that is not verbal, than to waste a lifetime trying to explain the 5% that is.

Lower Aspects of the Sixth Chakra

1. The Abstract Mentalist

"I think I feel that." As one of the greatest problems of the lower aspect of the sixth chakra dominant individual, mentalisms cause him to create mental images of emotional states. This is because the high vibration of the sixth chakra, similar to but an octave above that of the fifth (throat) chakra, leads him to simultaneously be out-of-body and in avoidance of a corporeal presence, due to the possibility of suffering pain when in the body. He would say, "I think I feel" instead of "I feel." This simple turn of words expresses the essence of the difficulty or challenge to be in the sixth chakra. Thinking is not feeling.

Thus, the strength of the sixth chakra is its weakness. The incredible power of knowingness from clairsentience creates an inverse relationship where there can be great difficulty in true feeling of the emotional state. Many sixth chakra dominant individuals have very little or no idea that they are a victim of their own mentalisms. They may assume that they are merely different, or can imagine that they feel a certain way without ever achieving the true feeling.

When one does perceive the true feeling, it is monumental and life-changing; an indicator that the individual is becoming balanced in the sixth chakra awareness. And, there is often a feeling of uniqueness that is so pervasive that the sixth chakra dominant individual feels there is no one to relate to, either on a level of basic understanding, or on the level of peer perceptiveness.

I reluctantly took a student to mentor for a week one summer. She is sixth chakra dominant and a very accomplished doctor and essential oil practitioner, and quite the clairsentient. She insisted, as I rarely take students singly to mentor. I relented, and upon our several encounters and healings I could see her inner struggle to understand this strange and nonsensical, ironic dimension she found herself in. I would patiently explain what I knew of the sixth chakra in relation to her life, and so often she would say, "I don't get it" afterwards. It seemed that no matter how I explained my opinions of her consciousness, her answer would be the same. These are all the effects of ungrounded mentalisms. The only real way for sixth chakra individuals to ground is to be focused on their heart center.

Often the sixth chakra individual may say, "Why don't I get it?" or "Why can't I figure it out?" with the exasperation of having heard the same old remedies again and again. Yet, when one thinks he is applying the cure, he is merely committing the act of abstract mentalism without connecting the emotional *receiving* that is so vital for true evolution of character. As you may know, this creates an emotional barrier, an emotionally unavailable sixth chakra individual absorbed in an inner world of abstraction and mentalism.

Without applying as much responsibility to receiving one's emotional goodness as to one's clairsentient disposition, the sixth chakra individual will repeat the lesson, including suffering, until it is learned. Because of the rarity of sixth chakra dominant individuals, the rest of us must raise our consciousness to help them ground their precious gifts to humanity.

2. Emotional Imbalance

This lower aspect is the imbalance of the emotions and of the tremendous responsibility of knowingness enshrined in the petals of the sixth chakra individual.

The emotional impact is due to the tremendous emphasis on "knowing" at the expense of truly feeling. The separation of thinking from feeling should only be regarded as two sides of the same coin; a healthy individual experiences both equally. With the negative aspect of the sixth chakra affecting mentalisms, there exists great separation (illusion) from the true emotional state, and this separation causes great suffering until the individual begins to emphasize the emotional aspect of his human nature. He must focus on the feelings, or feeling state, without subordinating his mind. This can be achieved through daily practice of the heart-centered meditation.

Sixth Chakra Relationships

A difficult negative aspect in relationships is the knowingness of the sixth chakra reality. The sense of singular knowingness can bear so heavily that the individual can experience feelings of intense loneliness, even within the most loving family. There is an inexpressible, ineffable longing filtered through a vague understanding, that can render the individual a feeling of a bleak future, or of a despondency that has no physical or logical component.

In fact, the feeling of repression of the ability to express the knowingness can result in a feeling of failure to achieve one's goals: a certain lofty yet unexpressed purpose in life does not yet become externalized to the conscious level.

There are many people who feel that by disguising their thoughts they can hide their true nature from others. Sixth chakra individuals don't even look at the thoughts, so they can see right through you and read you like a book. Your efforts to hide thoughts and issues are completely transparent to the sixth chakra individual. They are the pearl of great price, incarnated onto this planet to help us see a version of ourselves that no one has yet seen.

It would be of no use to you in a relationship with a sixth chakra individual to hide your true being. They see you, though many such sixth chakra individuals have been totally misread and misinterpreted by society as lacking in some way. It is quite the other way around, and so very difficult to be in relationship to the sixth chakra individual without immense patience and the desire to truly expose you to your Self through their great clarity of being.

Healing Issues for the Sixth Chakra

There can be neurological, psychological, and physiological effects from the quality of the sixth chakra, including myopia (nearsightedness), blindness, and other problems with vision (seeing what is really there). This represents an inverse relationship due to the individual's ability to "know" the future. He tries to see into the future and cannot, or sees it and reacts adversely, shutting down his vision.

Schizophrenia exists when more than one dimensional reality "bleeds" through into this dimension simultaneously, as more than one aspect of the individuated soul vies for prominence in the third dimension. As soul aspects struggle for simultaneous recognition and identity of "Self," the individual suffers a loss of identity or anchor to the original soul aspect incarnated. In some cases an individual will incarnate with simultaneous soul aspects active, and from the beginning, struggles with externalizing a coherent Self.

Autism exists when the mind is so affected by the influence of the sixth chakra, that externalization of the personality is shunted to the inner mind. Witness the mute brilliance of so many autistic individuals who have otherwise not been able to fit in with the consensus of social reality.

Imagine the sixth chakra lens like a polished sphere, where the inner surface is as a mirror. All energies directed outwards are reflected back to the inner Self; no externalization of the consciousness of the soul presence reaches the physical plane through the senses. There is a high amount of energy in the sixth chakra, but when it is all bounced back there is a with-drawal from the physical plane, though there is abundance of energy on the inside plane.

I have worked with children who exhibited many types of sixth chakra difficulties, including attention deficit disorder (ADD), mild autism, and abstract mentalism, and we have achieved remarkable success in only a day or two. However, some issues do not heal fully, and sometimes not at all. This is due to the soul's purpose and any karma that may ensue, regardless of the right action of the individual and any healers he brings into his life.

Other issues include:
- Neurological and psychological disorders
- Mental abstraction from reality
- The savant
- Down syndrome
- Epilepsy
- Paralytic conditions

How to Emphasize the Strengths of the Sixth Chakra
- Center in the heart
- Be with people who want nothing from you, who are tender with you
- Cherish your mind as brilliant, yet fragile. Be gentle with your Self
- Never underestimate your gifts of clairsentience
- It is OK to be who you are

Evolving the Soul-Group Consciousness

The soul-group for sixth chakra individuals is often the world as a whole, as their consciousness affects humanity on a very large scale.

So many people have suffered because they were sixth chakra persons in a world that had no capability to understand them. The autistic child, the savant, the genius; all affected by their sixth chakras.

The difficulty in understanding is similar to the parent/child relationship. Those who understand may not be able to explain to those who are not yet capable of understanding. The problem is that the lower mind of only practicality and rationality based in linear thought presumes itself to be dominant to the higher-inspired functioning of the sixth chakra. Instead of embracing it as a necessary mutual (collaborative) effort in raising consciousness, it is condemned to conform to the lower level of functioning. We, through mutual ignorance, have extinguished and caused to languish so many sixth chakra individuals because we do not have the capacity to understand the delicate gift offered us.

Humanity's history is full of individuals who have been committed to asylums and sanatoriums by those who had little or no capacity, due to their current evolution, to understand those whom they've locked up.

We must cherish, protect, and nurture the sixth chakra person. If you understand how the fifth chakra individual must suffer because "no one knows them for who they really are," then how much more exquisite the pain must be for the sixth chakra person, an octave above the fifth. It is up to all of us to work together by destroying any of our illusions that keep us separate from the Oneness in which we exist.

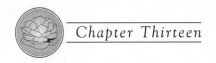

Chapter Thirteen

Seventh Chakra – Zero Point

The seventh or "crown" chakra is the gateway to other levels of consciousness and existence. The crown chakra represents the "God spot" or the point where everything and nothing exists. As no one lives in a hallway, no one lives in a gateway either, but rather in rooms. No one is consciously in their seventh chakra as they would be, say, in their second.

It is necessary to make the distinction of the first and seventh chakras from chakras two through six. Just as much as it takes a whole first chakra to have a physical body and presence in this dimension, it takes a whole seventh chakra to have any concept of a true multi-dimensional reality.

That our seventh chakra gives us a reference point to our multi-dimensional nature is saying a lot, because our concepts of many dimensions at best are flawed if you take as a first premise that we live in Oneness. If we live in Oneness, there is no seam between one thing and another.

But we live in illusion, and the illusion is a very good one.

Similar examples that are representative of the zero-point are black holes, which are stars that may once have been hundreds of millions of miles in diameter, but are super-condensed to the size of a basketball (*see Illustration #4-c*). Because they still have the same gravitational mass, they exert such a great pull that nothing within a few light years, not even light, escapes their pull.

It is my opinion that the energy of the seventh chakra is similar to a toroidal (donut shaped) energy field. It operates in much the same way as a black hole (or white hole) in that much of the higher dimensional energies are coalesced into the

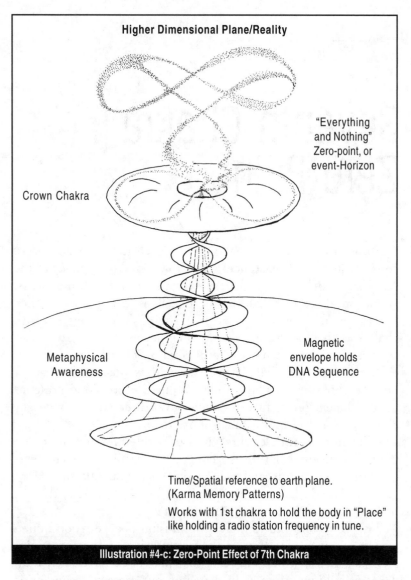

Higher Dimensional Plane/Reality

"Everything and Nothing"
Zero-point, or
event-Horizon

Crown Chakra

Magnetic
envelope holds
DNA Sequence

Metaphysical
Awareness

Time/Spatial reference to earth plane.
(Karma Memory Patterns)

Works with 1st chakra to hold the body in "Place"
like holding a radio station frequency in tune.

Illustration #4-c: Zero-Point Effect of 7th Chakra

physical plane through the lens of the seventh chakra. Nothing can escape the zero-point region because it represents the totality of reality.

In a way, all of the chakras are like the seventh. Perhaps they are all white holes of a form; localized space-time continuum portals that allow the consciousness that is us to access states of beingness. The "pull" is nothing less than the desire of

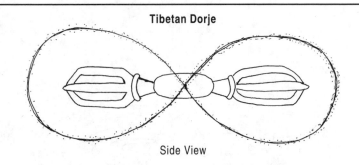

Tibetan Dorje

Side View

Energy Dynamic of a Dorje (also called Vajra)

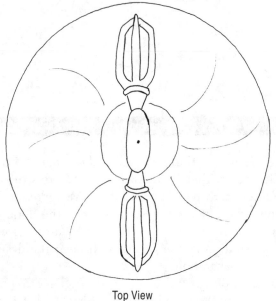

Top View

Toroidal Energy Field
Grasping the Dorje places one's hand over the zero-point, touching
everything and nothing in the same moment.
The field appears flattened into a doughnut shape, but is actually spherical.

Illustration #4-d: Tibetan Dorje and toroidal energy field

our consciousness to express as Self, and the universe enfolds
itself around our idea of ourselves, the primary motivation of
the power of the will as the first cause of creation in the collaborative leadership with All That Is.

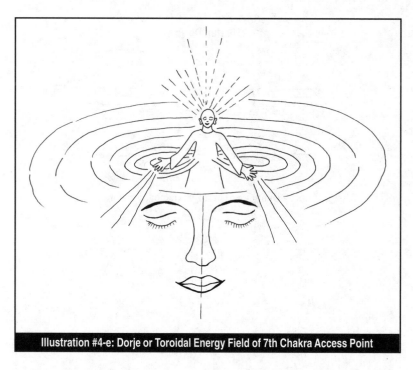

Illustration #4-e: Dorje or Toroidal Energy Field of 7th Chakra Access Point

In Tibet, the use of the dorje, *(see Illustration #4-d)* or vajra (meditation tools, that by their shape and construction represent hand-held zero-point physics devices), represents the same application, where closing one's hand over the dorje represents grasping the spot where everything and nothing exists, the seamless integration in the Oneness through the destruction of the illusion of separation.

The access point through the seventh chakra represents the point where everything and nothing exists, and it is the grasping of this point that allows the transcendence of the limitations of a physical existence into the seamlessness of the Oneness that includes a physical existence *(see Illustration #4-e)*.

Chapter Fourteen

Chakras 8, 13, 20 and 64

There exist chakras, localized events of consciousness threading through this dimension, as the seven main chakras you are familiar with. There are twenty-one minor chakras and tens of thousands of minute chakras throughout the physical body.

Again, the difficulty of discussing chakras is that they cannot directly be observed with third-dimensional senses or tools. To discuss chakras that are not even located on the body is even more difficult.

There are also chakras that function with the human energy system that are not perceived in physical reality, but nonetheless exist *(see Illustration #1-d)*. Think of these higher chakras as localized events of consciousness within the individuated human energy system, along an axial reference above the head (refer to the illustration).

Most are in line with the axis of the shushumna, but are not perceived in the physical plane as having any direct effect upon the mental, physical, spiritual, or emotional archetypes as the seven main chakras. These chakra centers are similar to chakras one and seven in that they are gateways of existence, and many may believe them to be successive in terms of rank or level of evolution.

I do not hold to that understanding but rather contend that these higher chakras represent equal opportunities (a two-way gate, if you will) for progress on the evolutionary spiral. Of course they are a part of our human existence, but are not normally considered in texts about the chakras because descriptions of them have been relegated to prior masters' teachings or channelings.

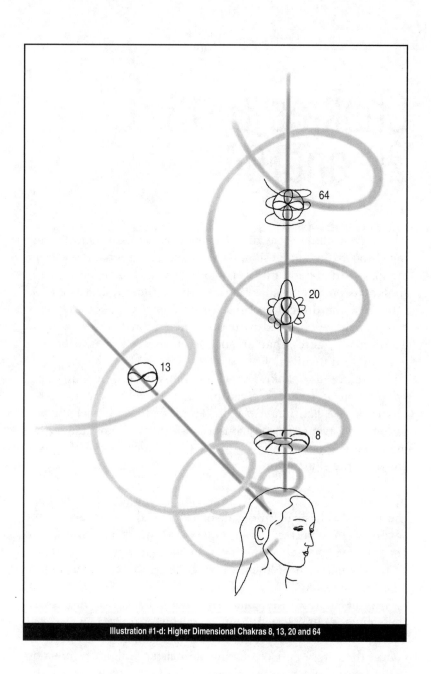

Illustration #1-d: Higher Dimensional Chakras 8, 13, 20 and 64

From my observations, there are four main higher-order chakras: eight, thirteen, twenty and sixty-four.

The Eighth Chakra

It has been said by others and in print that the eighth chakra is located at the rear of the head behind the crown and above the occipital area *(see Illustration #1-d)*. Also, it has been said that this is the "escape route" or exit-gate where the soul leaves the body for astral travel and to even higher dimensions. I do not agree with this.

My feelings place the eighth chakra above the head at a biometric distance exactly that of your own hand, from the wrist to the tip of your longest finger. That is the center of the eighth chakra, and it is fair to say that it is an entry point of higher dimensional realities if you continually view the chakra as a two-way street, that chakras *are* you, and that you are not separate from anything you observe.

Remember, it is all too easy to talk about chakras as if they are something separate, and that the dimensions in which they exist are separate as well. This is not so, but we are so inured in physical existence that we often can't help it. You are in One-ness. There is no separation.

The eighth chakra regulates the awareness of our auric fields, their emanation between bioenergetic and quantum states, and is a higher gateway working in conjunction with the seventh chakra. In it is the patterning for the auric-filed contents that emanate the grid to our physical reality. Your aura emanates you; you do not emanate your aura.

The Thirteenth Chakra

As the seven chakras are said to be our higher organs, the thirteenth chakra is like the endocrine system for higher awareness. If it could be located spatially, it would be behind and above your head, about the length of your arm extended out behind you at an upward angle at the fingertips *(see Illustration #1-d)*.

The endocrine system is also affected by the heart chakra, and there is an energetic exchange with the thirteenth chakra and the heart chakra that has to do with the immune system to energetic illnesses and anomalies. The endocrine system also has to do with hormonal activities from the various hormone-secreting glands in the body: pineal, pituitary, thyroid, thymus, adrenal, and ovaries/testes.

The higher patterning effect of the thirteenth chakra is like a grid template that has a symmetrical design embedded in it. It is used as a holding and transfer point for higher (be careful, you quantitative, analytical types) dimensional patterned energies to step down into the lower heart-centered endocrine system.

The Twentieth Chakra

The twentieth chakra is located an entire arm's length above your head, at the tips of the fingers (see Illustration #1-d). Think of it as the ever-watchful mother/father presence, reminding your Self that it is still you. It is through this chakra that we seem to see the face of God through our own monad. It is through this chakra that the presence of the soul is brought near the personality, that we might imbue the soul presence in our corporeal lives.

Through right action and right behavior we accentuate and develop the strength of the twentieth chakra to hold and accept the vibrational energies of the soul as it approaches (still us) the personality. Strengthening the twentieth chakra also increases our awareness that such parts of the whole human being even exist, without falling into the quantitative trap.

As we yearn for God by whatever name you know it to be, we strengthen the twentieth chakra, and thus the path the soul takes to imbue its qualities into our personality.

The Sixty-fourth Chakra

The sixty-fourth chakra is also located above the head, approximately five feet or so (see Illustration #1-d). It is the place of the monad, the highest possible expression of the existence of

Divine Mind, or God. The monad is what we seek to infuse into our personality ultimately, after the soul is fully infused. An example of a soul-infused personality would be a saint like Paramahansa Yogananda. An example of a monad-infused personality would be Jesus the Christ.

The best way to strengthen the sixty-fourth chakra is through spiritual practices that emphasize the Oneness of all things. But be careful that spiritual practices do not take the place of God-realization.

To put it succinctly in the words of Shunryu Suzuki-roshi, "All this talk about prayer and meditation. If we would just realize we were Big Mind, we wouldn't have to do any prayer or meditation." He also said, "If you are trying to attain enlightenment, you are creating a being driven by karma, and you are wasting your time on your black cushion."

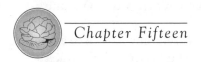

Chapter Fifteen

Reference Chakras

Dominant chakras can have an energetic *reference to* secondary chakras. In other words, your dominant chakra functions in concert with another chakra in a dynamic, externalized relationship. Just as there are relationships between thymus and thyroid, liver and gall bladder, so there are energetic relationships between chakras in all individuals. Some are much more pronounced and active than others.

Many individuals have reference chakras that affect their behavior in everyday life. Some have reference chakras that become involved energetically when there is stress or trauma to their dominant chakra. If there is enough stress in the dominant chakra, it begins to pull energy from its reference chakra. Eventually, problems of a mental, physical, spiritual, or emotional nature show up in both chakras.

Bear in mind that all your chakras are working and all interplay energies with each other. As one tends to predominate, there can be a reference to another chakra in both positive and negative manners. The relationship is ceaselessly interactive between the higher levels and the physical plane. Your mind is mostly unaware of these interactions.

The positive aspect of a reference chakra is similar to the dominant chakra in the coloring or filtration of perspective in life's experiences. As a secondary influence, the referent chakra is a major branch of the dominant chakra tree, or disposition towards life.

For example, a "5-2" individual (fifth chakra dominant, with a reference to the second chakra) is born as a communicator and teacher. That person may pull in the "lustiness" of having a referent second chakra: The great passion of creativity through the second chakra gives a fierce love of teaching through the fifth chakra as its dominant partner. The passion for life of the second chakra is imbued in the characteristics of communication however it may be externalized.

The positive benefits of having a reference to the second chakra is that the second chakra is the "visceral" chakra, the one most closely associated with our five senses. This offers throat chakra individuals the best opportunity to be grounded in physical reality, and to feel through the passions more of their presence in the moment.

The *negative aspect* of a reference chakra is that it can behave like a sympathetic dystrophy. There may be no inherent "problem" with the reference chakra, but its energy may be recruited by the dominant chakra to help with a life challenge. The dominant chakra is suffering, anomalous in its spin, and draws energy from a referent chakra (if there is one): Thus the disposition (mental, physical, spiritual, and emotional) from the referent chakra may increase difficulty in one or more of those archetypal areas of life. It's a double-whammy, you can experience a mix of externalized issues in both chakras.

As an example the "5-2" individual may be experiencing the stress of un-groundedness and frenetic behavior. The stress in the fifth chakra draws energy from the second chakra, producing corresponding issues of chaos, and loss of focus and inspiration that are related to second chakra function.

If the distress is great, the corresponding reference relationship also produces greater problems in the referent chakra.

Interestingly, an approach to healing for such an individual takes into account that if he is manifesting issues in the second chakra area, it is because he is *first* having a problem in the fifth (throat) chakra. For instance, if he is feeling chaotic or bland, he would seek to ground himself and address the healing of the fifth chakra, even though it is manifesting in the second.

In addition, healing the fifth chakra (in this case) heals the second chakra. The individual pays attention to the healing aspects of issues with the dominant fifth chakra, and it automatically addresses the issues in the second chakra. This is because of the interconnectedness of energies, as a link, between the two chakra influences with which the individual incarnated.

As far as I know, references are established for life, but there are variations as an individual experiences aspects of life related to all the chakras at different times. The dominant chakra, however, does not change, and neither does the referent chakra.

Chapter Sixteen

Stepping Through The Chakras: The Evolutionary Path

Many people wonder whether you rise up in a linear fashion through your chakras in succeeding lifetimes as you improve your spiritual standing through right action and right behavior (dharma). Does a person in his second chakra in the last life incarnate in his third chakra in this life, then the fourth in the next life, and so on?

The answer is "no." The concept of successive incarnations through the chakras in a linear fashion, accruing merit for the next lifetime to incarnate in a higher chakra, is relating the higher dynamics of the chakras to a *limited third-dimensional way of thinking*. It attempts to impose quantitative thinking of reality on qualitative reality. It does not happen in such a 1, 2, 3, 4... pattern. Individuals vary according to their experience

First of all, it would raise problems with the concept of a number of past lives, limiting your availability to higher levels of awareness.

Another part of the answer lies in the qualitative vs. quantitative aspect of human beings. It is logical to assume that you would make a linear progression through the chakras in successive lifetimes, but the experience of a chakra is non-physical translating into the physical (even though the true energy is always a two-way, seamless flow between levels of reality). The nature of the chakra itself, while still "you," is inter-dimensional, and not limited to third-dimensional space and time.

To think the higher number is better, is false, and does not embrace the qualitative aspect of our being. In fact, I have seen fourth chakra dominant individuals who were much less evolved than second chakra dominant individuals.

It is our desire to quantify that causes the mind to assume that one chakra is "better" than another: That, for instance, it is better to be in the heart chakra than in the second, or sacral, chakra. There are those who contend that to be in any of the lower chakras constitutes a lower level of awareness, and that we should concentrate on being in the higher four chakras.

It is my contention that all the chakras offer infinite levels of evolutionary access, with the proviso that chakras two through six must color the perceptions of the individual in accordance with certain spiritual laws that regulate the manner in which we incarnate in third-dimensional reality.

When you take an incarnation, you have a dominant chakric disposition that most closely fits the lessons, experiences, karma, and mission statement that you are to have in that lifetime. It is not a progression from one chakra to another - it is a qualitative statement of what is called "the experiential set." The experiential set is how many years you have been in this incarnation so far. That is, a statement of the linear, year-to-year expression of your life in the pursuit to build character through evolution of your personality, by infusing the qualities of your soul into that personality.

As you evolve, the experiential set is important but it is not the whole picture. You perceive beyond the confines of a linear and temporal/spatial awareness, and pull into a given lifetime the awareness that transcends your own physical and material being. You become "more than" the person in the body, but living in the inseparable Oneness that permeates all things.

As you evolve in spirituality and consciousness, the path is said to be an evolutionary upward spiral: The rise upwards indicates progression as a soul through time, the soul is infusing into the personality, and the circumference of one's awareness is rippling outwards through succeeding levels of increasing awareness.

Though looking at the illustration can only give you a linear sense of a non-linear quality, it is important to recognize that such illustrations are best conveyed in as many dimensions as possible *(see Illustration #16-a)*. Hence, this illustration must have a third coordinate. The ego and the feeling, or intuitive state, must balance through time for the spiral to maintain a circular, or balanced symmetry. Too much intuition or ego creates a "wobble" or imbalance in the upward spiral, thus the opportunity to create as well as overcome an illusion.

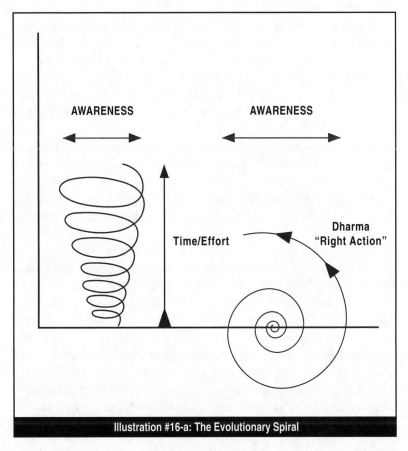

Illustration #16-a: The Evolutionary Spiral

Each incarnation presents an opportunity to experience life through not only the dominant chakra, but also the past life (karma), mission statement, and freewill conditions that apply in a given lifetime. Please refer to the chapter *"Dominant Chakra Positions of Famous People"* for examples.

In my opinion, Jesus the Christ was a second chakra dominant person. He was a healer, exorcist, passionate about his work and his love for his fellow beings. His main lesson was that we must love ourselves fully and hold strong to our faith. He was martyred for what he believed in and widely unaccepted. Those traits are very second chakra. Is it possible to be an evolved being and still have a dominant chakric disposition? What dominant chakra would he have evolved to if he took another physical incarnation?

We must separate ourselves from the notion of limiting a person's evolution to the placement of the chakra. It is better to focus on how much that person is evolved within the dominant characteristics of that given chakra than to think of the position of the chakra itself. Remember that chakras are still "us," and are our gateways to all other dimensional manners of existence.

If in the higher dimensions there is no space and time, it would be relevant for us within this dimension that uses the laws of space and time, to attempt to explain the phenomena of chakras in a third-dimensional framework. You can't blame a human being for trying, but in order to understand, you have to think in non-linear terms.

We are all given opportunities to far exceed the notion of who we *think* we are in favor of who we *feel* we are. Remember that the smallest feeling is greater than the greatest thought. Through the living of life in a given lifetime, you always have the inner tools to exceed your understanding of your physical environment. Thoughts are physical, limited to the third dimension. But feelings are transcendent, and they go beyond what your mind can think.

You must yield with your heart to what your mind cannot yet embrace. Add to that a certain amount of discernment and you have a perfect formula for dealing with the challenges of life from a position of strength.

Chapter Seventeen

Are We In Just One Dominant Chakra Our Whole Lives?

When I am asked whether you stay in your dominant chakra your whole life without changing or migrating to another dominant chakra, I am reminded of the story of the young man who goes to his local Army recruiting depot in a small town. As the sergeant is signing the young man up, he asks, "Have you lived in this town your whole life?" The young man replies "Not yet."

It is my opinion, based on years of research, that you would have only one major dominant chakra your whole life.

The work I've been doing for more than seventeen years is highly subjective, and in seeing people repetitively, whether for a "Flower Reading" or in a consultation, there begs the question of "being right." That is, when a person comes for repetitive intuitive counseling and healing, whether I will be "right" in assessing the dominant chakra and its characteristics. It is more correct to say that I am attempting to be "accurate" as much as possible, in that trying to remember exactly what I had said to a specific person in the past brings in a fear-based projection on the need to be correct every time. This effect also plays into the quantitative, sequential nature of what it is to have a human experience, and takes away from the qualitative aspects,

In addition, it is similar to being right-handed or left-handed. We have two hands but tend to favor one over the other for certain tasks. Even though both hands work, one will be used for tasks such as writing, painting, etc. The hand you used to write your name years ago is probably the same you use today, and will use in the future.

We have seven major chakras, and tend to "favor" one of chakras two through six as dominant over the others, even though they all are functioning and play a part in living our lives. It is better to say "I have two hands, and tend to favor my right" than to say "Is my right hand my dominant hand during my whole life, and is it so in every situation?"

We have issues through all of our chakras. At one time, perhaps, we have all had a money issue, or a flow of abundance. All abundance issues come from the second chakra, and while it may not be your dominant chakra, there may be lessons for you there as well.

Our sequential nature tends to lock us into a specific state of the understanding of reality that non-physical attributes such as chakras should be of fixed design. .

You can weave in and out of your chakras in a seamless mix of energetic dispositions, but the centrality of your dominant chakra will always tend to dictate the manner in which you perceive and respond to your experiences. The dominant chakra remains so, even though you are composed of all your functioning chakras.

Chapter Eighteen

Inverse Relationships -The Law of Reciprocity

Your Strength is Your Weakness

A reciprocal represents an inverse relationship: you tend to bring into your life those people who represent the inverse of what you represent as a given chakra dominant individual (*see Illustration #18-a*).

The energy is meant to set up a type of resistance so that through application of your weakness to the given resistance, you are helped to rise into the higher aspects of your Self. It is analogous to weight training, where the amount of weight and duration of training are similar to the life's lesson and chakric disposition.

The Law of Reciprocity brings the inverse relationships to mirror your issues in life. The mirror works in both positive and negative aspects, depending on the issues you are working on. The nature of the reciprocity depends also on the dominant chakra types involved.

For example, a second chakra individual, because he represents variety, would tend to bring into his life individuals whose lives are black and white, or individuals who have illnesses caused by the illusion that there are little or no choices in life. The charts below show sample inverse relationships through the Law of Reciprocity for a second chakra dominant individual.

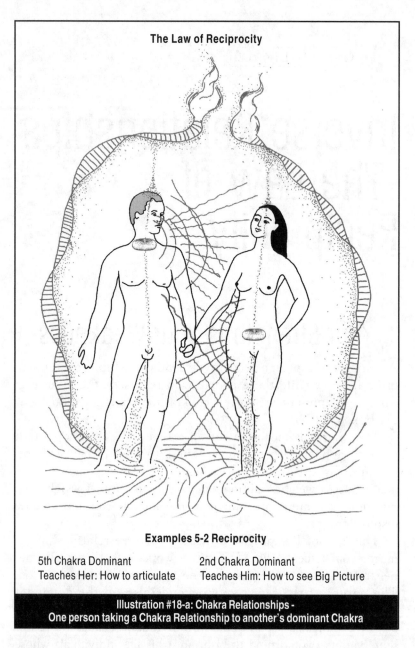

The Law of Reciprocity

Examples 5-2 Reciprocity

5th Chakra Dominant
Teaches Her: How to articulate

2nd Chakra Dominant
Teaches Him: How to see Big Picture

**Illustration #18-a: Chakra Relationships -
One person taking a Chakra Relationship to another's dominant Chakra**

The first chart is a negative inverse relationship. The second chart is a positive inverse relationship. There are many different types of reciprocities possible:

Sample Inverse *Negative Relationship* for a Second Chakra Dominant Person

Second Chakra Person's Energy	Other Person's Reciprocity
Variety	Black & white, no choice in life
Healer	Martyr
Creativity	Smothering
Accepts self	Passive-aggressive
Focus	Chaotic behavior
Flexibility	Rigidity
Infinite alternatives	Single-mindedness
Visionary	Pessimist
Faith	Hope

Note: *These relationships also work in the other direction as well. One who represents a black and white reality can call a healer into his life, and so on.*

Sample Inverse *Positive Relationship* for a Second Chakra Dominant Person

Second Chakra Person's Energy	Other Person's Reciprocity
Variety	Communication
Healer	Self-acceptance
Creativity	Inspiration
Accepts self	Collaborative leadership
Focus	Individuation of power
Infinite alternatives	Infinite love
Visionary	Teacher
Faith	Confidence

It is typical that our soul-group and familial interactions are based on a certain amount of reciprocity. As you progress through your life's lessons, the nature and extent of the reciprocity changes and evolves, often including an exchange of one soul-group for another, one relationship for another, and so on.

If you notice, the people around you are a loosely-affiliated sphere of your influences and contacts, and they are there in your life to reflect your current, yet ever-changing state of consciousness. As you evolve, your affiliations within and among soul-groups change as well. The reciprocity you encounter is always functioning at varying levels, at every moment.

Some individuals cycle in and out of your life very quickly, some more slowly. The periodicity is determined by your requirement for the life's lesson, the karmic attachment (positive or negative), and the rate at which you heal or become conscious of any limiting illusions.

To have an abiding respect for the interaction itself is to recognize the innate and Divine organizing principle that renders you both teacher and student, asker and giver of answers, inquisitor and font of all knowledge.

The Law of Reciprocity always provides the seed of the answer within the framework of your life's encounters. It is better to ask how many apples are in one seed than to ask how many seeds are in one apple.

You are guaranteed to experience this dynamic movement of energy. Being awake to its existence and a willing participant while knowing, in fact relying, that the answers are already there, empowers you and induces increasing alertness to the unfolding and evolving of your own flower of life.

Chapter Nineteen

Representation Through Relationship, and the Evolution of the Soul-Group Consciousness

As we take psychic relationships to each other, we do so on a subtle, energetic level of interaction in order to work out the details of our mission statement, karma, and freewill. These interactions are dynamic, in motion, play out through our choices, and are most heavily influenced by our given dominant chakra. *Remember that you engage energetically with others long before your mind thinks a single thought.*

If you knew why you interacted with people the way you do, wouldn't that be empowering to you? Wouldn't you then realize why you pick the people in your life? By understanding the way energy and consciousness works, you can change the effect by changing the cause. You can create a new outcome.

We all take a relationship to what another person represents energetically. This is called *representation through relationship*. We see others through the filtered reflection of our own understanding of the universe and how it works. It is this due regard for others in our lives that sets the stage for the development of our character. Those others in our lives are the soul-group with which we must interact to determine the choices we will make in this lifetime.

Representation through relationship is a circumstance of psychic connection, where the exchange of energies affects consciousness between individuals. The best example is that of teacher/student, where the student takes a psychic relationship to what the teacher represents as a more spiritually-evolved being. If the student exercises the will to be vulnerable to higher teachings, then the teacher's emanations of higher-evolved consciousness may imbue an increase in consciousness on the student.

The strongest effect the teacher has on a student is not through personal truths that are taught, but through the association, capability, and capacity the teacher has to hold higher, universal truths. It is the quality of emanation from the teacher that infuses the soul qualities of the student into his own personality, making his personality more soul-like. This emanation may also accelerate and activate the consciousness of the student simply because the teacher has now appeared in the student's life.

By holding the higher consciousness, the teacher becomes vulnerable to appear wherever he or she is required, by maintaining the representation through relationship status of consciousness.

If others are in the higher aspect of their given dominant chakra, we have a greater opportunity to evolve and grow in our consciousness by taking a relationship to what they represent as more evolved souls. Doing so also will tend to bring up all our "stuff;" our insecurities, fears, and issues.

The emanation of their evolved energies affects the way we think, feel, act, respond, etc. This, through the 95% of communication that is energy, is seldom understood or perceived by most of us, for we lack training in Western society in the understanding and application of metaphysics. Still, the energetic dynamic continues, just as gravity continues whether you are conscious of it or not.

If the other person is in the lower aspect of his dominant chakra, we will respond accordingly by having a less fruitful interaction, taking a psychic relationship to what he represents at his current level of soul's evolution. It also offers us the opportunity to be of service, whether taking the high road of elegance and graceful interaction, or taking the lower road of condescension and manipulation.

By making good choices for ourselves, by applying thoughtful and self-empowered interactions with others, we optimize the exchange of energies between us and hence optimize our soul's growth through the Law of Reciprocity.

In the chapters on each chakra, I have discussed the specific manner in which the soul-group takes a psychic relationship to the dominant chakra individual for the evolution of the entire group.

Evolving group consciousness through individual effort occurs as we serve the greater good of humanity in general, and the karma of our soul-group specifically. A soul-group is a loosely affiliated gathering of souls (people) who incarnate together for the purpose of mutual soul-infusion, reinforcement of spiritual goals, and the resolution of group karma through overcoming illusion and suffering. The people in the group may be your grocer, bank teller, gardener, etc. These are people you see from time to time, but don't know deeply. The soul-group also includes family and friends and those souls who come in from time to time for karmic ties and for spiritual teachings.

The more you recognize your succinct role in the evolution of group consciousness, the more you are able to empower your life to recognize why this soul-group is in *your* life. Remember, the Law of Reciprocity will bring inverse relationships into your life to evolve your strengths through an examination of your weaknesses. Without resistance, there is no opportunity for growth. Resistance training builds strength, so our lessons teach us to overcome our illusions of being separate.

In the evolution of soul-group consciousness, the relevant soul-group takes an energetic relationship to what the dominant chakra person represents. If you are that person living in right action and right behavior, and if you are exhibiting the higher aspects of your dominant chakra, your soul-group has the highest, most optimal possibility of evolving as a group. The playing field of the entire group is effectively raised in consciousness because of your dharma (*see Illustration #19-a*).

Everyone benefits from your right action. This is why monks in monasteries pray day and night for the benefit of humanity.

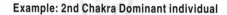

Example: 2nd Chakra Dominant individual

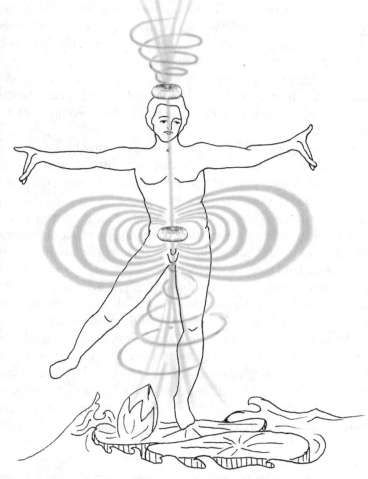

- Living in Dharma represents least illusions, most soul-purpose.
- Mere presence provides possibility of inspiring others through 95% non verbal, energy in communication
- Brings up issues in others in Soul Group to clear illusions
- Offers the larger vision to Humanity
- Example of Faith in Action
- Provides the greatest possibility of the evolution of soul group by Representation through relationship

Illustration #19-a: Chakra Dominant individuals living in dharma have the greatest possibility to affect their Soul Group

They know the metaphysical laws that help to raise the level of consciousness on this planet.

Something to remember is that we (in our higher desires) create the visionary, the charismatic leader, the teacher, and the prophet to come into our lives. This dynamic is in effect constantly, though many of us do not realize it.

For example, the teacher appears because a relevant soul-group has created the mild vacuum for him to appear. That is why the right teacher can express himself with the exact skill sets necessary to most efficiently and holistically articulate to the soul-group what it does not collectively and individually understand, but yet is ready to evolve to.

That does leave open the question of whether individuals in the group are going to exercise their freewill to make good choices, but you only have control over your own freewill. In making right action for your Self, you are accepting and fulfilling the reason why you incarnated in this lifetime, benefiting the entirety of creation, by being totally conscious, in harmlessness and in harmony with all things.

Having learned your lessons, your evolution helps the soul-group take a relationship to what you represent as an evolved being. As it is indeed their choice how to react to you, the relationship becomes most fruitful when all are making the most of the lesson. Knowing that not everyone carries the same level of metaphysical and spiritual understanding is not an impediment to growth. On some level of their being, everyone knows the Divine interaction and contracts existing in relationships.

This is why we take a psychic relationship to each other in the first place; in order to work through the relationships, have our necessary life experiences, raise our level of consciousness, and ascend from our limitations and illusions.

We are working in a collaborative leadership, where no soul is better than any other, where we must all work and agree to our highest potential: the resolution of all illusion.

Through your own spiritual self-empowerment, the desire to evolve, and the will to act, you stand in the best position to help your Self and others in your soul-group.

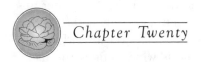

Chapter Twenty

Masking

Masking refers to hiding the external dominant chakra characteristics with those of another chakra. Like the chameleon, a reptile that attempts to look like the branch or leaf but is not, the person who masks is diverting energy from his dominant chakra in order to appear to have the dominant strengths of another chakra. This is typical of a defense pattern.

In most cases this is not a problem if you are only using the positive attributes of any given chakra. It only becomes a problem when you are hiding in another chakra in order to avoid facing dominant chakra lessons. Remember, the hardest thing you do is to overcome the weakness of your dominant chakra.

For example, you as a heart chakra dominant individual can migrate to your throat or sixth chakra in order to avoid feeling emotions too deeply, or, emotional overwhelm. You take on the characteristics of a more mentally active, perspicacious nature if you perceive a threat to being totally in your heart chakra. You may substitute a quick wit as a defense mechanism to avoid the deep emotional lessons that are part of the heart chakra existence. In order to avoid emotional overwhelm, you might become the "thinker" (sixth chakra), "aloof teacher" (fifth chakra), or "very controlling" (second chakra), for example, and there may be infinite variations.

The problem deepens if hiding in another chakra that is not dominant becomes a habit. It is in the unlearning of your point of view, the adoption of a more optimal experience of life through your dominant chakra that makes the lesson so very difficult.

To continue our example, could you just focus on unconditional love or on the Divine Presence to regain the sense of the heart chakra orientation, or to surpass the heart chakra in favor of a higher level of understanding?

In my experience, no. Being in the heart chakra is neither a good nor a bad experience, but it is an experience that you must have in order to evolve your soul. What you do with that relevant experience in a given lifetime is what defines the nature of your character and dharma.

It is important to note that masking refers to those who are hiding their real chakra dominance, not the normal shifting of energies and awareness between all chakras, that is part of the whole human experience.

Ultimately, you learn life's lessons from your dominant chakra, regardless of the masking, because your higher Self articulates lessons that will help to destroy your illusions and fears. As a grand and eloquent being, your temporary forays into third dimensional, linear thinking of resistance through fear is surpassed by your Inner Knower (still you on a higher level) that deftly helps construct the interactions necessary to overcome your illusion and fear.

Chapter Twenty-One

That's Just What a Chakra Would Say

There are certain attitudes, mannerisms, and sayings that serve to illustrate the point of your chakra's dominance in your life. While not exclusive to each chakra, I have noticed some general trends.

Second Chakra

- Whatever I do, it's never good enough.
- What's the use in trying?
- If I can't do it perfectly, I don't want to do it at all.
- I'm such a perfectionist.
- Me? In denial?
- I couldn't imagine not having lots of things to do, or many projects at the same time.
- Why is there so much chaos in my life?
- I should probably get another degree from school, even though I already have three. Then people will listen to me.
- I'll just work harder.

Third Chakra

- No one does what I say.
- Am I the only one in this room who knows what's going on?
- Nothing's wrong. I'm in charge.
- I have no peers.
- Why does this always happen to me?
- I'll put that off for later.

- Why do people treat me like judge and jury?
- All my boyfriends/girlfriends are ten years younger than I am.

Fourth Chakra

- Why am I so tired all the time? I have chronic fatigue.
- I feel emotionally numb.
- I feel like I don't give enough love to others.
- Oh, my muscles/joints hurt so much. I have fibromyalgia.
- I have not earned the right to receive love.
- I'd rather hurt myself than hurt others.
- I've explained my emotions but I feel I have not fully communicated after I'm done.
- I don't deserve love.

Fifth Chakra

- No one knows me for who I really am.
- No one listens to me, they don't understand. When I explain clearly, they still don't understand.
- I feel so alone and detached, so separate from others.
- My life is not productive or meaningful.
- I've explained it a dozen times, and they don't understand me.

Sixth Chakra

- I don't get it. Explain it to me again.
- I've done that over and over. Why isn't it working?
- I think that would feel great.
- I think I love that.
- Of course I understand, but I still don't get it.

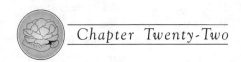

Chapter Twenty-Two

Dominant Chakra Dispositions of Famous People

Following is a list of some notable individuals and my assessment of their dominant chakras. Using what you've read in this book about dominant chakras, consider these famous people and see what *you* think.

Individual   Dominant Chakra

Individual	Dominant Chakra
Jesus the Christ	Second (Sacral) Chakra
Rumi	Second (Sacral) Chakra
Deepak Chopra	Second (Sacral) Chakra
Paramahansa Yogananda	Third (Solar Plexus) Chakra
Billy Graham	Third (Solar Plexus) Chakra
Joan of Arc	Third (Solar Plexus) Chakra
Mohammed	Fourth (Heart) Chakra
Saddam Hussein	Fourth (Heart) Chakra
Pope John Paul II	Fifth (Throat) Chakra
Buddha	Fifth (Throat) Chakra
George W. Bush	Fifth (Throat) Chakra
Mahatma Gandhi	Fifth (Throat)/ Second (Sacral) Chakra
Stephen W. Hawking	Sixth (Third Eye) Chakra, Second (Sacral) Chakra Reference
Albert Einstein	Sixth (Third Eye) Chakra

You can see by the table that these individuals had/have vary-ing levels of evolvement within their respective dominant chakra dispositions. Attempting to compare one individual to another is difficult, as we are each on our own path.

The method by which I arrived at my opinions of chakra dominance of these famous people is the same as I use in my spiritual counseling. It is a matter of tuning in to the conscious-ness of the higher Self of the individual, even if deceased, and ascertaining his soul's purpose and disposition.

As we live in oneness, not separate from all love, wisdom, and will, it is possible to discern, at the least, an opinion of anyone's chakra dominance. Since there is no time or space, the time since one has passed renders no obstacle to percep-tion.

Here are explanations of two examples from the table:

Jesus the Christ, second chakra dominant. Many would argue that he surely must have been heart (fourth chakra) dominant, rather than second. Jesus was a very perfected being, infused with the higher aspects of all of his chakras.

The second chakra has to do with a higher vision and ever-unfolding creation, a value of what is possible to achieve, many times through faith. Individuals who are dominant in this chakra represent the opportunity for us to see our potential if we are vulnerable in ourselves and courageous to achieve it, while demonstrating in a tangible way (performing miracles) a visceral connection with the Divine in each of us. "Ye are Gods" (John 10:34, Bible). "Greater things than these shall ye also do" (John 14:12, Bible). Jesus represented the essence of the healer, visionary, and martyr: all major aspects of the sec-ond chakra.

So, how could *Saddam Hussein* be a heart (fourth) chakra domi-nant individual, given what many feel about the emotional qualities of the heart? We expect kindness, gentleness, and abundant love. Granted we only know about Saddam what is printed in the press, but if true, how can a heart chakra indi-vidual behave in the manner ascribed to him?

Remember that life is about one thing: the development of

one's character. Saddam, through his freewill, may choose among alternatives how to express the desires of his heart. Those alternatives can be rooted in the lower aspect of the heart chakra. The lower aspect of a heart chakra individual can include the opposite of what it is to be yielding, kind, and loving. It can include the absence of compassion and a refusal to take part in the healing of the emotions of others.

When the populace takes a psychic relationship (representation through relationship) to Saddam as a potential emotional anchor, the psychic energy can be perverted into its darkest, most pernicious potential. What people may perceive initially as a healing experience psychically can be degraded into continual suffering and hardship.

The examples in the table are meant to stimulate your understanding of the archetypal dispositions relative to chakra dominance. The mental, emotional, physical, and spiritual aspects weave together a tapestry of the character of the individual, based on the choices represented by those dispositions.

Chapter Twenty-Three

Hand Positions and the Chakras

When you see people "talking with their hands" they are often activating or working with the energies of a given chakra (usually the dominant one) by their gestures. People use hand positions and movements most often unconsciously *(see Illustrations #23-a and b)*.

- Movement in front of the heart chakra to denote the expression and emanation of the quality of love. The hands wave in an outward movement; starting at the heart area and waving or gesturing outward.

- A male who hooks a hand in the belt loop, pointing the fingers towards the root chakra to denote survivability or existence. The hand or hands usually stay pointed in that direction to emphasize stability of the physical nature, permanence, or physical presence.

- The person who holds a finger or fingers to the third eye or temple to stimulate and emphasize the sixth chakra. This is used to stimulate conception of ideas, spontaneity, and transcendence of time.

- The person who stands or sits with palms over the solar plexus chakra, palms turned inward and covering the chakra in a defensive move to protect the Self and the idea of what the Self represents. This person has already reacted to the energies directed at him, and is defending because he has taken the energetics personally, as an attack on Self.

Movements are usually: (see Illustration #23-a)

- Defensive/Protective – Holding the hand or hands directly in front of the given chakra in a resting or blocking position.

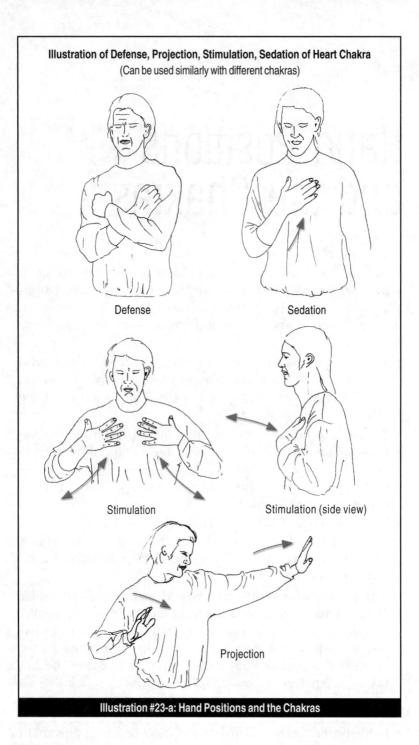

Illustration of Defense, Projection, Stimulation, Sedation of Heart Chakra
(Can be used similarly with different chakras)

Defense

Sedation

Stimulation

Stimulation (side view)

Projection

Illustration #23-a: Hand Positions and the Chakras

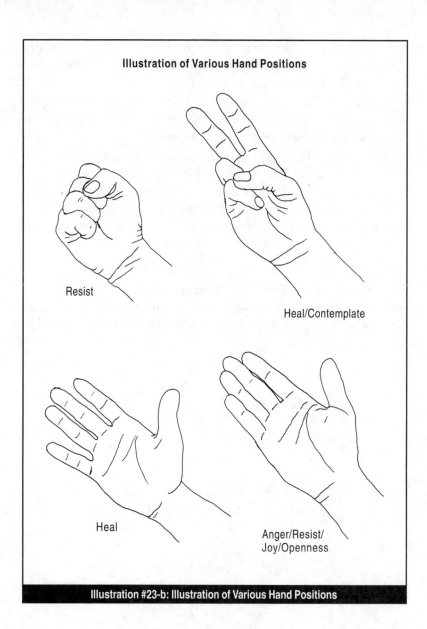

Illustration of Various Hand Positions

Resist

Heal/Contemplate

Heal

Anger/Resist/
Joy/Openness

Illustration #23-b: Illustration of Various Hand Positions

- Stimulating – Movement of the hand or hands to activate, emphasize, or stimulate the positive properties of the given chakra. Usually touching or waving
- Sedating – The hand movement is covering or gently stroking the affected chakra area to sedate or calm the associated energies it is experiencing in a situation.
- Projecting – The hand movement is projecting the energies of the given chakra outward, either to another person or a room of people. The legs can be employed as projective, also. The woman who wags her crossed leg is stimulating and emanating energies from her second chakra, self-creativity and sexuality.

Remember that we are elegant and magnificent beings, most often totally unaware of our sublime sophistication. When next you see someone using these body positions, see if you can match the gesture and motivation with the individual's possible dominant chakra.

Chapter Twenty-Four

Psychic Manipulation Prevention

Manipulation of others is something we all do, and on its own it is neither positive nor negative. We seek to gain advantage for ourselves in the world based on our wants, perceived needs, desires, and fears.

One who goes to a chiropractor or massage practitioner has been manipulated physically; one who goes to a psychologist has been manipulated mentally. Though neither is negative, it is manipulation of someone's perception of the environment.

Of course, manipulation *can* be a negative or positive event. The untimely call of the persistent telemarketer, the visit to the new car showroom, the first date, the new stock deal, the Ginzu knife offer, the well-intentioned in-law: we are all exposed to subtle and not-so-subtle manipulation on a daily basis. There are times when others will push their agendas onto us, to convince or persuade us to their points of view, based on *their* perception of need or priorities.

Since most all communication is energy, the amount of energetic manipulation that occurs on a daily basis is massive. It is so pervasive and constant that it is the underlying fabric of our energetic personality dynamics. Individuals are in constant energetic contact with one another, whether it is intimate, familial, professional, etc. Our energies interact, no matter the distance, with the greatest interaction based on our intimacies, family, and soul-group.

The best possible reaction you can make to either well-intentioned manipulation or negative manipulation is to respond from a place of absolute clarity and center. In this manner, all that proceeds has the least affect of coloring your perceptions due to the weakness of a given dominant chakra characteristic.

This chapter identifies ways in which each dominant chakra archetype can be manipulated by other dominant chakra archetypes, and the ways to prevent its occurrence. Remember that there are times that no matter what you do, you may fall prey to certain manipulations that are necessary for your soul's growth, maturity, and experience.

You are subject to the exigencies of life through all of your functioning chakras and thus may come into contact (a life lesson) with a manipulation from a chakra different than your dominant one.

There are times when you must engage in manipulation by others to experience a contract, mission, karma, or freewill choice. Hence, the following prevention techniques are offered with the caveat that, for these reasons, they sometimes may not work.

Many relationships suffer from this type of manipulation. The emotional wages are serious and can often result in suffering on many levels.

Manipulation by Chakra

Second Chakra Manipulation

The most pervasive and most common manipulation techniques are those applied against the second chakra, as these are based on guilt, validation, and self-criticism. In some instances, you need only imply guilt to the second chakra dominant personality and being creative, that individual will do all the rest.

The manipulation comes in the form of passive-aggression, codependence, or enabling, where the otherwise sweet and compassionate nature that generally emanates from the second chakra is seduced into supplication and subordination to the desires of another. This generally involves capitulation in order to do "the honorable thing."

The method is to make the second chakra dominant person feel guilty or obliged to create for the manipulator, using his feelings of abundant creation to shackle him to the manipulator's will. By using this "emotional hostage" technique, the manipulation can go on for years, until the second chakra person perceives enough self-love to see that the playing field is anything but level.

Second chakra individuals often assume that the other person will naturally engage in active limitation of desires and will stay within appropriate behavioral boundaries, not transgressing the goodwill of the second chakra person. This is one of the fundamental lessons of the second chakra person: that of healthy emotional boundaries, of responsibility to enact them, and not to rely on another's good graces to keep healthy boundaries for both.

Second chakra individuals can lose their perspective quickly through committing their creative abilities to the means and goals of another person or institution. This manipulation may have many names: love, loyalty, patriotism, team player, the greater good. But if it involves a sacrifice of the internal integrity of the second chakra dominant personality, the loss of the perspective will ensue quickly.

When you lose your perspective in life, the next thing to go is your identity. All too easy to lose, a little at a time, one day you awaken to a life of feeling you are in a trap that closed very slowly. It closed through your good intentions to give of that goodness to others, without respect of Self or perception of self-integrity.

Another way to manipulate the second chakra is through the creative chaos of usefulness. Having the second chakra person always create for others helps to keep that person in an endless loop of self-criticism, that nothing they do is good enough. The result is that the second chakra person just works harder, but never really comes to resolution.

The essence of this type of manipulation is to turn the creative aspect of the second chakra out of control, resulting in chaos. The second chakra person assumes he is creating wonderful lives for others, while slowly destroying himself from the inside out, because he is creating from emotional obligation and desire for approval.

Second Chakra Manipulation Prevention

There are a few very effective ways to reduce and prevent manipulation through the second chakra. Please remember that it is not enough to know that these techniques exist, you must *apply* them to be effective.

The first technique is "perspective through inspiration." Simply removing your Self physically from the event, relationship, or situation even for a few moments is enough to spark an awareness of Self through the use of personal will power. Separating your Self from unhealthy manipulation gives your feelings time to breathe, to recover from emotional inundation, and to gain a space around you that is safe and sacred.

It is in this space where you can receive inspired meditations that bring on vast amounts of love and sacredness to your existence. Inspired meditation can help you bring in a sense of self-value and identity by showing you the "big picture." Second chakra dominant individuals must learn to place a value on themselves, on their contributions to their health and integrity, and on their ability to receive as well as to give love.

As they begin to see the overview or big picture, they will gain a sense of perspective. The hidden benefit is that they will increase their sense of personal identity, knowing what they want and what they need. This is not selfish; it is the maintenance of integrity.

There are Shaolin priests who know fighting arts such as Kung-Fu, but their application of it is to maintain their safety and their integrity as monks, not to harm anyone. Likewise, healthy emotional boundaries are first served by having a sense of Self that can be discerned from perspective. This perspective is gained by making the time and space to become inspired.

Inspiration comes as a personal, sacred event. By its nature, it is immediate, holistic, and comprehensive. And it is private to the beholder. When you choose a space of vulnerability to become inspired, a sense of value is placed on Self and integrity. This is a necessary and fruitful step in the development of a self-empowered consciousness, one that is not dependent on the emotions of others for well-being.

Inspiration can be anything meditative: meditation itself, a walk on the beach, bowling on Tuesday night, or whatever evokes the inspiration of your soul and it's longing to be externalized as whole and complete through your personality.

Regular application of this separation, or time for your Self to become inspired, is the key to the prevention of manipulation of the second chakra. Building inspirational time into your life has many more benefits, but most of all gives a sense of integrity, perspective, and purpose - so vital to a productive and meaningful life.

A second technique to prevent manipulation through the second chakra is creating "healthy emotional boundaries." Ask your Self the following questions when you have a sense of manipulation:

1. Is this person taking power from me?
2. Am I giving my power away to this person/institution?
3. Have I spread my Self too thin?
4. Am I taking on too many things?
5. Are we both benefiting emotionally?
6. Am I giving to my Self as much love as I am giving to my partner?
7. Has my life become too chaotic?

If you answer "yes" to any of these questions, put up healthy emotional boundaries regarding what you will and will not accept. Then do the first technique, *perspective through inspiration*, and make sure that you perform the technique at regular intervals: daily, weekly, monthly, or whatever is most appropriate for you.

Third Chakra Manipulation

The essence of being manipulated through your third chakra must contain a distraction, diversion, or devaluing of the Self or a confusion of the emotions. As the third chakra is the "I am" chakra of individuated personality, the energy most others feel is some intimidation due to the individuation of truth through power that the third chakra represents.

If you can manipulate people by giving them the impression they have no personal power of their own, it will effectively prevent your growth, and will also help to hold the manipulated individuals in a lower aspect of their third chakra, causing them to internalize anger. The anger rests in the geographic area of the third chakra (solar plexus) and affects the internal organs there, as well as emotional, mental, and spiritual states.

The manipulation results from one's own fears of "what could be true *is* true." This chakra represents the individuation of truth at such a high level that the mind capitulates to the power of the third chakra. The result of the power of the third chakra is to daunt the mind of the individual to believe he really could *not* be that powerful, hence inviting others into his life to be abused through low self-esteem and self-worth.

This manipulation of Self can continue on until the third chakra affected individual becomes angry enough to make a change. Relationships like this, as with the second chakra, can go on for years, resulting in continuing devaluation of Self and the non-exposition of power through the third chakra. The individual will actually subordinate his truth as not important enough, if the manipulation by the other person is convincing enough.

One of the easiest ways to manipulate third chakra dominant people is to keep them emotionally confused. The hardest thing the third chakra dominant person does is to make emotional, qualitative decisions. It is the key weakness of the third chakra, because it plays on the individuation of truth and the dispensation of personal power.

Keeping a third chakra person confused emotionally is a powerful manipulative tool: the confusion "locks up" the individual's otherwise powerful ability to decide.

Third Chakra Manipulation Prevention

The best way to prevent manipulation of the third chakra is to emphasis the uniqueness of one's own life and skills. This can be much easier said than done, because if a length of time has transpired and the third chakra person has been in the lower aspect, it can be a difficult climb.

Individuation is the strength and the weakness of third chakra individuals. Often, they feel that if they externalize their truth, it creates separation through that same individuation because of the unique value of the truth they hold. They decide that if they give their truth, it will forever change energetic relationships between themselves and others. And, they are correct. This is the very action required for third chakra individuals to raise not only their vibration, but to present the possibility to the soul-group that the entire vibrational playing field could be raised in consciousness.

Hence, one becomes equally strong by individuating through truth, and desiring to dispense the truth in a compassionate and harmless manner. Remember that the third chakra is all about personal power; the individual who has this chakra as dominant must deal with issues of personal power over a lifetime. So often, they come for counseling and realize they've once again encountered an issue related to their dominant chakra, and wonder why they are still in those issues. They are *life* issues, as the dominant chakra is unlikely to change in a given lifetime. They can become stronger, but must still be tasked with the challenges relative to their dominant chakra disposition.

To prevent manipulation of the third chakra, individuation may mean getting angry enough to make the change. Anger has one positive attribute: it motivates change. Anger does not mean violence: it means externalizing lies and untruths; releasing them to prevent harm to your Self. Anger does not mean hurting another person. It means you love your Self enough not to hold a lie, and enough to tell another person what they really need to hear. Determining what that course of action is, and what you must tell the other person is best reflected in tact, diplomacy, and harmlessness, but you must have due regard for your ability to hold truth, as it emanates as a quality from the third chakra.

Asking your Self if you're living a lie, if you are deferring from the truth by picking up seemingly harmless addictions instead of facing and enacting the truth, is a great step towards ending manipulation. The more truthful you are with your Self, the greater liberation from manipulation by others.

Fourth Chakra Manipulation

The fourth chakra represents love itself, and many such individuals willingly give of themselves to others, thus creating most of their life lessons; that of healthy emotional boundaries.

The most fundamental energetic manipulation of the fourth chakra individual is similar to that of the second chakra. Using their own good and loving nature against themselves, with very little extra energetic manipulation from others, invokes a life of service to others but does not help to complete their self-fulfillment.

As with any chakra dominance, what one comes here to do is not the same as what one comes here to learn. The fourth chakra dominant person is here to learn to communicate the profundity of the heart chakra, and sometimes does so at the expense of negative manipulation by becoming the human pincushion for others.

As before, one's strength is also the weakness. Manipulation occurs by counting on the heart chakra individual's inherent goodness to spend emotional energy to hold together a relationship, a family, a soul-group, and so on. The amount of energy required to do this work is enormous. As you understand from the chapter on the fourth chakra, there are very few of them relative to other dominant chakra types, as these individuals are about four out of every hundred persons, or less. That energetic bonding to the emotional spiritual maturity of the relevant soul-group requires tremendous expenditures of energy, even though it may appear that the individual has a rather placid life.

By allowing the heart person to assume you are more emotionally complete than you are; by allowing him to hold the emotional energy of your non-commitment to your own emotional evolution; by transgressing the heart person's emotional boundaries, you are committing manipulation of the fourth chakra.

Fourth chakra persons struggle to see the purity that they have earned from several sequential incarnations in dharma. Helping to hide that purity from the fourth chakra dominant person is a terrible misuse of power and an effective negative manipulation. The fourth chakra person is struggling to communicate that purity through externalization to the outside world of a depth of emotions that has no physical way of being communicated. The act of effort helps to define the soul's growth through the fourth chakra; the effort of communicating feelings though limited by language.

If the framework of that communication has no healthy emotional boundaries, if another person is helping to keep hidden the fourth chakra person's purity, the manipulation continues.

Fourth Chakra Manipulation Prevention

Prevention of manipulation of the fourth chakra begins with healthy emotional boundaries. Through such boundaries, fourth chakra people can differentiate between their own feelings and that of others, thus defining their own identity.

Many fourth chakra persons suffer from loss of identity early in life, because they are empathically relating to the emotions of others. This can be to the extent that they *define* themselves according to the emotions of others, because the heart chakra is energetically feeling those emotions all too well.

Healthy emotional boundaries means using words like "no" to the full extent of their purpose: to set a boundary beyond which you will not cross and neither will the person with whom you are interacting. This takes the power of the will to enact and maintain the emotional boundaries. By having a boundary, you know your own limitations emotionally and thus begin to know your identity. It is all too easy to completely deplete your Self through your heart chakra, thinking that giving unbounded love with no expectation of any in return is enough. It is not.

Many sacred texts speak of the giving of limitless love, that it flows through you completely and effortlessly. But incarnation also involves life's lessons that are experienced as an individuated being. That means there are lessons you, as that unique being, must experience to evolve your consciousness and infuse your soul-quality into your personality. In order to do so, you must maintain the integrity of who you are and what you represent as that individuated being; no different than the example above of the Shaolin priest who practices Kung-Fu to maintain his integrity.

A given lifetime allowing love to fully flow through you is not enough if you are not fulfilling your purpose for being here. If you have the extra challenge of being dominant in your heart chakra, it is even more difficult to realize this very important rule of life: you must fulfill your Self. It is not enough to give to others, because you cannot fully affect humanity's evolution from a place of weakness. You must first make your Self strong spiritually; then, from a place of strength, help others.

It is all too easy to assume that fourth chakra beings help others to heal by their mere presence, and that that is enough. Thinking/feeling this way causes the serious diseases and emotional problems apparent to the fourth chakra dominant individual.

One of the best prevention exercises is the water exercise. This is because the mental faculties of the fourth chakra person are diminished when the emotional energy body is over-saturated with negative compressive emotional energy. Performing this exercise merely invokes the power of the will, but it is a highly effective means of purging excess negative emotional energy. When the emotions are clear, the mind is clear in the fourth chakra dominant person.

Follow the exercise for the fourth chakra, as illustrated in the "Exercises and Meditations to Build Strength in Each Chakra" in Appendix A.

Fifth Chakra Manipulation

Throat chakra dominant individuals can be easily manipulated, if you can keep them out of their bodies. Energetically speaking, you are "in your body" or "grounded" when you are aware of your metaphysical nature and your corporeal presence at the same moment. It is the essence of being "totally present." Out-of-body is another way of saying you are unaware of the grounding of your power, and your power to articulate.

Since we all take a psychic relationship to each other, there is also considerable latitude in your awareness of the energetic inter-dynamics between your Self and others. To a limited extent, at the very least, we all "know" certain techniques of engagement with each another.

Exciting a fifth chakra person, engaging him to resist feeling, facilitates his desire to be out-of-body to avoid visceral contact with his feelings and the gross (rough and uneven) vibration that can be experienced on the earth plane. Facilitating the detachment of the fifth chakra person from his grounded, corporeal existence, limits his ability to call in all his power, to feel coherent and complete, and accelerates feelings of detachment, alienation, and aloneness.

The fifth chakra represents communication and teaching. It is the chakra associated with articulating the ineffable information that comes from higher planes of existence into physical reality. Cutting off this connection is something that throat chakra dominant individuals do well enough as they incarnate to learn the lessons of communication and feeling. Doing so deliberately to another is like cutting off one's oxygen supply. Agitation, frenetic behavior, deliberately behaving in an ungrounded manner can cause the throat chakra person to lose the direct connection to the other persona, and to his grounded reality. This creates the possibility of engaging in mentalisms, which can be endless loops of pure mental energy, with no connection to his emotions or to earth.

Fifth Chakra Manipulation Prevention

The main emphasis on manipulating a throat chakra dominant person is by keeping him from being grounded or in his body. Interrupting the throat chakra potential to bring "as above, so below" cuts the individual off (in a sense of being present) from his whole-being integration.

By nature the throat chakra dominant individual tends to be ungrounded; as the mind capitulates to the tremendous multi-dimensional nature of the throat chakra. The mind attempts to keep up with the dynamics of the throat chakra, but cannot by virtue of comparing the linear mind to the multi-dimensional chakra.

Grounding, for the fifth chakra person, is exceptionally difficult because it is so very simple. Because of this, energy from the fifth chakra is near the jump-off point to the octave-leap to the sixth chakra. This is altogether different from the movements between the first and the fifth chakras that are made with single steps, like the notes on a piano. With these chakras, each step carries a vibrational quality relative to that chakra's ability to be grounded on the earth plane. More on this is written in the following paragraphs on the sixth chakra.

It is highly likely that because of the simplicity of breathing being an effective technique for grounding, that the throat chakra person will ignore its use and efficacy. This is not due to intellect but rather to the compelling, near-octave leap in frequencies to the sixth chakra, but only single-note equivalent frequency spacing to the lower chakras.

The fifth chakra is the horizon, where the earth plane meets the esoteric, higher-plane realities. The impending reality of this phenomenon looms over the entire consciousness of fifth chakra people; a dwelling of the higher states impels them to draw themselves out of body continually. Thus, the difficulty.

Yoga, Pranayama Yoga, Tai Chi, Chi Gung: these are all very grounding breathing techniques. Using the techniques in the appendix on exercises for the throat chakra are of great help in grounding.

I have done many healings on throat chakra dominant individuals, only to have them leap out-of-body instantly afterwards. Some begin babbling incessantly because they cannot resist their mind's tendency to embrace the esoteric values on the horizon of the octave-leap to the sixth chakra.

To prevent manipulation, throat chakra individuals must ground themselves, and must do it for the rest of this incarnation, as a mindful, daily practice. No one can do this full time, but the more you do, the more grounded, productive, and efficacious you become. It can be very difficult to remember to do this on an ongoing, daily basis, but that is the discipline.

Any grounding technique reminds throat chakra individuals "as above, so below," and unites their metaphysical nature with their corporeal being, thus making them totally present, focused, and grounded. Doing so prevents energetic manipulation.

Other grounding techniques are through mnemonic or intermediary devices, such as grounding materials. Worn on the body, they in themselves do no grounding, but because they have grounding properties, the individual takes a relationship to what they represent, and causes grounding to be enhanced. Here are a few stones you can use; size and shape are not as important as the stones themselves:

- Hematite
- Smoky quartz
- Obsidian
- Malachite
- Black tourmaline

Anything in, on, around, or near water is grounding. Getting your hands and feet into the dirt, ground, grass, sand, rock, etc., is grounding. Feeling your chair, the carpet, reminding your Self that they are made from earth, is grounding.

Sixth Chakra Manipulation

Manipulation of the sixth chakra person is similar to the fifth chakra ungroundedness, but remember that the sixth chakra is an octave above the fifth. The sixth chakra person is already functioning at a very high level of vibration. Sometimes, it is all he can do to remain somewhat functional on the earth plane; his mind is preoccupied with higher, cosmic circumstances.

The difficulty explaining the functioning of the sixth chakra is no different than a parent explaining something to a child. No matter the eloquence, if the child is not mature or evolved enough to understand, no explanation is possible. Rather, an abiding respect for the power of the sixth chakra is necessary, because there is so very much suffering in the world by sixth chakra dominant persons who are misunderstood.

It is hard enough for true communication to transpire with the sixth chakra individual's inherent difficulty of connecting to his heart feelings in this dimension. However, manipulation by using guilt and separation from feelings, as with heart chakra manipulation, makes emotional communication for the sixth chakra individual near to impossible.

Without being grounded, the sixth chakra dominant individual suffers internally by engaging in his own mentalisms, and this can be manipulated. If the sixth chakra person has been able to successfully externalize his mission and to be somewhat grounded, this represents the best possible means of protection from manipulation.

Sixth Chakra Manipulation Prevention

Prevention of manipulation requires first that the sixth chakra dominant individuals are sufficiently composed in this dimension to enact their will to prevent manipulation in the first place. This is not always the case.

Doing heart-centered exercise (see Appendix A) is the best deterrent to manipulation, because it unites the things most important to sixth chakra individuals: their metaphysical awareness, mental power, and heart-centeredness. Once this is done, they are very hard to manipulate because, like the fifth chakra person, they have united as above, so below.

Most sixth chakra people operate at such a high-energy level that their weakness of not being able to relate to the world can even be a part of a natural defense against manipulation, because the average person would not even know how to relate to them.

Chapter Twenty-Five

The Evolutionary Aspect of Truth

Truth is relative to the person experiencing it. As you grow in consciousness and expand in awareness, your understanding and exercise of truth, as you know it, is relative to your capability and capacity to hold it. For the moment you are quite sure of what you are feeling, what your truth is, until in the light of new evidence and experience you evolve a higher truth. The truths you hold now may not be the same a year from now, as they may have evolved to a higher level of understanding.

Did the truth exist before humans existed on the earth? Will it exist after our passing? Is the truth innate in each of us, equally accessible by all? I believe it is, or the argument that we live in Oneness with no separation would have no validity.

If it is true that we live in Oneness, then our aspiration to the truth provides the resistance that makes us strong, through due tribulation. As the Buddhists say, "God picks you, you do not pick God." It means that when you are ready to face your weakness or life's lesson, the truth will stand before you, and you've decisions to make. Will you stand in the truth, avoid it, ignore it, or misuse it? Will you use it to gain admission into a higher understanding of who you are and what you represent as a soul incarnate?

Suppose there were a three-year-old boy present, and a great truth of the Universe was read to him, one sentence in length. Next, suppose we again read that great truth of the Universe to the same boy at thirteen years of age; then again at thirty, word for word. We would have read the same great truth of the Universe to the same person, at each age. But his capability and capacity to hold, understand, and realize truth is very different at those three ages. He is not the same person, and yet he is the same. His awareness shifts with the inculcation of a higher truth; he grows into a new understanding of himself and his universe.

What we regard as true is constant only for the moment; we surpass our understanding of truth with time. And you could have two evolved people in a room, but their concept and understanding of a universal truth may differ. It is the same for larger groups of people as well.

Suppose you live in a three-bedroom house. You've lived there for a number of years. One day, you walk down your hallway and see a door to a fourth room that had not been there before. You would be extremely puzzled and bewildered at how you could have lived in that house for so long and never noticed the door, but would nonetheless (like us all) open the door.

Once inside you see all around you colors and shapes that you've never seen nor envisioned, yet there they are. Above and below you are openings, doors to other universes, and your mind and heart are filled with wonder at such visions.

Now suppose you leave the room after only five minutes inside, and never go back into that room. Would you remember what you saw? Would those sights, sounds, and images stay with you for the rest of your life? Of course they would. *This is how aspiring to greater levels of truth occurs in our lives.*

We live in an abiding understanding, for the most part, of our surroundings and circumstances, perhaps given a religious framework. When exposed to a truth that is out of the ordinary or transcendent, we are challenged to assimilate the truth into our everyday circumstances. But, like ripples in a pond, the water must radiate outward, not inward, and we must make our circumstances adapt to the higher truth, not the other way around.

As you progress through higher levels of consciousness, the outward radiating sphere of understanding encompasses everything that came before **(Illustration #25-a).** All your former experiences fit into your higher experience, *but you cannot make a higher experience fit into a lower one.* This is precisely the difficulty with metaphysics: that when you have an epiphany it is

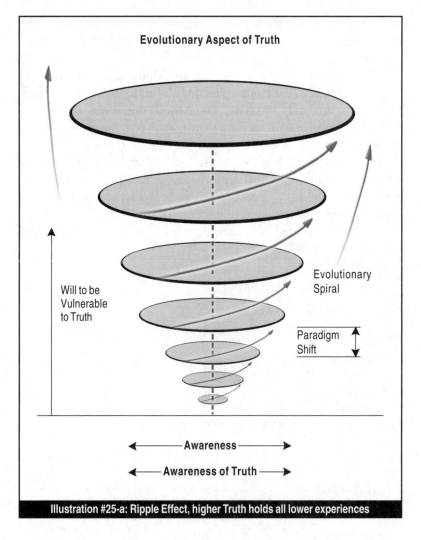

Evolutionary Aspect of Truth

Will to be
Vulnerable
to Truth

Evolutionary
Spiral

Paradigm
Shift

◄——— Awareness ———►

◄——— Awareness of Truth ———►

Illustration #25-a: Ripple Effect, higher Truth holds all lower experiences

very difficult to explain to others who have not yet transcended to that level of understanding. If you could fully explain an ecstatic moment or an epiphany, it would not be an epiphany. We write about it, talk about it, attend workshops on ecstatic (from the Greek *ex-stasis*, meaning "out of the normal") experiences, but the real experience can only be realized from the individual point of view.

This is part of the difficulty of imbuing the soul's quality through third chakra dominant individuals. They must individualize the truth through expressions of personal power, and must often hold higher levels of truth than their immediate contemporaries.

We can only approach absolute truth gingerly until we have had the experience for ourselves, for the nature of higher levels of truth is intensely intimate. Even then, our intimate encounters with truth are by levels according to our spiritual capacity to hold it, karmic influences, and mission statement.

Even though we may be exposed to higher levels of truth, we may choose not to dwell there for various reasons, but the experience nonetheless is a part of us. It is forever recorded in the subconscious and the cellular memory of our lives. To reject the lesson now is to create it later, perhaps in a more vigorous and less subtle way.

Chapter Twenty-Six

Quantitative VS. Qualitative Reality

Why is it so difficult to understand the field of metaphysics, its tenets, and functioning? For the Western world, it is because we are steeped in duality, the separation of one thing from another.

In Western society we are taught to believe we are separate from that which we seek. "I am here, God is there" - two separate and distinct phenomena, when in reality there is no separation between them. The separation causes the inception of a belief system that becomes very linear and quantitative. We see this so often in science, where the observer counts, divides, summarizes the subject of study.

The problem is similar to apples and oranges: Phenomena of a metaphysical nature has a physical, linear counterpart, but cannot be thought of in the same way. The flashlight is not the light, the map is not the topography, the menu is not the meal.

The nature of metaphysics is rooted in a qualitative state of being, rather than what can be quantified or counted. We often think of intuitives in terms of "Where did they get their information from?" or "How do they know that?" In essence they are tapping into a sea of consciousness that is not separate from them or their existence in any way. This is the manner in which all psychics work. They are merely accessing something that already exists, but that which most people feel is quite separate from their daily lives and activities.

If, one thousand years ago, you and I had a conversation and I told you of a wondrous energy that when run along two pieces of metal to a filament, the filament would glow like the sun, of course I would be talking about electricity. Logically we know that electricity has always existed, *but our awareness of it has not*. The relevancy of truth in our lives shifts with our awareness to grasp it.

Electricity exists now in our waking consciousness: Perhaps most people living in the world today know of it but think very little of it because it is ubiquitous. And yet, no one has *seen* electricity. We've seen streams of electrons as lightning bolts and sparks, flashlights and street lamps, but we've not seen the energy itself; just what it does and the effects it has.

Energy from higher dimensions permeates every space, every aspect of our lives, but we are mostly unaware of its existence because of our linear, dualistic approach to life. We see and hear, two of the most vital of our five senses that tell us what in the world is real. Our five senses are the way in which we reach out to our third dimensional physical existence - they inform us of our experiences here. We perceive and interpret differently, according to level of ignorance and understanding, awareness, karma, mission statement, and freewill.

Western science empirically measures and counts. And it has been said that the best way to teach the Western mind that metaphysics is real, in lieu of an instant epiphany, is to use the very same model of separation or reductionism. In other words, to use science and technology to explain a qualitative phenomenon that externalizes into a physical realm.

Recall the reference in Chapter 2 of inventions such as the AMI, created by Dr. Hiroshi Motoyama, Ph.D., that measures the functioning of the meridians with very small direct-current pulses applied at the terminations of the meridians on the fingers and the toes. The amount of time it takes for the signal to decay is converted into an analysis of the functioning of the meridian system through a series of computerized algorithms and displayed as a map, or radar chart, of the individual's health.

The AMI has been in use in Japan for over thirty years, and has been going through the FDA in the United States for licensure since 1992.

Another device invented by Dr. Motoyama is the Chakra Chamber, a radiation-proof copper enclosure, impervious to electromagnetic radiation, including light. A subject sits inside, and a device called a photon (a photon is the smallest particle of light, where light behaves like a wave and a particle at the same time) counter measures the amount of light (called biophotons) that is emitted by the human body.

Researchers found that the human body emits about 1 biophoton per cubic centimeter. However, when the device was placed over a person's chakra centers, researchers found an emission of between 100 and 1000 biophotons per cubic centimeter. Obviously, something is going on.

However, no matter how much research and analysis is done in this manner, it is not enough to bridge the gap in consciousness between the quantitative state and the transcendent qualitative state. It is, however, enough to pique the interest of those Western minds that would never accept a qualitative state of being that could not be empirically established.

There has to be the initial leaping-off point, where technology shows that there is *something there*. Another way to say it is that the best way to change a paradigm is from within itself. The best way to get the Western mind to understand that there really are qualitative states of consciousness that transcend our everyday lives is to use the very same duality that gives us the illusion of separation. In that way a chink in the armor of incredulity is achieved, where we first entertain the *mysterious* in order to get to the *real*.

The metaphysics of our lives cannot be measured directly through our five senses. We must use a part of our nature that is based in an inner knowing, a *trust*.

This is where we have the greatest opportunity and the greatest problem of all. If you were asked, "Do you love your mother?" you would most likely respond "yes." And if asked, "How do you *know* that?" you may respond that you "just know." Well, *how* do you know?

And if you were asked to produce this love, to set it on the table for all to see, you could not do it because that love is a qualitative state and cannot be quantified. Yet, the access to true consciousness is not in how many books you've read or workshops you've attended, nor is it in your intellectual capacity, but rather in your vulnerability to trust that not only do you live in a Oneness, not only is it accessible in any instant, but the way to achieve awareness is through your *feelings*.

We are taught that our feelings are fleeting and our emotions are based on transitory thoughts, but the reality is that our feelings are the keyhole through which we see and aspire. I've said before that "The smallest feeling is greater than the greatest thought" because feelings transcend the linear and temporal, qualitative state of being.

As the mind and heart must be balanced, so it is with metaphysics, wherein feelings alone cannot take the place of the discerning mind and critical thinking. However, if one were to be put before the other it would be "Trust what you feel, apply what you know."

To yield to the qualitative state is exactly what a psychic would do. To achieve a high state of consciousness, the guru or yogi must transcend the limitations of thought and mind to achieve the qualitative state of beingness.

It is the feelings that transcend the waking state of consciousness, not the thoughts, for the thoughts are borne of the experiential mind and linear existence, based in a third dimension of quantified existence. Here again, you must yield with your heart to what your mind cannot yet know. That is the inception and path of our true greatness and genius. It is the part of our minds that we are not using, the hidden part of the universe that cannot be seen but definitely can be *felt*.

We often have difficulty with this because we are not educated to trust our feelings, to have a high regard for our emotions, or to nurture and take care of our emotional well-being. It is through this avenue, though, that the greatest shifts in awareness can be achieved because it represents direct access to that sea of consciousness, a Oneness in which you already exist, where technology cannot embrace and thoughts cannot count it.

You must have the courage to trust with your heart through an abiding faith that what you cannot see exists nonetheless, regardless of religious tenet.

We must have a balance of mind and heart, of thoughts and feelings. The technologies we use can help us to achieve some success, but they are not the answer; no more than restructuring a gene sequence will automatically make us more enlightened, no more than doubling our brain capacity makes us smarter. The technologies can only help to point to the answer, for the answer is within us.

Chapter Twenty-Seven

Three Reasons Why People Do Not Heal

Healing is our constant endeavor. It is interesting that when we are ill our attention becomes very focused on the illness and its healing.

The illnesses we face can be caused by many factors, but usually it is because of the illusion of separation that we engage in suffering. The suffering is in direct relationship to the igno-rance and to the disposition of the related chakra.

With most illnesses, we wish to heal as soon as possible. When you visit a health-care practitioner, the practitioner is only a facilitator for a Divine blueprint of healing that already exists within us: *We actually heal ourselves.*

We all have that perfect Divine blueprint within us; our en-deavors in the world are externalizing circumstances and events that create the possibility of healing. That creative search for healing is constantly being mirrored back to us through everyone we meet, and in our daily affairs.

If we are aware, we recognize that the power of the healer helps us to enact our own healing process; a process that must be begun with vulnerability to growth and yielding to release illusory beliefs that do not serve us in our highest good. The effort to heal takes courage and will power.

Even when you have done everything right there are still reasons, mitigating circumstances why you may not heal. This can be the case even if you have seen your healing practitioner and followed all the prescriptions and healing practices.

*There are three reasons why people do not heal imme-
diately from their afflictions:*

1. Karma
2. Mission Statement
3. Freewill Choice

Karma can also be described as ignorance that Oneness exists.
In that ignorance is the embrace of separation and illusion,
which creates attachments representing incomplete or incoher-
ent levels of reality as it is. That complicated sentence means
that you can be ignorant without knowing you are ignorant.
Young children don't know they are not mature. Many adults
live their lives in ignorance that metaphysical laws of being exist, and that they are subject to those laws.

Your karma in a past life carried forward into this one can
cause you to have your infirmity or suffering a little while
longer until you absolve your Self from the karma, learn the
life's lesson, or pay fully the karmic debt. Healers may become
frustrated as to why a person does not heal in the face of remedies and an array of healing arts. Even in the process of releasing negative core beliefs, if the individual they are treating is
not yet karmically ready, the healing will not fully take place.

*The three greatest ways to overcome the influence of
karma are* **prayer**, **meditation** *and* **healing**:

- Prayer is an invocation, speaking to Divine Source and asking for specific relief.
- Meditation is being still and listening for the answer.
- Healing refers to spiritual healing work done by a qualified
  practitioner.

As you pray and meditate, you gain momentum towards evolution as a spiritual being, and your recognition and acceptance
of your Self as a multi-dimensional being grows through personal realization that it is, in fact, true.

Your *mission statement* is the contract that you incarnate to
accomplish. Some may have a mission statement that includes
being a paraplegic from birth. Steven Hawking, one of the
world's greatest astrophysicists, is a quadriplegic from multiple

sclerosis and it seems unlikely that he will "heal" from that condition. Measured in terms of success, he has a family, money, academic prestige, and notoriety. It may be that there is no healing required for that aspect of his physical life, but that his mission statement set the precedent that he incarnate in that manner.

A mission statement does not *have* to include any illnesses or suffering, but those experiences are enacted to help the personality grow and infuse its soul characteristics. Mission statements are life-long, but the possible illness and suffering may not be: those are essentially a part of the life-path of the individual. That means that the length of an illness, if it is part of the mission statement, may be in force only as long as is needed to learn the life's lesson. The illness will not heal immediately if the mission statement lesson is not yet learned.

Freewill choice includes those who, given the option to heal, refuse it in order to continue in a lower level aspect of behavior. Some who are martyrs, chaotic people, and manipulators may reject any healing in favor of continuing a path that avoids personal responsibility of Self.

Usually this is because of negative self-reinforcing belief systems, or negative philosophies, based on illusions where the individual sees more merit in being ill and suffering than in healing. Freewill also means that you can engage in negative behavior leading to suffering if you believe you do not have to take responsibility for your life.

There have been cases of those who perpetuate the chaos in their lives, bringing in a string of qualified healers to no avail, because those individuals perpetuate the business of being sick. It gets them the attention they desire and defers real healing until they garner the courage to be vulnerable to a greater level of truth than they now hold.

Although not perfect, using freewill to remain ill is a functional way to avoid responsibility, create self-loathing, procrastinate in one's mission, and to perpetuate an interdependence on others. Many times this originates, though not exclusively, in the second chakra.

There are times when individuals have come to me for spiritual counseling/healing and have not achieved the healing results they were after. These same people may have been attempting to heal from various afflictions for years. The answers are twofold:

1. A life's lesson is just that. It could be that you must continually struggle to work on certain issues in order to strengthen your resolve to overcome some major illusion or karma related to your mission statement.

2. You are not ready to heal fully from the affliction.

It is most important that you do make the effort to heal. The effort itself is even more important than the goal, *for the nature of our character is defined by the effort we expend in each moment.*

The Universe operates on two principles: *Desire* and *effort.*

- Desire is the active participation of the emotions.
- Effort is our will in motion or action.

Once set in motion, the universe enfolds itself around us to assist in a collaborative, co-creative effort steered jointly by our soul expression and Universal Mind.

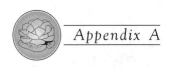

Appendix A

Appendix A-1

Recommended Reading For Each Chakra

Chakra Number	Recommended Reading
2	*The Prophet*, Kahlil Gilbran Any writings by Rumi, the 11th Century poet *The Inward Arc*, Frances Vaughan, Ph.D. *Polyamory*, Dr. Diane Anabol *The Four Agreements*, chapter on "Do your Best," Don Miguel Ruiz
3	*Spiritual Emergency*, Dr. Stanislav Grof *I and Thou*, Martin Buber *The Power of Now*, Eckhart Tolle *The Four Agreements*, chapter on "Nothing is Personal," Don Miguel Ruiz *Bhagavad-Gita*
4	*The Inward Arc*, Frances Vaughan, Ph.D. *Fibromyalgia*, Marjorie Haynes
5	*I and Thou*, Martin Buber
6	Any writings by Rumi, the 11th Century poet

Exercises and Meditations to Build Strength in Each Chakra

Doing exercises and meditations strengthens your awareness and abilities with respect to your true metaphysical nature. The results are often subtle. Hidden benefits accrue that are not readily noticeable, but extremely positive. An example is the sense of contentment that a second chakra individual will experience when exercising composure and calmness around chaotic friends.

Please do not underestimate the power of these exercises; they are very powerful and effective. *Energy follows wherever your attention goes.* If you apply your Self with positive attention, you will achieve results.

With the application of these exercises and meditations, the abilities may dawn on you like a gentle mist or growing awareness. Some of you may even have sudden, revelatory experiences.

If at any time you feel any discomfort or disorientation, stop your meditations or spiritual practices until you feel it is safe to continue. Consult with your inner knower and inner trust, with your spirit guides, or a spiritual counselor.

Conditions to remember:

1. You are in charge of your life, and you make the decisions by your freewill.
2. You always have a choice.
3. Prepare for these exercises with the highest intent for your greatest good. Be deliberate, and use them as a ceremony to celebrate your being.
4. Always call in your guides, masters, and angels to surround, protect, and guide you.
5. Place your understanding in a Divine Presence (whatever your belief system) such that you feel totally in the embrace of that Divine Presence, head to foot. If you have no such belief system, imagine a perfect triangle or another geomet-

ric shape, and focus your energy on how perfect and balanced that form is. Place your energies within the perfection of that geometry.

6. If you feel ungrounded, nervous, or out of sorts doing any of these exercises, STOP. Close the book, rest, and relax. Start again when you feel ready.

From these conditions you are, by the power of your will, "commanding the blessing," as it says in the Bible. That is, you are using your will to be in your power, your integrity, and your safety. You are calling your higher Self into this place and this time. From this place of centering, you may proceed with the following exercises and meditations.

This chapter is divided into three sections. Some of the exercises repeat for certain chakras. You can do any or all of these exercises on a daily basis, or as you feel the desire.

Chapter sections:
Section One: **Simple Exercises to Increase Intuitive Abilities**
Section Two: **General Energy-Balancing Exercises**
Section Three: **Specific Exercises for Each Chakra**

Section One: Simple Exercises to Increase Intuitive Abilities

1. Grounding Exercise/Meditation **"As Above, So Below"**
Grounding is the realization of your metaphysical and corporeal nature in the same moment, the absolute blending of the two, to one.

Close your eyes and breathe.

With three slow breaths, imagine you are pulling white light energy down through the crown in your head, through your neck, and that the white light energy is swirling and mixing all through your torso and limbs. Feel the connection to all that is.

With three slow breaths, imagine you are pulling earth energy up through the soles of your feet, through your ankles, calves, legs, and that the earth energy is swirling and mixing all through your torso and limbs. Feel the grounding effect.

Pause for a few moments to feel the mixing of the white light energy and the earth energy.

When you are ready, open your eyes.

2. Heart-Centered Exercise/Meditation

Close your eyes and breathe.

Imagine a beautiful ball of energy, about the size of a tennis ball, floating weightlessly inside your forehead. See or feel it as a platinum color, silver-white. Allow it to descend slowly, past the back of your eyes, your nose, your mouth, and experience it descending slowly until it comes to rest inside your chest, just above your heart.

As you experience the pureness of this platinum ball of energy, feel the sight of your physical eyes moving into it. Imagine your physical eyes are now in the platinum ball of energy, and it is as though you actually "see" from just over your heart, inside your chest. With those eyes, look out at your surroundings and experience what you "see." Note that you do not have to move your head.

With these eyes, look over the top of your head. You could not do this with your physical eyes, but with these eyes you can see anywhere, on any plane, in any place. You can see into the future and the past. You can see what cannot be seen.

Imagine your physical ears, your sense of hearing, is now located in the platinum ball of energy floating in your chest weightlessly above your heart. It is as though you actually hear from over your heart. Listen. What do you really hear? With these ears, you can hear the truth; you can hear what one is *really* saying.

Now move your sense of touch, taste, and smell into the platinum ball of energy and experience your world.

Lastly, move your ability to speak into the platinum ball of energy. It is as though the sound of your voice actually comes from deep in your chest, just over your heart. And when next you meet someone, experience that person from this place, over your heart, and respond with your senses and speech in that ball of energy.

When you are ready, open your eyes.

(Note: When you are ready, this meditation should eventually be done with your eyes open. You can do this anywhere, anytime you wish. However, not recommended while driving a car.)

3. Clearing the Energy Fields Exercise/ Meditation

After finishing any healing effort, it is always a good idea to clear your energy field of any negativity or clinging energies. This you accomplish through the power of your will. Remember, you are in charge.

Close your eyes and breathe.

Imagine a rain of silver-colored droplets descending from a beautiful sky. The soft, cleansing rain touches you at the crown of your head, and expands into a purifying mist. The mist drapes over your body and slides off to the ground, carrying with it any and all negativity, thought forms, and energies that are ready to release.

The mist magnetically pulls any of these energies out of you, leaving cells, molecules, and atoms clear and refreshed. The mist cleanses the emotional body, the mental body, and the light and desire bodies. All negativity harmlessly slips from you into the earth, where it is transmuted to neutral energy.

Breathe in and out for a few moments to feel and experience the cleansing action.

When you are ready, open your eyes.

4. Clearing the Mind Exercise/Meditation

Close your eyes and breathe.

Imagine a comb, like a sweeping hand, is moving through your mind, gently catching and removing any errant thoughts, any discordant thinking, any doubts or fears. The combing action sweeps through your entire mind three times, thoroughly removing anything that is ready to release, even if you don't know what that is.

When you are ready, open your eyes.

5. Gratitude Prayer

An essential part of a healthy spiritual existence is a recognition and acknowledgment of those beneficial forces in the Universe that are beyond our mind's comprehension, but within the flickering grasp of our hearts.

A gratitude prayer:

"I reach out with my heart, passing understanding, to that place of yearning in my soul. I embrace with an open heart my Divine heritage in the Oneness; there is no separation. I give thanks that it is so and recognize my place as an individuate being of light in the heart and mind of the Creator, whole and complete. And so it is."

Section Two: General Energy-Balancing Exercises

1. Initiation Prayer

"I now align my chakras to their most perfect function and greatest clarity. I do this in the name of the All That Is in my highest and greatest good. Any and all impurities, impediments and lower level beliefs, as Divinely appropriate, effortlessly dissipate and evaporate. Each chakra, from my root to my crown, is in perfect alignment with my metaphysical and corporeal nature. Each chakra is in perfect relationship to all my chakras, through which Divine Life-Force flows."

"I release the highest, most loving desires of my soul to the universe, knowing them to be true and good, and give gratitude that it is so. I command the blessings of these desires in the name of the All That Is. And so it is. Amen."

2. Governor Vessel/Conception Vessel Exercise/Meditation

Very gently breathe fully, deeply, in and out for a few moments, being deliberate about pulling the air down to the bottom of your stomach. Allow your stomach to rise and fall, filling it first with air and then expanding your chest as you inhale. When you exhale, expel the air from the lungs first and the stomach last.

For women (female energy flow): Imagine a loop of energy, flowing down your back, through the shushumna, and up the front of your body.

While you inhale, very gently begin an imaginary "pull" of limitless, Divine universal energy up the front of your body. Let it rise to the crown of your head. As it reaches the top, begin to gently exhale and let it crest over and begin to spill down the your spine, through the shushumna and through the lenses of each chakra, and gently "push" it down to the perineum (between anus and genitals, where the legs meet the body) where it pauses only briefly before going back up the front of your body. This is one cycle.

Gently and deliberately keep the energy going in a slow loop, pausing only briefly as a roller coaster would as it goes over the top. Do not speed up, but keep the cycle going, with your breathing, gently and deliberately.

For men (male energy flow): Imagine a loop of energy, flowing down the front of your body, and up the back, through the shushumna.*

While you inhale, very gently begin an imaginary "pull" of limitless, Divine universal energy up the spine, through the shushumna and through the lenses of each chakra, and let it rise to the crown of your head. As it reaches the top, begin to gently exhale and let it crest over and begin to spill down the front of your body, and gently "push" it down to the perineum (between anus and genitals, where the legs meet the body) where it pauses only briefly before going back up the spine. This is one cycle.

Gently and deliberately keep the energy going in a slow loop, pausing only briefly as a roller coaster would as it goes over the top. Do not speed up, but keep the cycle going, with your breathing, gently and deliberately.

Do this exercise for a few minutes, or about seven cycles. Breathe evenly and gently for a few minutes after finishing.

*Note: this flow of energy is not exclusively male or female. If you are a female, and feel the energy flowing down the front and up the back, that is perfectly good. The energy flows differently in each of us.

3. Shushumna Exercise/Meditation

This exercise is meant to strengthen the shushumna, the column of light that goes up and down your spine. The shushumna shines through the lenses of all seven chakras.

Sit comfortably, hands in your lap. Men, left hand resting on top of right, palms up, thumbs lightly touching. Women, right hand resting on top of left, palms up, thumbs lightly touching.

Breathe deeply and slowly. Pull the air down to the lower abdomen, push out gently with stomach, with mouth closed, tongue touching the roof of your mouth.

Close your eyes, and imagine two shafts of brilliant white light, shining from infinitely above your crown and infinitely below your root, coming together and meeting at the lens of the fourth chakra, the heart chakra. The columns of light shine through the lenses of each chakra and meet at the heart chakra.

As you breathe, imagine a pulse, or cycle of breath, that is moving through the now single-column shaft of light. Move into the column of light as you breathe. Experience the feel of the infinite nature of the light, infinitely upwards and infinitely downwards. Be in the light, feel its own pulse and rhythm. Breathe rhythmically.

Experience the cleansing and purifying feeling from Divine Source moving through all levels and dimensions of the column of light. See or feel it moving effortlessly through chakra four, three, five, two, six, one, and seven. Feel the column of the light balancing itself automatically through the chakras. Feel its infinite length.

Focus on the column of light. Allow it to be as intense as Divinely appropriate. Effortless. Breathe. Relax and open your eyes.

Breathe easily for a few minutes.

4. Chakra Balancing Exercise/Meditation

This exercise balances the seven chakras, and brings into alignment chakras eight, thirteen, twenty, and sixty-four.

Sit comfortably, hands in your lap. Men, left hand resting on top of right, palms up, thumbs lightly touching. Women, right hand resting on top of left, palms up, thumbs lightly touching.

Breathe deeply and slowly. Pull the air down to the lower abdomen, push out gently with stomach, with mouth closed, tongue touching the roof of your mouth.

Visualize and/or feel your chakras as pulsing lenses of pure consciousness. Give them a quality of color, sound, texture, etc., that feels right to you. Call your guides, masters, and angels in to witness and hold energy with you for your perfect and effortless alignment and balance of the chakra system.

Ask for a bubble of golden light to surround you, enfold you, and permeate your being with its purity to hold a space of sacredness.

Hold your will to infuse your soul-quality into your personality, through the lenses of each chakra:

"I now infuse the quality of my soul into and through my *first chakra*, as Divinely appropriate and in my highest and greatest good."

"I now infuse the quality of my soul into and through my *second chakra*, as Divinely appropriate and in my highest and greatest good."

"I now infuse the quality of my soul into and through my *third chakra*, as Divinely appropriate and in my highest and greatest good."

"I now infuse the quality of my soul into and through my *fourth chakra*, as Divinely appropriate and in my highest and greatest good."

"I now infuse the quality of my soul into and through my *fifth chakra*, as Divinely appropriate and in my highest and greatest good."

"I now infuse the quality of my soul into and through my *sixth chakra*, as Divinely appropriate and in my highest and greatest good."

"I now infuse the quality of my soul into and through my *seventh chakra*, as Divinely appropriate and in my highest and greatest good."

"I now infuse the quality of my soul into and through my *eighth, thirteenth, twentieth and sixty-fourth* chakras, as Divinely appropriate and in my highest and greatest good."

"As above, so below. So I now command the blessings of Mother/Father God, as an individuated aspect of the creative force of the universe. I see, feel, and experience all of my chakras in perfect alignment and balance."

Allow the golden light to soothe, adjust and balance each chakra and among the chakras as a whole. Feel and experience the balancing provided by the perfect symmetry of the All That Is.

Sit with this experience for a few moments, until you feel a "complete" feeling.

Rest and relax for a few minutes.

Section Three: Specific Exercises for Each Chakra

1. First Chakra (Root Chakra)

Prayer
"Divine and Heavenly Mother/Father God! I give thanks that my root chakra touches my feet upon the earth, allowing me to embrace the sky and to behold the canopy of Heaven. May my physical existence here in this plane of experience be of your holy purpose, of benefit to my Self and humanity."

Exercise/ Meditation
Breathe deeply and slowly. Pull the air down to the lower abdomen, push out gently with stomach, with mouth closed, tongue

touching the roof of your mouth.

While focusing on the location of the first chakra at the perineum where the legs meet the body, feel your physical presence in the world. Listen to your breathing, experience the blood flowing in your veins, your weight upon the floor. Visualize and/or experience the energies in your first chakra in harmony with the vibration of earth and physical reality, in harmony with the third dimension.

Sit with this experience for a few moments, until you feel a "complete" feeling.

Rest and relax for a few minutes.

2. Second Chakra (Sacral Chakra)

Prayer

"Divine and Heavenly Mother/Father God! Thank you for my visceral experience, for my five senses and my corporeal experience. May my senses be filled with your Divine will. May my suffering bring due reward of the evolution of my consciousness. May I, through my example and vision, bring an end to suffering in the world."

Dropping into the Second Chakra Exercise

This exercise is similar to one that I teach to martial arts students.

Stand, feet at shoulder width. Feel your center of gravity focused precisely in your second chakra, your lower abdomen. Ever so slightly, flex your knees forward, almost imperceptibly. While you stand, the slight flex in your knees will pronounce the feeling in your lower abdomen.

Now, rotate your hips slightly, so that your butt rolls, tucking your tailbone even further under you. This makes the pelvic bone protrude and emphasizes the center of gravity and awareness even more in the second chakra, the visceral chakra.

Hold this pose for about 3 - 5 minutes, gently, while breathing rhythmically.

Rest and relax for a few minutes.

Second Chakra Builder Exercise

Imagine, as you breathe, that you are also breathing through your second chakra, in and out. Feel an inner rhythm as you focus your attention on your lower abdomen, and as you do, feel absolutely connected to all love, all wisdom, and all will.

While rhythmically breathing, feel the infinite, unending abundance of love and creative power from the All That Is, flowing in through your second chakra and flowering the infinite possibilities of your being within you. Feel that unseverable connection between your inner trust and The All That Is. Breathe. Breathe. Breathe. Rest and relax for a few minutes.

Exercise/Meditation

Breathe deeply and slowly. Pull the air down to the lower abdomen, push out gently with stomach, with mouth closed, tongue touching the roof of your mouth.

While focusing on the location of the second chakra below your navel, feel your five senses as they experience third dimensional reality. Hear, smell, taste, touch, and see your physical experience in the world. Take your time.

Now feel your heartfelt sense of trust; that sacred and holy part of you, private and secure, that trusts. Allow that trust to nurture, slowly, the five senses with love and sensitivity to experience and discern what is real.

Feel your sense of infinite creativity and alternatives flowing to you, and through you, from Divine Source: ever evolving and unfolding, effortlessly creating.

Feel acceptance and acknowledgment of your passion and desires by Divine Source.

Visualize and/or experience the infinite energies in your second chakra in harmony with the vibration of trust and your five senses, harmonizing with the third dimension.

Sit with this experience for a few moments, until you feel a "complete" feeling.

Rest and relax for a few minutes.

3. Third Chakra (Solar Plexus Chakra)

Prayer

"Divine and Heavenly Mother/Father God! Thank you for gift of my freewill and the individuation of my personality! May the Divine power and truth that flows through me be an instrument for your will. May I infuse my soul-quality through my uniqueness to empower myself and all humanity."

Making Emotional (Qualitative) Decisions Exercise: The Thirty Second Rule

As third chakra individuals are not known for their patience, thirty seconds may seem like a long time, but you have to use all thirty for a reason in this exercise. It is designed to help you make emotional decisions, and also to sit with the feeling of authenticity for your Self: that you have the right to be right with your feelings. It is much more difficult than it would seem for the third chakra individual.

Take thirty seconds off your watch. Breathe and place the emotional question at the front of your mind and heart. For the *full* thirty seconds, ask your Self the following repeatedly, "What am I feeling now? What am I feeling in this moment?"

At the end of thirty seconds, it may be vague, but you will have an answer.

Now, you must trust what you feel, and *apply* the answer. That means, it is not enough to just hold the answer, you must *act* through the power of your will.

Let's use the worst-case scenario, where the emotional answer you receive is vague, like "I'm angry." OK, what about? "It's not fair (a third chakra judgment)." What's not fair? "I'm allowing this to happen, again. I've been acting powerless."

You see? From this simple exercise, you can derive an answer to an emotional question. But, you must be willing to accept the fruits of your emotional decision. You must be willing to accept your power and apply the action to the decision. You accept the successful evolution and upward spiral of your consciousness, because once you do, it can change interpersonal relationships instantly, and sometimes drastically as you accept your power. You must be willing to be powerful, a succinctly third chakra experience.

Little Spiritual Epiphanies

The reason this exercise works is because it has two main parts in "What am I feeling now:"

1. When you say "I" in "What am I feeling now," your energies and awareness instantly go to the "I am" chakra, your third chakra. Your energy is now focused in your personality.

2. When you say "now" or "in this moment," you are pulling in all of your power, spread across space and time, into this moment.

When you put them together, it puts you into that qualitative state in the moment, where all of your power is located.

Exercise/Meditation

Breathe deeply and slowly. Pull the air down into the lower abdomen, pushing it out gently with the stomach. Keep your mouth closed, with tongue touching the roof of your mouth.

While focusing on the location of the third chakra in your solar plexus, feel your personality, and the individuation (uniqueness) of your freewill. Sit within absolute truth and feel your Self transcend limiting beliefs and lower truths. Feel accepting ultimates of truth, the will to choose it, and the power to enact it. Feel Divine Source flowing will and power through your inner truths; feel your Self accept your own authenticity and authority. "I am in my power, I choose freely, and I know the truth."

Sit with this experience for a few moments, until you feel a "complete" feeling.

Rest and relax for a few minutes.

4. Fourth Chakra (Heart Chakra)

Prayer

"Divine and Heavenly Mother/Father God! Thank you for the gift of love from the heart of the Divine Presence. May I accept the purity my heart represents, and may I hold the ocean of love that effortlessly pours through my being. May I be a representative of Divine compassion for humanity and may humanity heal by humbly accepting your endless love!"

No-Stick Teflon Exercise

When in a gathering of people, an empath can often feel claustrophobic due to the many chaotic emotional energies characteristic of mixed gatherings that press into the feeling sensitivities of the fourth chakra person.

Knowing what Teflon does for cookware, imagine and project the no-stick qualities of "No-Stick Teflon" in your energy field.

Your energy field will not filter any goodness that comes through, but will tend to fend off any negative emotional energies, hooks, or tubes from others. You may still take on certain things, as you must, if it is within your path's learning.

Invisibility Exercise

Similar to the exercise above, this exercise is used where the feelings of having your emotional energy field over-saturated may create distress or discomfort.

Imagine that you are invisible to energies that are coming your way, such that when you feel them approach, they pass right through you and stick to nothing.

This is the essence of non-attachment, and this exercise, rather than the one above that uses protection, requires much less energy. It takes more energy to protect than deflect. It takes even less energy to be totally invisible. It is the power of your will to be in equanimity, choosing not to take on chaotic energies, even though everyone around you may be very much in chaos. Remember, it is a choice.

Water Dispersal of Emotional Energies Exercise

Whether you shower or bathe, imagine the water as magnetic. Knowing what a magnet does, imagine the magnetized water pulling out of you, as appropriate, any negative emotion, thought or feeling. You don't even have to know what the negativity is, just think "*Release, release, release*," as the negativity goes out into the water, the water goes down the drain, and you are clear.

The earth then transmutes the negative energy into neutral

energy. If you cannot get to a shower or bath, hold your hands under running water and think *"Release, release, release."* If you cannot get to water at all, just imagine it running over the back of your hand. The power of your will helps to clear you.

You can do this exercise as often as you want every day. It will help to keep your emotional energy field clear. Water is a great conductor of emotional energy, and most empaths always live near water or love being in water.

Exercise/Meditation

Breathe deeply and slowly. Pull the air down to the lower abdomen, push out gently with stomach, with mouth closed, tongue touching the roof of your mouth.

While focusing on the location of the fourth chakra in your heart area, feel love, absolute and total love. Feel no seam between you and your heart's desires. Feel the love of Divine Source and your love melding into that seamless Oneness.

Feel your Self transparent, like glass. Now, experience the love from Divine Source, shining as though light through seven perfectly colored filters. Experience through your heart chakra the Divine compassion of awareness of all seven of the chakras in your Self, and in those of humanity. Divine compassion flows and flowers, to you and through you.

You accept the purity that you've earned, and you accept the perfect love that imbues your every action. You allow others to heal by your presence. As transparent, you take on nothing of their suffering but that which is Divinely appropriate for you in helping you to destroy any of your illusions of separation. Rest in perfect love.

Sit with this experience for a few moments, until you feel a "complete" feeling.

Rest and relax for a few minutes.

5. Fifth Chakra (Throat Chakra)

Prayer

"Divine and Heavenly Mother/Father God! Thank you for allowing me to breathe in the air of earth. May I represent Heaven on earth by uniting my metaphysical and corporeal na-

ture. I pray you will hold my feet to the ground, that I may better infuse your teachings into the group soul consciousness of
the world. I give thanks that it is so, and release any
mentalisms that hold me in separation from your Divine plan.
And so it is."

Grounding Exercise: "As Above, So Below"

Grounding is the realization of your metaphysical and corporeal
nature in the same moment, the absolute blending of the two
into one.

Close your eyes. Take a deep cleansing breath.

Imagine a brilliant shaft of white light running up and down
the length of your spine. See it extending infinitely upward to
the Creator above and infinitely downward into the earth.

Begin to breathe. With a deep inhale, feel your Self bringing
the white light of the Creator from above into your body
through your head. As you inhale, feel the white light coming
in and going to all parts of your body, energizing, connecting all
parts of you to the Creator. Do this *three* times. Each time, you
bring the energy into your body.

With a deep inhale, feel your Self bringing the energy of the
earth up through your legs and into your whole body, mixing
with the white light energy from above. The earth energy is
grounding, focusing you and centering you in the earth plane of
activity. Do this *three* times. Each time, you bring the earth
energy up and throughout your body.

Pause to feel the energies mixing: As above, so below. So you
are connected to all things at all times. As you reflect inward
upon your Oneness, you will feel that special place of
centeredness.

When you are ready, open your eyes.

Rest and relax for a few minutes.

Exercise/Meditation

Breathe deeply and slowly. Pull the air down into the lower
abdomen, push out gently with stomach, with mouth closed,
tongue touching the roof of your mouth.

While focusing on the location of the fifth chakra in your
throat, feel your connection to all knowing and your connection to the earth plane.

You are the lightning rod, buried partly in the ground, and partly exposed to the electrified atmosphere of the Divine Presence. Through you flows the communication, the articulation and the emanation into the earth plane.

Feel your common bond with humanity, know that your presence illuminates and elucidates what humanity cannot yet know. Feel that you are seen and known, on the highest levels, by your soul-group, and that you are seamlessly connected to all higher wisdom from Divine Source. Feel the acknowledgment of your presence in the third dimension by Divine Source.

Sit with this experience for a few moments, until you feel a "complete" feeling.

Rest and relax for a few minutes.

6. Sixth Chakra (Brow or Third Eye Chakra)

Prayer

"Divine and Heavenly Mother/Father God! Thank you for the gift of my many-faceted mirror to the universe through the lens of my sixth chakra! I pray for Divine guidance that your heart is my heart, that your will is my will. May I be the instrument to ground the new paradigms for the ever-unfolding understanding of humanity's purpose in Divine will."

Breathing/Meditation Exercise

Breathe from the Hara (lower abdomen), in through the nose, out through the mouth. Concentrate on visualizing the air going as deep down into the torso as possible. Do this breathing for a few moments. If you feel any discomfort, stop. Feel the comforting guidance of God through this exercise.

Now, focus your eyes upwards, and inward towards a spot about a quarter inch above your eyebrow, imagining that you are looking about an inch back into your head, behind the forehead. Raise the eyes up, and in, almost but *not* to the point of being uncomfortable. Hold there for a breath, and then relax. Do this for about three minutes.

Now, close your eyes, and continue with the same breathing style. Imagine a shaft of titanium-white light extending from infinity down through the crown, meeting at your brow chakra.

And, imagine a shaft of titanium-white light extending from infinity up through your legs and back, meeting at the brow chakra.

Focus *gently* on the center of where those two shafts of light meet, and see them simultaneously feeding your sixth chakra. See the energy building and reaching to connect to your heart chakra. Feel your emotions connecting the sixth chakra to the heart chakra. Feel those emotions nourishing your heart chakra. Do this for only a few moments.

Now breathe, as before, deeply. Slowly bring your Self to full focus of the room and your awareness of it and your physical surroundings. Breathe to feel focused, centered, and grounded as you open your eyes. Continue to breathe a few breaths until ready to arise.

Heart-Centered Meditation/Exercise for the Sixth Chakra Individual

Close your eyes and breathe.

Imagine a beautiful ball of energy, about the size of a tennis ball, floating weightlessly inside the lens of the sixth chakra. See or feel it as a platinum color, silver-white. Allow it to descend slowly down the shushumna, past the back of your eyes, your nose, your mouth, and experience it descending slowly where it comes to rest inside your chest, just above your heart.

As you experience the pureness of this platinum ball of energy, feel the sight of your physical eyes moving into it. Imagine your physical eyes are now in the platinum ball of energy, and it is as though you actually "see" from just over your heart, inside your chest. With those eyes, look out at your surroundings and experience what you "see." Note that you do not have to move your head.

With these eyes, look over the top of your head. You could not do this with your physical eyes, but with these eyes you can see anywhere, on any plane, in any place. You can see into the future and the past. You can see what cannot be seen.

Imagine your physical ears, your sense of hearing, is now located in the platinum ball of energy floating in your chest weightlessly above your heart. It is as though you actually hear from over your heart. Listen. What do you really hear? With these ears, you can hear the truth; you can hear what one is *really* saying.

Now move your sense of touch, taste, and smell into the platinum ball of energy and experience your world.

Lastly, move your ability to speak into the platinum ball of energy. It is as though the sound of your voice actually comes from deep in your chest, just over your heart. And when next you meet someone, experience that person from this place, over your heart, and respond with your senses and speech in that ball of energy.

Open your eyes when you are ready.

(Note: When you are ready, this meditation should eventually be done with your eyes open. You can do this anywhere, anytime you wish. However, not recommended while driving a car.)

Use this meditation to stay focused in your heart. You'll lose nothing of your mental abilities but rather will achieve a very healthy balance by focusing on your heart and feelings.

Exercise/Meditation

Breathe deeply and slowly. Pull the air down into the lower abdomen, push out gently with stomach, with mouth closed, tongue touching the roof of your mouth.

While focusing on the location of the sixth chakra in your brow center, feel your Self as a multi-faceted prism, collecting and refracting/reflecting energies from Divine Source. Feel energies of paradigms humanity has not yet experienced moving smoothly and effortlessly to and through your sixth chakra, with no desire to understand them, but rather to feel their import. Allow them to pass through you to humanity's higher purpose, knowing that when oil pours through a funnel, a little always sticks to the sides. There is no separation.

Cherish your heart, your love, your desire to serve Divine will and to act as an instrument of prophecy to the third dimensional world. Feel and be in your heart, passing all understanding, to that place of contentment in experiencing the mind and heart of the Creator.

Sit with this experience for a few moments, until you feel a "complete" feeling.

Rest and relax for a few minutes.

7. Seventh Chakra (Crown Chakra)

Prayer

"Divine and Heavenly Mother/Father God! Thank you for the gift in me where everything and nothing exists. I am nothing, and therefore everything. May your Divine Presence hold the template of my temple to creation whole and complete, without end. Amen."

Exercise/Meditation

Breathe deeply and slowly. Pull the air down to the lower abdomen, push out gently with stomach, with mouth closed, tongue touching the roof of your mouth.

While focusing on the location of the seventh chakra at the crown of your head, feel that you are everything and nothing. You are in Oneness with All That Is. The crown of your head is a place where everything and nothing exists in the same moment, your leaping-off place to all dimensional planes of experiences, and all universes of connectivity.

Feel no seams, no boundaries, only an infinite continuum within Divine Source. God's mind is your mind. God's heart is your heart. God's will is your will, whole and complete.

Sit with this experience for a few moments, until you feel a "complete" feeling.

Rest and relax for a few minutes.

Summary

These exercises, prayers, and meditations represent the accumulated knowledge and instruction of many lectures and workshops. Doing them is like going to the chakra gym. You cannot just look at the weights and accomplish the workout. This is a dimension of *effort*. You must apply your Self, until there no longer is a need to do so.

If you are willing to give these exercises your best, you'll be giving your Self your best. You will be open and vulnerable to true spiritual growth, which can only come from within.

Appendix A-3
Essential Oils That Help Heal Each Chakra

Contributed by Sabrina Dalla Valle, Master Distiller

"Open wide the door for us, so that we may look out into the immeasurable starry universe; show us that other worlds like ours occupy the ethereal realms; make clear to us how the motion of all worlds is engendered by forces; teach us to march forward to greater knowledge of nature."

– Giordano Bruno (1548 – 1600)

The primal engagement between cosmically engendered forces and specific characteristics in nature is one of the great mysteries that Giordano Bruno, a Renaissance thinker, risked his life to elucidate. His wisdom was inspired by an awareness of forces in what we now call *astrophysics*.

The movement of heavenly bodies shows us that the solar system abides by regular rhythms and patterns. Astrologers have used these planetary cycles to reveal personality traits, life destinies, and personal biographical landmarks of individuals. Cutting-edge scientists have worked with the mathematical rhythms and geometrical patterns of our moving solar system as a way of determining a cause for plant morphology.

It is the understanding of some that plant forms in their full metamorphosis from germinating seed to flowering bud are influenced by such cosmic patterns, and that these same planets exert a force upon plants that influences their energetic qualities. If humans are linked to the universe through a system of chakras, why shouldn't a plant do the same?

This chapter is a brief introduction to the value of essential oils as healing agents for both the physical body and the emotions. It lists a few oils for the strengthening and balancing of each chakra. The selection has been made based on the chemical value of the oils as well as a psychically intuitive perception of their activity. Hopefully, this will incite the reader to begin personal research on the use of essential oils for chakra balancing.

The Use of Essential Oils

The use of plant-derived essential oils as personal links to universal patterns of energy is on the frontier of holistic healing today. More people are seeing how essential oils influence levels of energy within our different physiological systems and emotional states as they are related to our chakra organization.

Mechanically speaking, topical use of essential oils penetrates the skin through osmosis by way of infrared vibrational frequencies. These enter the blood stream and lymphatic system, releasing oxygenating molecules as well as 30,000 aromatic chemical compounds.

One grand characteristic of the vascular system is its all-pervasive mobility, circulating blood and lymph throughout the body. It is a perfect transportation system reaching the entire body at the cellular level. And as it is with all things, it too needs to be maintained by keeping the fluids clean, like changing the fluids in your car. In a way, essential oils and the vascular system are in a kind of symbiotic relationship: the vascular system allows oils to permeate our entire body, while essential oils help to keep the vascular system healthy.

Essential oils are healing no matter how we use them: alone, in solution, externally or internally. However, many practitioners have experienced them to be most effective when used in combination with reflexology, an ancient hands-on massage technique originating in Tibet. This method focuses on specific target points related to a person's weakness. It also helps to draw essential oils into the body focusing on reflex points located on the hands, feet and along the spine and on the face. Pressing reflex points creates an electrical impulse that releases energy into nerve pathways in our electrical circuit and breaks down blockages caused by toxins, oxygen loss, or damaged tissues.

The most important thing to pay attention to when using essential oils is *quality*. Only 100% pure plant distillations have therapeutic value, and only low-steam, long-duration distillations are exact enough to distill a full spectrum of molecules from each plant. In any distillate, whether for alcohol or essential oils, molecules are divided into three groups: small, medium, and large size. Each group has its functions: anti-inflammatory, coagulant, analgesic, anti-viral, etc.

Many books are now published on the use of essential oils and on reflexology. These should be consulted to learn more about the effectiveness of this method, since such explanations are beyond the scope of this book.

Application of Essential Oils

Essential oils may be applied directly to the chakra area, and to meridian points. Applications must be frequent if they are to be effective. As far as I know, there are no contraindications of using more than one oil at a time. Please consult with a qualified practitioner of essential oils.

Two rules for using essential oils:

1. Never touch the reducer at the top of the bottle. Let the oil drip onto your hand or skin.
2. Never let the oils get too hot, like being left in the car on a hot day.

General Instructions

Place one drop on each chakra to open the energy centers and balance the electrical field of the chakras. Start with the feet and work up to the top of the head.

- *Harmony:* harmonizes energy between chakras and helps to even out emotions
- *Lavender:* used for its nervine (nerve)-sedative properties, brings harmony to chakras
- *Rosemary:* a piercing and stimulating oil that opens chakras
- *Sandalwood:* a sedative with an antispasmodic effect on the heart. This is one of the oldest known oils used therapeutically, distilled from the heartwood of the tree. This oil is distilled in different parts of the world, although the most therapeutic variety comes from trees grown in Mysore, India.

Essential oils recommended for each chakra:

1. First Chakra
Peppermint   Juniper
Sandalwood   Fennel

2. Second Chakra
Tangerine   Patchouli
White Angelica*   Marjoram
Acceptance*

3. Third Chakra
Di Tone*   Forgiveness*
Juva Flex*   Humility*

4. Fourth Chakra
Peace and Calming* Aroma Siez*
Frankincense*   Bergamot
EndoFlex*

5. Fifth Chakra
Gathering*   Geranium
Grounding*   White Angelica*

6. Sixth Chakra
Helichysum   Clarity*
Rose   Aroma Seiz*
Brain Power*

7. Seventh Chakra
Dream Catcher*   Harmony*
3 Wise Men*

* Note: These are "blends" of oils, made by Young Living Oils. You can use the separate constituents of the blends as well.

Following are a few of the companies that have very pure oils:

Young Living Essential Oils
250 South Main Street
Payson, Utah 84651
1-800-371-3515
http://www.youngliving.us

Diamond Lotus Essential Oils
Diamond Lotus Ranch
Attn: Internet Inquiries
Montague, Ca. 96064
http://www.diamondlotusoils.com

Simplers Botanical Co.
Phone: 707-887-2012
Toll Free: 1-800-652-7646
E-mail: info@simplers.com
http://simplers.com

Primavera Life
Phone: +44(0)1420 520530
Green and Organic Ltd.
Unit 2 Blacknest Ind Est
Blacknest, Nr Alton
Hampshire,GU34 4PX England
E-mail: info@primaveralife.co.uk
http://www.greenandorganic.co.uk/pvl

Tiferet Aromatherapy
P O Box 325 EL
Twin Lakes, WI 53181 USA
800 TIFERET
www.tiferetonline.com
tiferet@lotuspress.com
Pure premium quality organic
and wildcrafted essential oils.

Nature's Alchemy
P O Box 325 EL
Twin Lakes, WI 53181 USA
800 824 6396
www.naturesalchemy.com
lotusbrands@lotuspress.com
High quality aromatherapy grade
essential oils and carrier oils.

Modern alternative medical culture in America has just begun to unveil the guarded mysteries behind the use and extraction of volatile oils from plants, which are themselves volatile to external planetary forces as so fervently perceived by persecuted healers of the past.

For those who do not have the ancient way of identifying plant signatures and their uses, it is lucky that we have advantageous forms of technology (Gas Chromatograph/ Mass Spectrometers) to identify the different chemical structure of essential oils. Thus the utility of herbs, and the use of essential oils for healing, is available for all, without prior knowledge of alchemy.

Sounds That Help to Heal Each Chakra

This chapter covers sounds and recommended sources for auditory methods of balancing and healing the chakras and the whole body system. Some people respond better to sounds than other healing modalities. Sound is but one path, but it is incredibly powerful, as sound vibrations are not only heard by the ears, but by your *whole body*.

We tend to believe that we only hear with our ears. There are glands in our heads, just behind our ears, called saccules. In recent years science has proven that these glands are able to respond to ultrasound (higher than normal human hearing, 20 to 20,000 Hertz). There are devices, like the Neurophone, invented by Dr. G. Patrick Flanagan, that interpret any sound input into ultrasound through two metal pads that can be placed anywhere on the body. It lets the mind "hear" without using the normal hearing mechanism.

The body responds to sound through a "piezoelectric effect." That is, sound vibrations against the skin create small currents of electricity in your nervous system. If the sound is "pulsed" at specific frequencies, it can create a shift not only in consciousness, but in healing of the body/mind as a whole. The mental, physical, emotional, and spiritual aspects of a human being can be healed by using your own voice as the sound medium.

Researchers such as Dr. Jeffrey Thompson are pioneers in the field of psychoacoustics (see below); using the sound of one's own voice (a Biotuning note) being played back to the ears and the whole body to achieve balance and the healing of infirmities.

Music

Why do we instantly respond to music, knowing whether we like it or not? Partly because music goes directly to our feelings and emotions; no thought is required. Music helps us attain that qualitative state of being that cannot be quantified.

Most of us have experienced extremes of our emotional reactions to different types of music, from Mozart to heavy metal, from rhapsodies to rap. We have the capability to discern not only the harmonic symmetry of music, but also the nuances of timing beats and harmonic relationships.

Harmonious and symmetrical music seems to have an elevating effect on our emotions and helps to create an increased sense of well-being. Music that is discordant seems to have the opposite effect, though there are infinite variations.

There are two types of harmonics: octave and resonant.

Octave harmonics are exemplified when one hits the middle "C" note on a piano and observes that all higher and lower octave C notes also vibrate. Frequencies are measured in cycles per second, or Hertz (Hz). There is a fundamental octave relationship in frequencies, not just in notes on a piano, because after all, the sound of a note is a frequency (e.g., note "A" = 440 Hz).

A *resonant harmonic* is a third, fifth, or seventh note from the fundamental major note (e.g., E, G, and B are third, fifth and sevenths of the major note C). When heard together, they create a unique type of sound. The most ancient of these can be heard in the Indian ragas, when listening to the tabla (a stringed instrument) in the background.

We even sense "colors" in our music, setting the mood. "Blue" music may sound moody or melancholic, "red" music may be sensuous and passionate, and so on.

There are many artists who have used their intuition to produce albums of music designed to create a healing and balancing effect to the chakras. Use your intuitive discernment in choosing the appropriate album for you. As a rule, if you do not feel a resonance with what you hear, the music is probably not for you.

Crystal Bowls

Crystal bowls are very popular in healing for two reasons:

1. Crystal bowls make the purest sound that can exist

2. Crystal bowls, when played two or more at a time, create "binaural beats"

Sound from crystal bowls has a unique property: it is perfectly sinusoidal. That is, the bowls create sound as a sine wave, the most fundamental, pure sound that can exist. We gravitate towards perfection in all its forms, and the crystal bowls create that perfect in an auditory experience.

The crystal bowls come in sets of seven or more, and are tuned to the following notes to match the chakras.

Please note that the actual chakra may have a different specific frequency than the general key note assigned to it. (It is the same with colors that are assigned to chakras. The heart chakra may be one of millions of shades of green.)

These are the notes assigned to the crystal bowls:

Chakra	Name	Note	Frequency (Hz)	Color*
7	Crown	B	495	Violet
6	Brow	A	440	Indigo
5	Throat	G	396	Blue
4	Heart	F	352	Green
3	Solar Plexus	E	330	Yellow
2	Sacral	D	297	Orange
1	Root	C	264	Red

*not related by 40 octaves to the sound in this usage.

Crystal bowls are played either percussively, or by gently rubbing a mallet against the top rim in a circular fashion, holding steady pressure until the bowl starts to "sing." The bowl is rested on a thin rubber ring to harmonically isolate it from the surface on which it sits. The player can easily intuit the speed of the movement of the mallet to create the optimum humming sound that crystal bowls are known for.

Some healers who use crystal bowl therapy place the bowl directly on the skin (sans rubber ring) of their patients, usually over a chakra center, and "play" the bowl for a short length of time (a few minutes). This is done to pass the resonating tones of the bowl directly into the body through the piezoelectric effect, to resonate the physical and etheric bodies together.

Some healers have their patients positioned lying on the floor, with seven or more bowls placed around the body. One or more persons "tone" the bowls, playing them in different combinations, to affect healing to the physical and ethic bodies and the chakras. When two or more bowls are played in this manner, the binaural beats are also created.

Toning

Toning is a specific type of healing activity ascribed to individuals who intuitively sense the appropriate sounds to create, then use their voice to "tone" (not singing so much as holding a sung note) over the major chakra centers. The toners sometimes cup their hands over the chakra centers either on the front or back of the body.

Toners are active participants in the healing process. They use their intuitive abilities to sense the note, location, length, and duration of the sound. This is meant to resonate the etheric and physical bodies together and to balance and tone the chakras. Toning various vowels stimulates and balances the organs, brain functions and nervous system, besides the chakras.

Toners can also "overtone." They have the ability to resonate within their sinus, nasal, and throat cavities second and third notes related to the first. This is a very powerful and effective form of toning. Two very good examples of this type of toning are provided by Jerry DesVoignes and David Hykes.

There are CD's you can buy that have the toning already established in a progressive healing protocol, or you can visit a toner for a live session. The live sessions are much more interactive, dynamic, and effective. As in the last section, use your intuition to decide on which toner most suits you.

Mantric Chanting

Mantras are the singing of prayers, usually of Sanskrit origin, in specific phonetics, cadences, and sequences to achieve a "standing wave" of sonic energy that is meant to help the chanter and listener achieve transcendent states of consciousness.

The consistency of the chanting of a mantra is a key to its effectiveness. Mantras can be sung singly or in groups. Remember that when listening to these sounds, your body is receiving the sonic energy as well.

Bio-Acoustics

There are devices that analyze a sample of your voice, then "play" back to you any missing frequencies via synthesized sounds. The rationale is that your voice is your consciousness, and within it are the frequencies of your mental, physical, emotional, and spiritual health. Measured by bio-acoustics, frequencies missing from your voice indicate what might be missing from your body.

For example, zinc has a specific atomic weight in the periodic table of elements. Zinc has a specific frequency in its resting state. The theory is that if your body is deficient in zinc, the bio-acoustic device can detect this through the absence of zinc's frequency. The device then plays back to you the sound (specific frequency) of zinc to help you reconstitute it in your body.

Ostensibly, this theory works for specific frequency deficiencies in the chakras. The only problem is that the idiosyncrasy of one's given suspect chakra is not directly measurable. This follows the problem of assigning a general color to a specific chakra. It can be close, but often not close enough.

Cymatic Therapy

The science of cymatics is the organizing effect of specific single and complex frequencies on malleable substances. Originally, a plate is horizontally suspended over a speaker. On the plate is sand. Specific frequencies are played through the speaker, and the sand organizes itself to make a visual representation of the sounds.

There are cymatic healing protocols established for various types of infirmities. One of the world's foremost researchers and pioneers was Swiss medical doctor and natural scientist, Dr. Hans Jenny (1904-1972). For fourteen years he conducted experiments animating inert powders, pastes, and liquids into life-like, flowing forms, which mirrored patterns found throughout nature, art, and architecture. These patterns were created using simple sine wave vibrations (pure tones) within the audible range.

What you see is a physical representation of vibration, or how sound manifests into form through the medium of various materials. The theory is that specific wave patterns will cause your cells and organs to harmonize. The sound creates the form.

Binaural Beats

The ancient Tibetans knew that striking two bells together (Ting-Shas) would create a third beat called a "binaural beat." They made the bells so that each bell creates a specific frequency. When stuck together, the difference between the two frequencies would be "heard" by the mind. The hemispheres of the mind, when interpreting the differences in frequencies between the two bells (usually in the theta brainwave state, about 4 to 7 cycles per second, or "Hertz") would "hear" the wavering, even though the wavering sound does not physically exist!

*Here are the frequencies associated
with brainwave states:*

RHYTHM	FREQUENCY	PSYCHOLOGY
Beta α	14 – 20 Hz and higher	Awake, aware, attentive, active
Alpha β	8 – 13 Hz	Relaxed, meditative, low arousal
Theta δ	4 – 7 Hz	Hypnogogic, dreaming, low arousal
Delta Θ	Less than 4 Hz	Deep sleep, lowest mental arousal

Binaural beats are the foundation of a whole science of entraining the mind to more meditative states of consciousness using sound frequencies. The mind entrains itself to exterior pulses, and this is the foundation of a science of behavior modification, brain/mind research, psychoacoustics, and neuroacoustics.

Pioneers in the field of psychoacoustics are Robert Monroe, Jeffrey Thompson, and Anna Wise. Robert Monroe popularized the therapeutic effects of "hemi-synch" (the process by which the brainwave frequencies of the hemispheres of the mind are balanced and harmonized). All three researchers have produced many CD's to help with relaxation, meditation, balance of body/mind, and more.

Following is a list of recommended websites for healing music and sound:

- Brain/Mind Research http://body-mind.com/
- Center for Neuroacoustic Research (Dr. Jeffrey Thompson) http://www.jeffthompson.com/
- Sound-Remedies.com http://store.yahoo.com/sound-remedies/index.html
- Applied Music & Sound http://www.thepowerofsound.com/appliedmusic.html
- The Power of Sound http://www.thepowerofsound.com/powerofsound.html
- The Anna Wise Center http://www.annawise.com/
- Tom Kenyon http://www.tomkenyon.com
- The Healing Music Organization http://www.healingmusic.org/
- Music Qi Gong, Inc. http://www.musicqigong.com/
- American Music Therapy Association http://www.musictherapy.org/
- Canadian Association for Music Therapy http://www.musictherapy.ca/
- British Society for Music Therapy http://www.bsmt.org/
- The Academy of Sound, Color and Movement http://www.tama-do.com/
- Advanced Brain Technologies http://

www.advancedbrain.com/

- Colorado State University Center for Biomedical Research in Music http://www.colostate.edu/depts/cbrm/
- Chalice of Repose Project http://www.saintpatrick.org/chalice/
- University of California at Irvine Music Intelligence Neural Development (MIND) http://www.mindinst.org/index2.html
- The Monroe Institute http://www.monroeinstitute.org
- Sound Mind & Body http://www.soundmindandbody.com/
- The Tomatis Method http://www.tomatis.com/
- New Mind Machines http://www.new-mindmachines.com/

Overtoning

- David Hykes http://harmonicworld.com/

Cymatics

- Hans Jenny http://www.cymaticsource.com/

Appendix A-5
Light and Color That Help Heal Each Chakra

This chapter covers light and recommended sources for approaching chakra balance through visual, body, and meridian application. The use of light to heal may be as old as the use of sound, but today we have the ability to create frequencies of light that were not available in times past.

Using light as a healing medium makes even more sense if you apply what you learned in the preceding section on sound about the octave relationships of frequency. If you were to take the frequency of middle "C" on a piano and double it (octaves) 40 times, you would have the frequency of yellow-orange color.

The fundamental harmonic relationship of octaves and resonance to frequency means our consciousness responds in a recursive manner. In other words, no matter how far in or out the microscope pans, the universe endlessly repeats its symmetry. Whether very large or very small, all levels are symmetrically similar.

This is why we respond to the harmonics of sound and light. And why we respond with our emotions to paintings and their use of color to convey a state of being. Our natural ability to respond to and create symmetry through light and sound is the manner in which we reflect back to the physical world our inner state of being.

To give you an idea of what it takes for our eyes to "see" color, please look at the chart on the following page.

In order for you to "see" blue, its frequency must be oscillating at 6.82×10^{14} cycles per second, or Hertz (Hz). That means, the frequency must be moving at over 60,000,000,000,000 Hz for you to see it. Its wavelength (the distance for the wave to make one cycle) must be 440 nanometers (nm) or 440 *billionths* of a meter.

Your eyes are standing wave receptors for these very specific frequencies and wavelengths of electromagnetic energy. There

Number	Light Color	Frequency (Hz)	Wavelength (nm)	Sound Freq.(Hz)
1	Red	4.35 x 10^{14}	690	395.43
2	Orange	4.62 x 10^{14}	650	419.73
3	Yellow	4.69 x 10^{14}	640	426.37
4	Green	5.88 x 10^{14}	510	534.97
5	Blue	6.82 x 10^{14}	440	620.09
6	Indigo	7.26 x 10^{14}	413	660.65
7	Violet	7.41 x 10^{14}	405	673.66

are millions of colors that can be observed in the visible spectrum. Those lights that are purest are of single wavelengths only.

Pure Colors

The late Dinshah Ghadiali was far ahead of his time in using colors as healing protocols. His term "Spectro-Chrome Healing" became the fundamental groundwork for Colorpuncture (see below) and Chromopathy (healing with light). Research and experiments by Dinshah Ghadiali proved that the body could be tuned or adjusted from disease to health by systematically exposing it to colored light.

Today, there are entire protocols for healing specific infirmities by using "color wands" that emit very pure light in the visible spectrum, and wands that use ultra-violet and infrared light.

Coherent Light

Coherence of light is the wavelengths lining up neatly on top of one another to produce a single frequency. We best know coherence through the use of lasers. As the crystal bowls produce the most fundamentally pure sound that can exist (the sine wave), lasers produce the most fundamentally pure light that can exist (phase coherence).

This is why we respond to laser light shows the way we do. Your average pen pocket laser is about 2 MW (milliwatts, or 2/1000 of a watt). Your average light bulb of about 40 – 100 watts is much less efficient because there is no coherence of the wavelengths of light from its incandescence. Lasers are highly efficient, and the amount of wattage you see at a laser show is most times about 4 watts or less. The beam does not spread out because of the coherence of the wavelength phases.

We become "coherent" when all of our consciousness is in alignment with our higher selves. That is, the distractions (chaos) of lower aspects of our chakras have been overcome by the coherence (higher aspects) to keep in phase (intuition) with our higher expressions.

Used as a healing tool, lasers are very potent at helping us externalize the perfection that exists within us. Simple red handheld lasers are used as pulsed and steady to stimulate or sedate meridian points, as used by an acupuncturist.

Colorpuncture

Esogetic Colorpuncture™ is the creation of Peter Mandel, a German scientist and naturopath. He has conducted over twenty-five years of intensive empirical research to develop this unique system of healing. Colorpuncture involves focusing colored light on acupuncture (and other) points on the skin in order to energize powerful healing impulses in our physical and energy bodies.

In a Colorpuncture treatment, frequencies of colored light are focused on the skin using a hand-held light tool with specially designed, hand-made interchangeable glass rods that emit different colors of light through a focused tip. Each color consists of different wavelength frequencies of light and therefore communicates different energetic information.

Treatments include a specific set of points in a sequence using a prescribed pattern of colors. As the light is absorbed by the skin and is transmitted along energetic pathways or meridians deep into the body, it stimulates intra-cellular communication which supports healing.

Binaural Light Beats

There are a number of resources that use oscillating LED's (Light Emitting Diodes) fitted into a pair of glasses, meant to be worn with the eyes shut, that use the binaural beat patterns we learned about in the last chapter to harmonize the hemispheres of the brain, balance and tone the chakras, and heal infirmities.

The LED's are usually synchronized to sound sources supplied with the glasses, and some have prerecorded routines that one uses as a daily meditation and balancing exercise.

Mandalas

Mandalas are visual representations of whole systems. A mandala (man-DAH-la) is an integrated structure organized around a unifying center. It is a "whole world" or "healing circle." It is a representation of the universe and everything that ever was and will be.

Khyil-khor is the Tibetan word for mandala and means "center of the universe in which a fully awakened being abides." Circles suggest wholeness, return, healing, order, unity, the womb, completion, and eternity.

The mandala, or circular pattern, is used in most forms of religion, prayer and meditation to bring us to that sense of wholeness and completeness. Many cultures use mandalas to represent their religious beliefs and cosmologies.

Several mandalas are based on representations of creation stories or of perfected geometries. When you look at a mandala of perfected geometries while you are in a meditative state, it is meant to help you externalize the perfection within you. Such forms are called "non-personal" in that the form is not telling you what to think or feel, but causes you to yield to that which is perfected.

Here is a list of recommended sites for
light therapy and devices:

- Colorpuncture, Peter Mandel http://www.colorpuncture.com
- Foundation for Light Therapy http://www.fflt.org
- Full Spectrum Solutions http:// www.fullspectrumsolutions.com/
- Ganzfield Light Therapy http://www.morningstarlight.com/ meditation.html
- Light Therapy for PMS http://www.lightmask.com/

Yoga Exercises for Each Chakra
Contributed by Madhu Honeymann, Yoga Instructor

HATHA YOGA:
It's Purpose and Power

This offering is dedicated to revealing the importance of practicing Hatha Yoga as a means to nurture optimum health and to attain our human potential as conscious, compassionate beings.

The knowledge and practice of Yoga is thousands of years old. It is impossible to share all of the comprehensive teachings on Yoga in one chapter. Please note this is an introduction for beginners. Further study with a qualified teacher is recommended and is most often essential for safe practice and the most advantageous progress and benefit.

What is Yoga?

Yoga is a Sanskrit word meaning "union" or "to yoke". The goal of Yoga is often described as realizing one's True Self, resting in one's True Nature, or Oneness/Communion with the Divine. To seek and find the Source of happiness is to realize one's True Self **as** the Source of happiness. A famous line from one of the Vedic scriptures is "Thou art That!" Being established in this consciousness of union with the essence of all Life, is what we call Enlightenment.

There are many paths along the journey to Self Realization. "As many minds, as many gods." Ultimately, whatever works for you in creating a contented life that is heart-full, kind and genuine, with fulfilled purpose, no matter what name you give it, is Yoga. In this way, the Yogic teachings are non-sectarian and may be useful to anyone of any faith.

What is Hatha Yoga?

Hatha Yoga is one branch of several within the Tree of Yoga. It focuses on the art and science of achieving physical health and mental purity through the practice of postures (asanas), breath control (pranayama), cleansing processes (kriyas), deep relaxation (yoga nidra) and consciously directed mental attention (dharana).

Other Branches of Yoga

Hatha Yoga may stand alone as one branch of Yoga or may be found as one of the eight limbs of Raja Yoga, the Royal Path (also known as Ashtanga Yoga - literally meaning eight limbs or rungs – not to be confused by the **style** of Hatha Yoga also called Ashtanga).

Raja Yoga is a comprehensive approach to understanding, purifying, integrating and transcending the mind. Other common branches of Yoga are Bhakti Yoga (emotional - creative worship, love and devotion), Jnana Yoga (intellectual - discrimination and deductive insight), Karma Yoga (relational - integrity and selfless service), Japa or Nada Yoga (absorption - use of mantra - sacred sound). An integral practice of a combination of all these branches is recommended to serve the balance of all aspects of our humanness. Intuition is a natural element of success for all of the above.

Why Practice Hatha Yoga?

The body and mind are powerful and precious instruments. When the body and mind are fine-tuned they become instruments of extraordinary vitality and clarity, capable of creating profound personal fulfillment and wellbeing. They may be likened to a well-tuned musical instrument capable of creating beautiful, awe-inspiring music. You may achieve this through the practice of Hatha Yoga.

The goal of Hatha Yoga is not only physical health and mental purity, but on a deeper level, to balance the Life Force* energies, which includes the Chakra system, allowing optimum conditions for Self Realization to occur.

In the Sanskrit word Hatha, "Ha" means Sun and "Tha" means Moon. These sounds, and the meaning they convey, are symbolic references to the polarized forces of the primal Life Force energy within ourselves and all of Nature. Hatha refers to the balance and harmony of these forces. We may experience, observe, or conceptualize (by way of feeling, seeing or intuiting,) these forces on different levels: the physical, psychological, social, mythological - archetypal, psychic, esoteric, intuitive. Examples of how they are experienced or perceived in our world are: attraction/repulsion, health/disease; cooling/heating; water/fire; static/dynamic; negative/positive; feminine/masculine; light/darkness; creation/destruction; success/failure; union/separation; knowledge/ignorance; joy/suffering.

One attribute, or result, of attaining the highest goal of any Yogic practice is the integration, balance, or poise, as pure awareness, with the polar opposite forces of conscious and unconscious existence and non identification with all the mind's resultant impressions and false identities in response to these forces. When this balance, or "Samadhi", is attained one enjoys being established in their true nature of peace. Practiced with the right approach, Hatha Yoga becomes an effective tool for supporting the attainment of this balance and peace.

How does Hatha Yoga work?

We are all familiar with the adage "As you think so you become".

The maturity of your consciousness will reflect itself through your mind and the purity of your mind will reflect itself in your body. Conversely, your body will in some way reflect your mind and maturity of consciousness. As the Life Force is more subtle than the Chakra system, and the Chakra system is more subtle than the mind, and the mind is more subtle and not as easily controlled as the body, we begin with the body, which includes the breath. In this way, we begin with Hatha Yoga as a natural, practical approach.

Life Force refers to the mysterious power of the universal Source that creates and perpetuates all forms and cycles of life.

If you are mentally agitated it will be impossible for you to have an authentically relaxed body no matter how great of an actor you are. Likewise, when the body is relaxed and healthy it is easier for the mind to be calm and clear. With a calm and clear mind the balanced state develops naturally. In addition, a healthy, pain free body is easier to relax than a diseased, pain-ridden body. For these reason, aside from the benefits of stress reduction and other obvious benefits, it is important for beginners to learn how to effectively *relax the body* and improve or maintain their health. With physical health and mental harmony, everything becomes easier, more possible, whether it is worldly success, spiritual success, or both.

There are seven distinct ways in which Hatha Yoga may achieve and maintain optimum health and differs from other forms of health oriented forms of physical activity.

1. The main, traditional Chakras are in vertical alignment with the spine. In Hatha Yoga special attention is given to maintaining the flexibility of the spine through a balanced combination of backward bends, forward bends and spinal twists. The spine is originating home for the central nervous system as well as the subtle nervous system (made up of Life Force currents i.e. nadis and the nadi vortices i.e Chakras) in the subtle body. The nerve plexuses in the physical body are believed to be parallel in location to the Chakras. Both the gross and subtle systems work together as the chief communicators responsible for distributing information (stimulus/response) throughout the body and brain. In other words, our functions of health are all controlled by the natural vital energy flow that, in turn, is daily determined by how good the efficiency of the communication is of this energy through the gross and subtle nervous systems.

The Life Force is often referred to as Prana in Yoga or Chi (Qi/Ki) in Martial Arts. One of the ways we receive life giving Prana for the body is through oxygen, which is distributed through the bloodstream.

Increased and maintained flexibility of the spine affords a more abundant, thorough blood supply to all the nerves. As the flexibility of the spine directly affects the healthy functioning of the nervous system it also affects Prana's flow and function through the nadis and chakra centers. Hatha Yoga will maximize this Prana flow to both the gross and subtle nervous system. They will be able to function as healthier more efficient communicators thus serving the attainment for optimum health.

2. Traditional Yoga poses are slowly entered into and then **sustained** for a period of time depending on the individual's health and level of experience. They are performed easefully, mindfully, without strain, with short rest periods in between poses. Traditional Hatha Yoga is **not** referred to as exercise. Exercise, commonly understood, implies quick, repetitive movements with a measure of strain.

Held poses apply sustained pressure on specific areas of the body, unique to each pose. When pressure is released, blood rushes through again, stimulating oxygen supply to the organs, endocrine glands, nerves and nerve plexuses, as well as the muscles and other tissues (similar to the effects of massage). In addition, this assists in eliminating toxins, dispersing physical and emotional tension, as well as loosen and shift blocks in the Prana flow affecting the psyche and function of the Chakra centers.

3. At the end of a Yoga session, a progressive deep relaxation is entered into, usually for a minimum of fifteen minutes. This allows the body and mind to go deeper into releasing physical and mental tension. This kind of profound relaxation allows Prana to flow and function at its optimum healing and balancing capacity, thereby maximizing the benefits of all the poses.

Through the power of Prana, the body is self-healing. When the body and mind is afflicted with tension and stress, it restricts the natural movement of Prana. When the body is relaxed, the natural power of Prana is able to do its best work. Research results on the benefits of stress reduction substantiate this capacity.

As the physical relaxation deepens, the mind becomes calm and reflects a natural state of inner peace. This communion with inner peace is most restorative and also allows the portals of consciousness to open and gain access to intuitive knowledge. This natural chain reaction will promote a joyful presence of contentment in your life and satisfying relationships with yourself and others.

4. Mindfulness, by way of adopting an inner view as a "silent witness" or "observer" in alignment with consciously directed mental attention, is encouraged throughout an entire Yoga session. As the yogic saying goes "Where the mind goes, the Prana goes". By gathering the rays of the mind in this way it creates a body – mind connection that attracts, focuses and maximizes the healing potential of Prana. When the mind is concentrated (location and intention), the Prana and its beneficial power automatically increase to serve the intention of the concentration and/or its natural healing ability.

It may be likened to the use of a magnifying glass with the sun with the Prana as the sun and the mind as the magnifying glass. When the magnifying glass is tilted a certain way in relationship to the sun it suddenly has the focused power to be able to create intense heat, then combustion with a flammable material i.e. a form of transformation. By focusing the mind with a positive conscious intent or neutral presence, the power of Prana automatically intensifies and naturally heals and purifies the body and mind.

5. Hatha Yoga utilizes conscious use of the breath. The movement of our breath, the movement of the smallest particle of matter, the movement that makes a seed sprout and create new life, even the movement of our thoughts is made possible and directed by Prana. For human beings, on a tangible level, Prana is most powerful in it's life giving capacity through the movement of the breath. We are sustained by Prana through food, liquids, the sun, breath, even prayer, but we need to be able to breath and receive oxygen more than we need to eat or drink. Therefore, the profound power of life sustaining Prana is most directly observable through the breath.

The body thrives on oxygen. More Prana becomes available

when there is a greater intake of oxygen. Oxygen, after it is absorbed through the walls of the lungs, is distributed throughout the body by the bloodstream. Regular, automatic breathing only utilizes on average about a seventh of our lungs capacity. By consciously increasing the inhalation through deep three part breathing (see section on practice) you can utilize the full capacity of the lungs and increase the oxygen intake and therefore increase the flow of Prana. In addition, by calming and controlling the breath by breathing slowly, especially on the exhalation, the mind automatically becomes more calm and controlled, thus giving Prana an opportunity to achieve its greatest potential. This is important to remember. You can utilize this practice at any time of the day, wherever you are.

6. All of the above has a profound effect on the endocrine system of the body. The performance of the endocrine glands plays a very important role in preserving the healthy functioning of the body and mind. The hormone secretions are stimulated by the vibration of Prana, which in turn create our thoughts, which in turn direct our physical activities and determine our emotional stability. and ability to live a life of harmony. The secretions affect our state of being and our state of being affects them. Albert Einstein said, "Even our destiny is decided by the endocrine glands."

7. The flow of Prana and its vibrational quality will directly effect the purity and balance of all your Chakras in being able to be effective, transformative transmitters of the universal consciousness that creates all life and awakens our Self Knowledge. In this way, our ability to enjoy conscious awareness and harmony with all life is determined by the Chakras. As you can see, Hatha Yoga can be a powerful aid to expand your capacity for achieving this.

Preparation for Practice:

• If you have any health concerns or have had surgery, it is best if you consult with your doctor before beginning a practice of Yoga. If a practice is sanctioned, it is best to attain the guidance of an experienced yoga instructor that is knowledgeable on how to tailor a gentle practice for beginners, with modified poses if needed.

- Practice on an empty stomach. Wait two hours after a light meal, three to four hours after a heavier meal.
- If possible, have a bath or shower soon before practice.
- Wear loose comfortable clothing.
- It is best not to practice where there are drafts or distractions (i.e. people moving in and out, ringing telephones, mosquitoes, pets yearning for a walk, direct hot sun, etc.)
- Practice on a towel or blanket that has some padding underneath such as a carpet or padded yoga matt. It is conducive to use your towel or blanket only for yoga.
- For women during their monthly cycle it is recommended to suspend practice or at least practice more easefully. No poses with pressure on the abdomen.

General Instructions:

- Stay safe. Learn your limits. Never strain or cause pain. If you are shaking or your breath is labored then you are straining. Rest whenever you need to. Never take your body for granted.
- Enter and exit a pose slowly and mindfully.
- Practice keeping your attention on what you are doing and notice how you feel. Thoughts of other things will come and go, this is natural, but gently bring the mind's focus back to the moment with mindful observing each time it wanders away. Easy mind. Easy does it.
- In general, when entering a pose, you will inhale when you are moving the body open and out, and exhale when the body is folding forward toward itself. During and in between poses allow the breath to be easeful, though it may naturally deepen while holding a pose. If the breath becomes labored while holding a pose, ease up on your effort or come out of the pose and rest. Allow the breath to return to normal before repeating the pose or going on to the next one.
- Take a deep breath whenever there is a natural urge to do so. Your body knows when it needs one. Feel the relief/release as you exhale and, if possible without strain, deepen your relaxation into the stretch. Effort without strain. Cultivate the experience of enjoying the stretch, letting go of resistance.

- The rest period between each pose is about 10-15 seconds but if you need more time to bring the breath back to normal please do so.
- A good way to count for holding time is to mentally repeat "Om 1, Om 2, etc".
- The mental focus indicated for each pose is either a physical location or Chakra. You actually have four choices as to where to focus your attention; on your breath, an area of the body most dramatically affected by the pose, the benefit(s) of the specific pose, or a specific Chakra. However, for beginners I suggest you become familiar with the form of the pose first and focus on your breath. When you have discovered the most easeful rhythm for your breath in each pose then you may choose another area of focus.
- For more detailed descriptions for the physical benefits of each pose please see one of the resources in the recommended reading list at the back.
- To warm up the muscles and joints before your Yoga session you might consider a brisk ten minute walk or moving continuously to some nice music for ten minutes.
- It is generally not recommended to listen to music during your Yoga session as it may take your mind's attention away from listening to your body and your mindfulness practice. However, if you find it helps you to relax if your mind is particularly active, some soothing music may be played during the practice of the poses but not during the Deep Relaxation at the end. Becoming comfortable with silence is most often essential for achieving the best results.
- Deep Relaxation is called Yoga Nidra, or Yogic Sleep, but please refrain from falling asleep. It is okay if you do, however, as you deepen your practice, Yoga Nidra will give you even more restoration of energy than if you fall asleep.
- It is recommended to practice your poses in the sequence outlined below.
  - Backward bends
  - Forward bends.
  - Backward bends.
  - Spinal twists.

- Deep relaxation.
- Deep Three Part Breathing (Pranayama).

- The time suggested for holding a pose may be increased as you become stronger. Especially hold the backward bends for less time than the forward bends in the beginning.

- It is not common to assign a particular Chakra focus for a yoga pose, though this is becoming increasingly more prevalent. However, upon practicing, you will find that the reason for the Chakra chosen for each pose is obvious. You will feel it. There *is* room for your own creativity and intuitive choice but preferably after you have become familiar with an established practice. The element assigned to each is pose is traditional for the Chakra named. You may find it beneficial to work with the elements or not. Your choice.

- Using visualization/affirmation techniques during a pose can be deeply personal. They can be very powerful tools for healing and advancement in your practice. For example, if you want to work with the qualities of the second Chakra, you could engage a noticing practice or visualization technique to enhance your engagement, experience and healing with this Chakra. You may also engage the professional assistance of a therapist, an experienced yoga instructor or someone adept in working with the Chakras, for developing a visualization and/or affirmation practice for each pose and Chakra. Eventually your own intuition will be your guide.

- Notice mental resistance. If it is a persistent uninvited guest, acknowledge it and feel it. Give it what it wants: your attention. You may breath into it as you give it your full attention. Open and allow. The resistance will most often disperse, not to mention the possible arrival of new insights in relationship to the resistance.

- Please allow 45 – 60 minutes for the following sequence. However, a regular practice will yield the best results. If you don't have this much time, even ten to fifteen minutes practice is better than nothing. In this case, you may choose a few poses of your choice. I recommend one backward bend (eg. cobra pose), one forward bend (eg. full forward bend), spinal twist and deep relaxation – even if for only five minutes.

Start with what is comfortable and doable for you. If you are working with the full set but one day you do not have as much time, just practice what you do have time for – even if its just rolling over onto your stomach and doing a cobra pose before you fall asleep at night!

• The suggested time range for holding a pose is indicated for each pose. Start with the short end of the range and as your flexibility improves gradually increase the amount of time you hold the pose. If you feel sore the next day you have likely held your pose for too long or have gone too far into the pose. Easy does it.

Instructions for Yoga Poses for Beginners

Based on Integral Yoga style of Hatha Yoga – see recommended reading.

1. Relaxation Pose. Most Important.

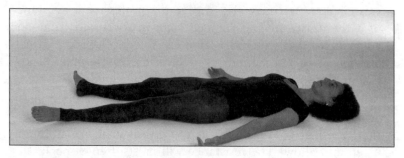

Lie on your back with feet about hip width apart. Arms away from your sides. Palms facing up. Mouth and eyes closed. Take a two or more deep, slow breaths and allow yourself to settle, center and relax, especially as you exhale. This is the position to enter into while resting in between poses and for the deep relaxation at the end of the sequence of poses. When you are on your stomach the relaxation position is the same with the exception that your head is turned to the side, cheek resting on the floor. Alternate cheeks resting on the floor from pose to pose.

Cultivate an experience of loving presence with yourself, nourishing and healing, throughout the session. At the beginning of the session, inform your mind that it is now having the great honor and privilege of being present during your Hatha Yoga healing time. You are giving and receiving a Gift for yourself. Creating this kind of conscious intention, with clear direction and gentle, firm commitment, will open the way for the best Prana flow and thus the best results. For example, "My precious Mind! How wonderful! We now get to do Yoga together! Let us now enjoy and stay focused in the moment and notice everything I do and feel. Enjoy, my Friend!" The mind likes this kind of attention and direction. The results are most satisfying. Stay with it as best you can, bringing the mind back to loving presence, and you will get better at staying focused. Eventually, this practice of directed loving presence is engaged in at all times during your waking life, no matter what you do. Easy does it.

2. Cobra Pose - Backward Bend. First Chakra. Earth.

From the relaxation pose, mindfully turn over onto your stomach. Bring your heels together. Forehead to the floor. Place your palms 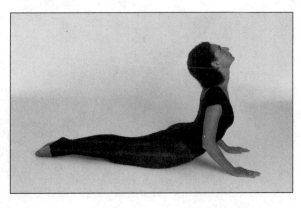 flat to the floor beneath your shoulders, fingers pointing toward the direction of your head along the floor. Elbows are close to the body and upper arms are more or less parallel to the floor. Stretch your chin over the floor. Be aware of the upper back as you slowly curl back the head and gently follow with curling back the head, neck and chest off the floor. Keep the elbows bent. Please use the back muscles to support the pose and not the arm muscles. Mmmm.

Physical Focus: Upper back and neck.

First Chakra Focus: The buttocks will be naturally squeezed together a little bit. The pubic bone is pressed into the floor and you may focus on the perineum area.

Hold the pose 5 – 60 seconds. Slowly curl out of the pose by lowering the chest first, while keeping the head back, then bring the chin to the floor, then forehead to the floor. Turn your head to the side, let your heels separate, keep your palms in place and rest for at least 10 – 15 seconds. Notice how you feel. Repeat. Rest in the relaxation position on the stomach. Take a deep breath or more. Ah!

3. Half Locust Pose – Backward Bend. Second Chakra. Water.

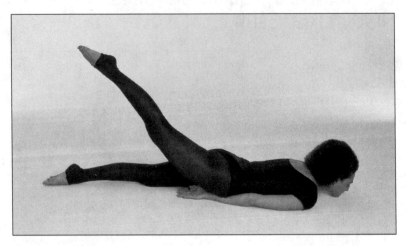

Bring the chin to the floor. Bring your arms underneath your body so that your arms are straight, elbows touching or close together, and your palms facing your thighs. Bring the feet together. Take a deep breath and raise the right leg while keeping it straight, both hips touching the arms and toe slightly pointed. Breath naturally.

Physical Focus: Lower Back.

Second Chakra Focus: Focus on pressured area between the pubic bone and your navel.

Hold for 5 – 60 seconds. Slowly lower the right leg and repeat for the left leg. Then rest with your cheek to the floor and let your heels separate. Repeat again for both legs. Then take the arms out from underneath you. Return to the relaxation position on the stomach for 10 – 15 seconds while taking one or more deep breaths. Ah!

4. Full Locust Pose – Backward Bend. Second Chakra. Water.

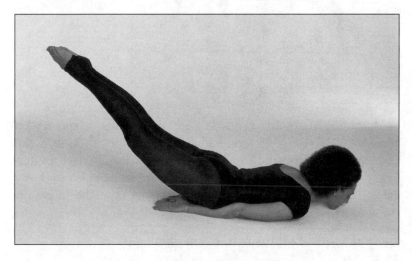

Same as # 3 but with both legs raised at the same time. Bring the chin to the floor. Bring your arms underneath your body so that your arms are straight, elbows close together and your palms facing your thighs. Bring the feet together. Inhale through the nose. Stiffen the entire body and raise both legs at the same time, even if it is only an inch or two. Keep the legs straight and together. Keep breathing.

Physical Focus: Lower back.

Second Chakra Focus: Same as #3.

Hold the pose steady for 5 – 60 seconds. Slowly lower the legs. Take the arms out from underneath you and rest with your head to the side. Take deep breaths. Let the air rush out of your mouth as you exhale. Rest. Ah! Repeat a second round if you are able.

5. Bow Pose – Backward Bend. Third Chakra. Fire.

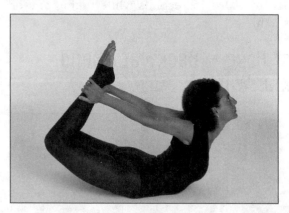

Separate the knees wide apart and bend them. Reach back with both hands and clasp the ankles or feet. If it is difficult to reach the feet or ankles, grabbing your pant legs or holding rubber exercise bands looped around your ankles is also acceptable. Bring your forehead toward the floor. Stretch the chin over the floor and slowly raise the head and chest up and back as in the cobra pose. Look up (helps keep your head back). If possible, gently pull on the legs to raise the knees off the floor. Keep the arms straight. Please do not strain.

Physical Focus: Entire length of the spine.

Third Chakra Focus: There is a lot of pressure on the navel/solar plexus area. Breath into it, let go of resistance and relax a little more each time you exhale while still holding the arch.

Allow the breath to find a deep natural rhythm while holding the pose for 5 – 60 seconds.

The body may naturally rock a bit, backwards and forwards, as the lungs fill and empty or simply hold steady. When *slowly* coming out of the pose, keep the head back as you release and lower the legs, lower the chest and then forehead to the floor.

Rest with your cheek to the side in the relaxation pose on the stomach. Take two or more deep breaths. Let the breath return to normal. Repeat two or three times if you like.

After your last repeat, take a big, deep breath as you turn over onto your back and exhale as you assume the relaxation position. This is one of my favorite breaths. Take a few extra moments here to thoroughly relax from head to toe with as many deep breaths as is necessary to release and relax. Let the breath return to normal. Allow the body to become soft and heavy as if it is sinking into the floor. Feel the nourishment from this conscious relaxing as you give permission for every single muscle to feel completely safe and supported in surrendering itself to the Earth/floor. Ah!

6. Head to Knee Pose – Forward Bend. Fourth Chakra. Air.

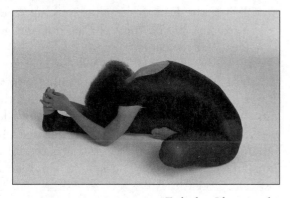

Bring the feet together and stretch the arms straight over- head along the floor with your thumbs inter- locked. Stretch your body out along the floor, take a deep breath and then come to a sitting position. Exhale. If your ab- dominal muscles are not strong enough to do a sit up then please feel free to come to a sitting position in the most direct and simple way that is most easeful for you.

Stretch the right leg straight out in front of you. Bring the left foot in so that the sole of the left foot is flat against the inner right thigh or knee. Right foot pointing up. Interlock your thumbs and stretch your arms up toward the ceiling, straighten- ing the back while inhaling. Look up. Exhale while hinging for- ward from the hips, arms straight and alongside the ears. Reach out toward the right foot and then grasp the shins, ankles or foot with the hands. Whatever is most easeful for you. Usually the best grasp is with the fingers under the leg with the thumbs on top. Keep the right leg straight but knee soft. The elbows are slightly bent toward the floor and head toward the right knee. Keep the shoulders relaxed. Keep the eyes closed and relax into the pose with the breath. As the leg and back muscles stretch out you may pull gently with your hands to extend the stretch a bit more. Easy does it.

Physical Focus: Posterior/sacrum area.

Fourth Chakra Focus: The head and shoulders are folding forward, creating pressure around the sternum area. Focus on the middle of the chest.

Hold the pose for 15 – 60 seconds. When coming out of the pose, interlock the thumbs and reach toward the foot. Inhale while reaching up with the arms straight and along side the ears. When the back is straight, look up, then lower the arms as you exhale. Stretch the right leg out and gently roll the legs. Rest for a few moments.

Repeat the same way with the left leg extended forward and the right foot tucked in. Upon coming out of the pose, when the arms are reaching up overhead, extend the right leg out to join the left while exhaling. Now with both legs together, with the arms still over head, take another deep breath and as you exhale slowly lower your back down to the floor. Lower your arms down by your side and assume the relaxation position and rest. Deep breath. Ah!

7. Full Forward Bend.
Fourth Chakra. Air.

Again bring the feet together and stretch the arms overhead along the floor with your thumbs inter-

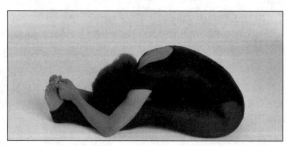

locked. Stretch your body out along the floor, take a deep breath, and then come to a sitting position. If your abdominal muscles are not strong enough to do a sit up then again feel free to come to sitting position in the most direct and simple way that is easeful for you. Lower your arms down and breath normally as you adjust yourself to sit comfortably on your buttocks with both legs outstretched on the floor in front of you. Bring the feet together. Stretch your arms overhead. Interlock your thumbs and stretch up. Look up. Inhale. As you exhale hinge forward from the hips and reach the hands toward the feet. Clasp the shins, ankles or feet with the elbows bent toward the floor and head toward the knees. Legs straight with soft knees. Do not strain. Keep the eyes closed and relax into the pose with the breath. The breath becomes nicely deeper. Gently stretch a bit more into the pose with each exhalation, as is comfortable.

Physical Focus: Posterior/sacrum.

Fourth Chakra Focus: Same as #4. Middle of the chest.

Hold the pose for 15 – 60 seconds. To come out of the pose, release the legs, hook the thumbs together, bring the arms along side the ears and stretch forward. Inhale and reach the arms up toward the ceiling as you sit up with the back straight. Look up. Exhale while lowering the back down onto the floor, arms down along the floor over head. Lower the arms down by your side and rest in the relaxation position. Take a few deep breaths. Ah!

8. Shoulder Stand – backward bend. Fifth Chakra. Ether.

*It is very important that you do the full pose slowly and carefully. If you have any doubts, or if you have high blood pressure, please go to the alternative modified version below until you have the guidance of an experienced instructor.

Bring the feet together. Bend the knees with feet flat to the floor. Bring the arms close to the body with the palms facing the floor. Clear the throat and make sure there is nothing bunched

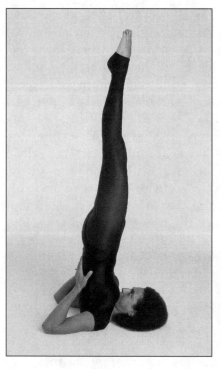

up under your neck and back. Press the palms to the floor and swing the legs overhead until the legs are parallel to the floor. Grasp your back with your hands to support the back's vertical position, more or less perpendicular to the floor. Palms are pressing against your back with your fingers pointing up toward the ceiling. Adjust your shoulders if needed. When you feel stable, raise the legs up toward the ceiling. Adjust the shoulders again and hand positions if needed so that you feel as stable as possible. Allow the breath to find its most comfortable rhythm. Hold steady. Do not cough or swallow in this position as there is a lot of pressure on the throat. If you need to do so please slowly come out of the pose.

Physical Focus: Upper back and neck or throat.

Fifth Chakra Focus: The chin is pressing into the hollow of the throat, creating pressure on the thyroid gland – parallel to the fifth Chakra location. Focus here.

Hold for 15 – 60 seconds, up to three minutes, depending on your capacity. DO NOT strain.

To come out of the pose, slowly lower the legs down overhead until they are parallel with the floor again. Bring the palms down to face the floor and while pressing the palms to the floor slowly lower the back down to the floor. Try not to raise your head off the floor when you lower the back down. Then lower the feet to the floor with the knees bent. Take a deep breath or more. As the lower back is likely to be tender do not rest but go directly to the Pelvic Tilt or Fish Pose.

Pelvic Tilt: With the knees still bent, soles of the feet flat to the floor and hip width apart, tilt the pelvis so that you are pressing the lower back flat to the floor. Press and hold for 10 – 15 seconds or more. Relax the pelvis. Repeat. Lower the legs and gently roll the head, arms and legs from side to side. Take a deep breath or more. Go directly to pose #9.

Alternate Pose to the Full Shoulder Stand: You may also do this pose in addition to the shoulder stand. Bend the knees so that the soles of the feet are flat on the floor and about hip width apart. Arms are close to the body with the palms facing the floor. Press the hips up toward the ceiling. Choice of focus is the same as in the full pose. Breath comfortably.

Hold for 10 – 30 seconds. Lower the hips back down to the floor and rest with your knees remaining bent. Repeat. Perform the pelvic tilt as many times as you like (see above). Lower the legs and gently roll the head, then arms and legs, from side to side. Take a deep breath. Go directly to the next pose.

9. Fish Pose – backward bend. Fifth Chakra. Ether. Sixth or Seventh Chakra.

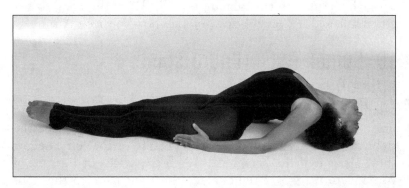

Bring the feet together. Grasp the thighs so the arms are straight and fingers under the thighs. With the elbows pressing down into the floor, bring the upper body up to a half seated position, looking toward the feet. Arch the back and place the top of the head on the floor. Look up toward the forehead. Create a slight smile with the mouth. Breath deeply through the nose.

Physical Focus: At the base of the throat, in between the eyebrows or the top of the head.

Fifth, Sixth or Seventh Chakra Focus: The thyroid gland is being stretched out here so you could continue the focus on the Fifth Chakra as in the Shoulder Stand. However, since the Head Stand is not recommended for beginners – you may focus on the Sixth Chakra, in between the eyebrows as you look up, or on the Seventh Chakra where there is pressure on the top of the head.

Hold for 15 – 60 seconds. To come out of the pose, press the elbows into the floor again and raise the head up so that you can look at your toes and then slowly lower your back down to the floor. Assume the pelvic tilt if desired. Repeat pelvic tilt as often as you like or needed.

As in after the backward bends, you may relax a bit longer after the fish pose. Gently roll your head, arms and legs back and forth. Let the body relax as if it is sinking into the floor. Take a few deep breaths. You may either let the air rush out of the mouth on exhaling for a releasing breath or slowly exhale through the nose for a calming breath. Allow the body to become soft and heavenly heavy. Notice how you feel. Ah!

10. Spinal Twist. Entire spine. Full Chakra range.

Mindfully come to a sitting position. Stretch both legs out in front of you, feet together. Bend the right knee and place the right foot flat to the floor on the outside of the left knee or shin. Straighten the back and stretch the arms out in front of you and turn to your right. Place the right palm to the floor behind you, fingers facing away from you. Have the right arm close to your back to support its vertical straightness. Lower the left arm down in between your chest and upraised knee. Press the knee aside. If possible grasp hold of the left leg with your left hand. Straighten up the back again and slowly turn to your right to look over your right shoulder. Keep the chin parallel to the floor and both b u t t o c k s touching the floor.

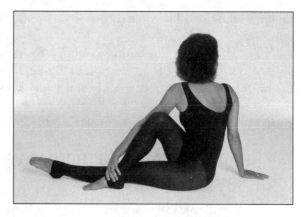

If needed, study the photo of the pose to assist you in finding the position.

Physical Focus: Entire length of spine.

Chakra Focus: Full range from the base of the spine to the top of the head or which ever Chakra you would like to give special attention to.

Hold For 15 – 60 seconds. Slowly come out of the pose, leading first with the head and releasing the arms and legs. Gently shake out the arms and legs and take a deep breath. With both knees bent, hug the knees with your arms wrapped around them. Let the head bend forward to rest on the knees. After a few moments, stretch the legs out along the floor again to pre-pare for the spinal twist in the other direction.

Keep the right leg stretched out along the floor. Bend the left knee and place the left foot flat to the floor on the outside of the right knee or shin. Straighten the back and stretch the arms out in front of you and turn to your left. Place the left palm to the floor behind you, fingers facing away from you. Have the left arm close to your back to support its vertical straightness. Lower the right arm down in between your chest and upraised knee. Press the knee aside. If possible grasp hold of the right leg with your right hand. Straighten up the back again and slowly turn to your left to look over your left shoul-der. Keep the chin parallel to the floor and both buttocks touching the floor. Hold for the same amount of time as the first twist.

Follow the same directions as above for coming out of the pose. After hugging the knees, mindfully lie down on your back in the relaxation position. Gently roll your head, arms and legs side to side. Relax with a deep breath or more. Bring the breath back to normal. Notice how you feel. Ah!

11. Deep Relaxation: Progressive with seven levels.

Your body will cool down in the Deep Relaxation so you may want a blanket over you. If you have a sensitive lower back you may want to put a pillow under your knees. Make sure you will not be interrupted for at least fifteen minutes. Listening to a deep relaxation tape will be helpful until you are able to do this effectively for yourself.

First Level: Progressively relaxing physical parts of your body by tightening muscles groups and then releasing, relaxing them. When the instruction "DROP" is given, do not use your muscles to lower down or release but simply drop and let go of the muscle tensing.

Cover yourself with your blanket and place your pillow under your knees if desired.

Assume the relaxation pose.

- Stretch out your right leg. Inhale and raise the right leg two or three inches off the floor. Hold the breath for 3-5 seconds as you squeeze the leg tightly from hip to toes. Open the mouth. Let the air rush out of the mouth as you exhale *at the same time* as you DROP the leg to the floor. Gently rock the leg side to side and then let it rest.

- Stretch out your left leg. Inhale and raise the left leg two or three inches off the floor. Hold the breath 3-5 seconds as you squeeze the leg tightly from hip to toes . Open the mouth. Let the air rush out of the mouth as you exhale *at the same time* as you DROP the leg to the floor. Gently rock the leg side to side and then let it rest.

- Stretch out your right arm. Spread the fingers apart. Inhale and raise the arm up two or three inches. Hold the breath for 3-5 seconds as you squeeze the arm tightly, shoulder to fingers. You may curl the fingers if you like. Open the mouth. Let the air rush out as you exhale *at the same time* as you DROP the arm to the floor. Gently rock the arm side to side and then let it rest.

- Stretch out your left arm. Spread the fingers apart. Inhale and raise the arm up two or three inches. Hold the breath for 3-5 seconds as you squeeze the arm tightly, shoulder to fingers. You may curl the fingers if you like. Open the mouth. Let the air rush out as you exhale *at the same time* you DROP the arm to the floor. Gently rock the arm side to side and then let it rest.

- Inhale and squeeze the buttocks and pelvis area. Squeeze tightly. Tighter. Hold for 3-5 seconds. Open the mouth and exhale as you release. Repeat.

- Take a deep breath into the lower section of the lungs by extending out the lower abdomen like a balloon and hold the breath for 3-5 seconds. Open the mouth and let the air rush out.

- Take another deep breath and fill the entire lungs with as much air as they will hold. Hold the breath for 3-5 seconds. Open the mouth and let the air rush out to empty the lungs completely. Repeat if you like.

- Squeeze the shoulders up toward the ears. Then press them down toward the feet. Squeeze them toward the ceiling. Then press the shoulders down into the floor, bringing the shoulders back and squeeze the shoulder blades toward each other. Relax and adjust the shoulders so that they feel comfortable.

- Screw the whole face into a ball that meets toward the tip of the nose. Relax. Repeat.

- Open the whole face, looking up toward the forehead, sticking the tongue out with the mouth wide open. Relax. Repeat if desired or simply stretch your face out and around in any way you like. Relax.

- Make any final adjustments to your position so that you are most comfortable and preferably will not have to move for the rest of the relaxation.

Second Level: More subtle. Without moving, mentally relaxing specific parts of your body, using the power of mental suggestion.

- Bring your awareness to the toes and mentally give permission for them to relax.
- In the same way, mentally relax the bottom of the feet and all across the top of the feet.
- Mentally relax the ankles.
- All around the shins and calves.
- Up, around and through the knees.
- All around and through the thighs.
- Mentally relax all around the pelvis and hip area.
- As you relax up through the abdomen chest and area, imagine even the internal organs relaxing more deeply. Reproductive organs and kidneys. Intestines and stomach. Even the heart and lungs relaxing more deeply.
- All across the top of the chest and color bone area.
- Now bring your awareness to the base of the spine. Imagine relaxation flowing up, relaxing the lower back. The middle back. All across the upper back, including the shoulder blades.
- Relax all around the neck and throat.
- Let the jaw soften.
- Chin.
- Lips.
- Even the teeth and tongue.
- The nose.
- Cheekbones.
- Ears.
- Allow the eyes to become soft. Let the eye lids become soft and heavy.
- Mentally imagine even behind the eyes relaxing.
- Eyebrows.

- Across your forehead.
- Temples and sides of your head.
- Mentally relax the back of your head.
- Bring your attention to the top of your head. Mentally relax all around the top of your head.

Third Level: More subtle. Observing the breath.

Bring your awareness to your breath. Become a silent observer to the breath. Become a Silent Witness. Simply observing. Do not try to control it. Feel the natural flow of the rhythm of life; flowing in and flowing out – receiving and giving. Do this for one minute or more.

Forth Level: More subtle. Observing the mind.

Bring your awareness to your thoughts. Remain as the Silent Witness. Watch as you would watch clouds passing by through the sky, coming and going. Thoughts are coming and going through the window of your awareness. You are not the thoughts that come and go. You are the Silent Witness. Do this for one minute or more.

Fifth Level: More subtle. Resting in the Presence of Peace. Resting into effortlessness.

Going deeper. Let go of all effort. Rest deeply into the Presence of Peace. Going deeper. Become the Presence of Peace. Resting in your own True Nature as Peace.

Simply "Be" for at least three to five minutes.

Sixth Level: Emerging.

When it is time to come out of your Deep Relaxation, take a few deep, slow breaths. Feel new life-giving vitality flow into every single cell as you inhale. Feel the Gift and Grace of Life with new gratitude. Become aware of where you are and your surroundings. **Slowly**, gently roll your head side to side. Your head feels very heavy. Gently roll your hands, feet, then arms and legs side to side. Bend your knees, soles of the feet to the floor and about hip width apart. Let your knees rest against each other. Bring your hands to your belly or your heart.

Allow your Heart to open and feel grateful for the gift of your body, the gift of who you are and being consciously alive.

Invite and entertain loving gratitude in whatever way opens your heart and allows you to feel held, nourished, whole, connected and satisfied. For example, think about what you really love about yourself and fill yourself with self-love. If the mind wants to wander away simply bring it back to your nourishing contemplation. Be here for as long as you like. Mmm.

Seventh Level: Arising.

When you are ready, roll over onto your right side and slowly, mindfully, come to a sitting position. Find a comfortable seat for yourself with your back straight but relaxed as best can be.

This may take the form of sitting in a chair or on a pillow or bench. Become quiet again. Take a deep breaths or more. Notice how you feel. Be here for a few moments and enjoy how you feel.

12. Deep Three Part Breathing.

This is a simple but profound technique. It utilizes your full lung capacity for air intake. If you become light headed, dizzy or sense a headache coming on while practicing, it is most likely due to the fact your nervous system may not be used to the extra oxygen. In this case, you will have to prepare your nerves to receive more "voltage" from the powerful Prana intake by developing your practice more gently and slowly. If this happens, please suspend the practice until your next session or sit quietly for a few moments and resume the practice while reducing your volume intake of air. In any case, be mindful not to over do it and rest when you need to.

To prepare, sit in a chair with both feet on the floor and a straight back that is not touching the back of the chair. Or, if you are comfortable enough with sitting in a cross legged position, please do so, again without your back touching anything. Sitting on the edge of a pillow or rolled up blanket, so that the pelvis is slightly tilted, assists in helping to keep the back straight with minimum effort.

Exhale all the air out of your lungs by pulling your lower abdomen in at the end of the exhalation.

First Part: Let the abdomen relax and automatically you will begin to inhale. As the lower lungs fill with air the abdomen expands.

Second Part: As you continue to slowly inhale, you will notice the rib cage expanding as the lungs continue to fill up.

Third Part: When you inhale to the capacity of the lungs the shoulders and collarbone automatically rise slightly. You will feel a slight, and often satisfying, pressure as the top of the lungs as they press up against the collar bone.

Exhale in the opposite way. As you exhale, and empty out the air from the top of the lungs, the shoulders and collar bone slowly lower down. Then the rib cage slowly contracts. And finally, using the abdominal muscles, pull the abdominal muscles in snugly at the end to gently but firmly squeeze out all the remaining air from the lungs. Relax the abdomen. You will naturally begin to inhale to start the next round.

As you start out, I recommend performing five of these breaths. After exhaling in the last round, bring the breath back to normal and notice how you feel. Really notice how you feel. If it feels right, do another five deep breaths. Rest again. If it feels right, do another five breaths. When your nervous system builds up its stamina to be able to enjoy the extra "voltage" of Prana and oxygen, then work up to a continuous deep three part breathing session that lasts five to fifteen minutes depending on your time allowance and comfort.

When asked what *one* practice to do, if there was limited time, my Beloved Guru would respond with "Pranayama". The reason being, by calming and controlling the breath, the mind is made calm, centered and clear. When the mind is calm, your intuitive wisdom is more accessible and the body relaxes. When the body is relaxed, the maximum amount of oxygen and Prana is utilized to the best benefit. By increasing the intake of air you will purify and detoxify the body as fresh oxygen is brought in and more carbon dioxide (waste) is released from the body via exhalation. You can practice Deep Three Part Breathing while in the deep relaxation position as well.

Take a few moments to sit quietly and notice how you feel after your deep breathing. There is deep sense of Peace and well-being. Try not to miss this. Just a few moments of this profound Peace can make all the difference. Your communion with your own reliable Source of inner happiness ~ Peace ~ will deepen and improve the quality of your life in every way. Develop a regular practice. Even if it is just a few minutes a day. Regular practice has accumulative effects. This is most often the best way for the best results. This will also be one of the best ways to contribute to arising Peace for all created kind that we share life with. We are not alone.

We also create Peace together, for ourselves and each other. Practice. Relax. Observe. Feel. Heal. Intuit. Realize. Adjust. Balance. Be. Whatever combination works for you. Repeat as needed.

May you practice your Hatha Yoga well and enjoy the great benefits. Dedicate yourself to the best you are and it will be so. Intention directs your destiny. You are alive and well in your own Soul. All will be well.

Peace Be. Be Peace. Om Shanti. Shanti. Shanti.

Recommendations

Please do not confuse the term Hatha Yoga as a "style" of Hatha Yoga.

More than once upon asking a Yoga instructor what style of Hatha Yoga they teach the response is "Well...Hatha Yoga!" Styles of Hatha Yoga are **different approaches** to the practice of Hatha Yoga presented and taught by various Yoga Masters or current contemporary teachers. Due to the renewed popularity of Yoga there is a wide range of styles offered in most cities.

It is my opinion that they may be categorized into two camps. Traditional and non-traditional, or what I may call "westernized" Hatha Yoga. Examples of different traditional styles are Hatha Yoga taught by Integral Yoga, Sivananda Yoga, ViniYoga, Babaji's Kriya Yoga Hatha (as taught by Sri Swami Yogananda's disciples, Ananda Ashram Teachers, Marshall Govindan and others).

There is also a wide range of competency and knowledge base among the teachers that are available to you, depending on their training and continued study and personal practice. Especially for beginners, I recommend you find an experienced traditional Hatha Yoga instructor that has at least some general knowledge and understanding of the other branches of Yoga, in particular Raja Yoga. I recommend first becoming familiar with practicing a traditional style of Hatha Yoga before experimenting with other styles.

References:

- The sequence and recommended duration for poses and pauses are based on the Integral Yoga style of Hatha Yoga. For more information on teachers in your area who teach this style of Yoga you may contact the Integral Yoga Teachers Association at iyta@iyta.org. If you cannot find Integral Yoga audio or video tapes at your local bookstore, or yoga studio, you may order them from Integral Yoga Distribution, 1-800-262-1008.

- Photos of yoga poses feature internationally acclaimed Yoga Instructor Extraordinaire, Meenakshi Angel Honig. Meenakshi's excellent Integral Hatha Yoga videos, and other teaching jewels, may be obtained by ordering through 1-800-FOR-YOGA or www.AngelYoga.com.

Madhuri Honeyman, the author of this offering, has been a disciple of Swami Satchidananda, Founder of Integral Yoga, since 1971. As an artist, ceremonial leader and teacher, she lives happily with her husband, Steffan in peaceful Point Roberts, WA. They own and operate Terra Spirita ~ Forest Home Retreats. You may contact her at honeyman@whidbey.com.

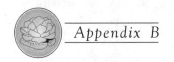

Bibliography and References

Bhagavad-gita as It Is, A.C. Bhaktivedanta Swami Prabhupada, Bhaktivedanta Book Trust, January 1998, ISBN: 0912776803

Bible, New International Version, Zondervan Publishing, Grand Rapids, MI, September 2002, ISBN 0310923077

Chakras, Balance Your Body's Energy for Health and Harmony, Patricia Mercier, Sterling Publishing Company, Incorporated, New York, NY. September 2000, ISBN: 0806966114

The Chakras, C. W. Leadbeater, The Theosophical Publishing Company, Wheaton, Il, March 1972, ISBN 0835604225

The Chakras and Esoteric Healing, Zachary Lamsdowne, Ph.D., Red Wheel/Weiser, Boston, MA, August 1983, ISBN 0877285845

The Chakra Handbook: From Basic Understanding to Practical Application, Shalila Sharamon, Lotus Press, WI, June 1991, ISBN: 094152485X

Chakras and Their Archetypes, Ambika Wauters, The Crossing Press, Inc., Berkeley, CA September 1997, ISBN: 0895948915

Eastern Body – Western Mind, Psychology and the Chakra System, Anodea Judith, Ph.D., Ten Speed Press, Berkeley, CA. October 1996, ISBN: 0890878153

The Four Agreements, Don Miguel Ruiz, Amber-Allen Publishing, San Raphael, CA, November 1997. ISBN 1878424319

I and Thou, Martin Buber, Simon & Schuster Adult Publishing Group, May 1976, ISBN: 0684717255

The Inward Arc, Frances Vaughan, Ph.D., Random House, Incorporated, New York, NY, 1st edition, January 1986, ISBN: 0877733244

Karma and Reincarnation, Hiroshi Motoyama, Ph.D., Piatkus Books, London, England, October 1998, ISBN: 0749919167

The Prophet, Kahlil Gilbran, Alfred A. Knopf, Inc., Random House, New York, NY, May 1976, ISBN 0394404289

Rays and Initiations, Alice Bailey, Lucis Publishing Company, New York, NY, September 1995, ISBN: 0853300224

Reference Guide to Essential Oils, Abundant Health Publishers, Toronto, Ontario, Canada, 1998, 888-718-3068.

The Sevenfold Journey, Judith Anodea, Ph.D., The Crossing Press, Inc., Berkeley, CA, April 1993, ISBN 0895945746

Spiritual Emergency, Dr. Stanislav Grof, Tarcher/Putnam, East Rutherford, NJ, September 1989, ISBN: 0874775388

Tapestry of the Gods: Psychological Transformation & the Seven Rays, Michael Robbins, University of the 7 Rays; New Jersey, 3rd edition (1997), ISBN: 0962186929

Theory of the Chakras, Hiroshi Motoyama, Ph.D., The Theosophical Publishing Company, Wheaton, Il, November 1981, ISBN 0835605515

Towards a Superconsciousness, Hiroshi Motoyama, Ph.D., Asian Humanities Press, Fremont, CA, November 1990, ISBN: 0895819147

Vibrational Medicine, Richard Gerber, M.D., Inner Traditions International, Limited, Rochester, Vermont, March 2001, ISBN: 1879181584

Wheels of Life: A User's Guide to the Chakra System, Judith Anodea, Ph.D., Llewellyn Publishing, St. Paul, MN, 2nd edition, July 1987, ISBN: 0875423205

Website References:

- California Institute for Human Science, www.cihs.edu
- Valerie Hunt, Bioenergy Fields Foundation, www.bioenergyfields.org/
- Abundant Health, www.abundant-health4u.com
- Young Living Essential Oils, www.youngliving.com
- Diamond Lotus Essential Oils, www.diamondlotusoils.com/
- Essential Dynamics, www.essentialdynamics.biz

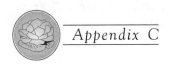

Appendix C-1

About the Author: Dr. Richard Jelusich

Richard Jelusich holds a Ph.D. in Human Science from the California Institute for Human Science ", where he is on adjunct faculty. A gifted psychic from birth, he is a renowned spiritual healer, spiritualist minister, speaker, researcher and author. After many years of engineering, managing, and consulting in various highly technical fields including space launch systems, he realized his true heart's desire to accomplish two goals:

- To de-mystify metaphysics.
- To profoundly heal, and help self-empower individuals, on multiple levels.

Dr. Jelusich has studied behavioral psychoacoustics, bioelectromagnetics, clinical biopsychology, consciousness expansion, transpersonal psychology, and Eastern-Western philosophy. His Ph.D. dissertation is: *"Psychophysiological Effects of Frequency Octave Related Light and Sound."*

He is most interested in helping the individual to heal on all levels in a philosophy he calls "The Whole Human Being." The pathway includes education about our metaphysical nature, and the information and realistic tools that assist us in understanding our multi-dimensional nature. Dr. Jelusich creates a philosophical and experiential environment for students of energy healing through his Institute for Chakra Studies and Esoteric Healing.

Having the ability to "see" the subtle energies in and around our bodies enables Dr. Jelusich to discern life path strengths and weaknesses, and dominant chakra dispositions, through the four archetypal energies: *mental, physical, spiritual, and emotional.* Through intuitive counseling and energy work, he facilitates qualitative healing on all four levels and helps us understand and integrate our life issues. Dr. Jelusich has received many testimonials on the beneficial effects of his healing abilities. He travels extensively, combining a busy schedule of healing work, lectures, and workshops.

Dr. Jelusich has appeared on numerous radio and TV shows, and has been featured at holistic health expos, national healing events, and many private gatherings. He has produced twenty-two public-access television shows of "Metaphysics 101," a TV series now airing in the southern California area. His keynote addresses and speeches include keynote speaker for the Universal Church of the Master annual convention, presentations to IONS (Institute for Noetic Sciences) groups in the U.S. and Canada, and presentations on metaphysics and technology at Langara College, Vancouver, Canada

He created the publication, "Light News," a newsmagazine dedicated to the blending of science and metaphysics, published monthly for seventy-five issues. "Light News" is now an on-line magazine on Dr. Jelusich's website, http://www.lightnews.org. Dr. Jelusich is a prolific writer, and has published many of his essays online, and is also published in newsletters, quarterlies, and magazines.

Through "Flower Readings," meditation groups, and workshops, Dr. Jelusich has counseled and facilitated the healing of thousand of individuals worldwide. Dr. Jelusich is the President and CEO of Light News, Inc. (USA) and Northern Light News, Inc. (Canada), companies actively engaged in creating products and media that enhance the consciousness and self-empowerment of individuals. He has developed unique energy tools that aid healing and spiritual understanding, and has an extensive catalogue of energy products and tools, tapes, and

CDs. One of his popular CDs is "Crystal Bowls of Tibet," a compilation of healing tones of crystal bowls, nature, and other healing sounds.

Dr. Jelusich has sought to show the blending of science and metaphysics. He produces *"The Mandala of Life,"* an interactive lecture/seminar series on the integration of light, sound, color, and brainwave entranement techniques as healing to the mind-body. From ancient Tibetan bells and tones to the science of "cymatics," to current research on lasers and their application in brainwave entranement techniques, Dr. Richard incorporates ancient and current wisdom in an enjoyable seminar/experiential setting for the public.

One of Dr. Jelusich's goals is to promote learning seminars on a world-wide basis, incorporating an audience-involved experiential setting that includes mind and emotion stimulating sounds, colors, and shapes, using:

- ancient Tibetan bells
- voice toning
- ancient instruments (didgeridoo), and
- light and sound techniques for brainwave entranement, including:
  * cymatics
  * recorded primordial sounds of earth and planetary objects, and
  * lasers that are tuned to light/sound/brainwave patterns.

More Books by Dr. Richard Jelusich

Coming Soon! Dr. Jelusich's books in progress:

Flower Reading Oracle Deck and Workbook Set

The set includes a very unique deck of oracle cards that may be used as a daily meditation, to answer simple questions, or as a full life-reading instrument for insight and inspiration, accompanied by an instructional workbook.

The Flower Oracle combines the essence of Dr. Jelusich's Flower Readings and his work on the Psychology of the Chakras in a divinatory deck of cards. The cards combine beautiful pictures of flowers and major and minor aspects of the chakra influences on our character.

The accompanying workbook includes a basic philosophy of our chakra systems and how our lives are influenced by our chakra disposition, plus a description of the cards with easy instructions for sample layouts.

The Book of Reciprocity: Why We Pick the People We Do

The follow-up to *Eye of the Lotus*, covering why we choose the relationships we do, how we take psychic relationship to certain people, and how the dynamics of the energy in the relationship tend to play themselves out on interpersonal levels.

This book is a guide on how to respond to and optimize your relationships through a thorough understanding of the fundamental energetics taking place, with an emphasis on how and why we take *inverse relationships* (mirroring) to others to bring about our own challenges and growth.

It will discuss the various types of relationships (e.g., a third chakra dominant person with a second chakra dominant person, or a fourth chakra dominant person with another fourth chakra dominant person), and will include many illustrations and case histories of chakra interactions.

A Head in The Game

An indispensable book for those in the beauty industry, explaining why you choose this type of work, the subtle energy influences and exchanges that occur between practitioner and client, and methods for nurturing those energies to enhance your effectiveness and your career. Instructions are given for practitioners to protect and nurture your energy, how to flow gentle healing energies to your clients, and how to clear your energy fields.

A Hand in The Game

This book is designed for those in the massage and body-work industry, and for healing professionals. Included are discussions of the fundamental energetics of consciousness and qualitative healing, along with analysis and inventory techniques built on Dr. Jelusich's years of experience as an energy healer and teacher of energy healing techniques. His effective techniques for energy work, clearing, and cleansing are revealed.

The Book of Healing

Based on Dr. Jelusich's many years of teaching energy healing techniques, this book is first a fundamental treatise on the philosophy of our qualitative being, followed by unique aspects of healing techniques that address the whole human being in four archetypes: mental, physical, spiritual, and emotional.

This book is designed for healers who wish to understand and apply various techniques of advanced healing work, including *axialtonal alignment, out-of-body healing,* the *shushumna, soul-infusion,* and several more.

The Empath

This dynamic book addresses the urgency to understand our true nature and our need to grow spiritually. Dr. Jelusich answers the following important questions, among others: *Why are we increasingly sensitive to others and their emotions? Why are we feeling so deeply, but with no context to explain the intensity of those feelings?*

The Quality of Mind

Dr. Jelusich explains he different states of attachment as they affect human consciousness and motivation in this thoughtful book. Included is a discussion of the basic state of qualitative being, methods of attachment and protection vs. availability with respect to energetic interaction with humanity.

This book helps the reader understand how we take a relationship to our perceptions, the nature of our experiences with regard to the attachment we assign to them, and the process by which we can choose the "middle state" of *beingness*.

Speak for Your "Self"

Channeling is a very popular method for delivering Divinely-inspired information from spiritually-developed disincarnate beings. This book challenges and raises the question of its necessity, and discusses the power of the Self's vulnerability to all love, wisdom and will in oneness as a *unique path*, vs. our need to associate with each other in a *spiritual collaborative* that can include seeking the influence of higher consciousness beings.

Metaphysics for the Rest of Us

An easy-to-understand primer on metaphysics, its pervasive nature in our consciousness, and how a basic understanding and application of its principles will empower you. It is designed for the beginner who has had no exposure to subtle energy or metaphysics.

Flower Readings

This book is a fascinating owner's manual, with anecdotes, of the popular "Flower Reading" sessions that Dr. Richard Jelusich has been doing for 11 years. The premise is a group setting, where each participant brings a single flower and anonymously places it with the others.

In a safe and loving environment, and not knowing who brought it, Dr. Jelusich reads the impressions left on the flower from each individual's energy field. Dr. Jelusich explains: "You leave an imprint of your soul's history on everything you touch: The history of your past, present, and future reveals deep insights into each person's life's strengths, weaknesses, and motivations."

This book is a compilation of some of the most interesting readings, anecdotes, and their outcomes, as well as the philosophy and methods used in Flower Readings.

Workshops/Products Offered by Dr. Richard Jelusich

Healer's Training Workshops

Dr. Jelusich teaches seventeen levels of workshops in healer's training at the soul level, from the "whole human being" perspective. Dr. Jelusich creates a philosophical and experiential environment for students of energy healing through his Institute for Chakra Studies and Esoteric Healing. His methods are based on his teachings about dominant chakras affecting our mental, spiritual, physical, and emotional dispositions. Beginning to advanced training available in six US and Canada cities: whole program takes two years. Please see online calendar for Healer's Training schedule. **www.lightnews.org**

Lecture/Workshop Topics

• The Mandala of Life – a multi-sensory, multi-media presentation illustrating the blending of Western science and Eastern philosophy
• Psychology of The Chakras
• Your Chakric Relationships
• Sacred Geometries
• Healing Technologies for the New Millennium
• De-Mystifying Metaphysics
• Past Lives, Karma, and Reincarnation
• Experiential Healing, the Integration of Self
• Healer's Training Series

Audiotapes and CDs

• Crystal Bowls of Tibet – a wonderful CD of the sounds of crystal bowls, created by Dr. Jacob Hans and Dr. Richard Jelusich
• Healing Technologies for the New Millennium: The Blending

of Western Science and Eastern Philosophy
- De-Mystifying Metaphysics
- Psychology of The Chakras
- Past Lives, Karma and Reincarnation
- Inner Peace, and Journey to Knowledge – meditation tape
- Meditations – guided imagery set to music
- Lectures from Healer's Training Workshops

Private Sessions (in person and by telephone)

Private sessions seek to determine your soul's purpose in this lifetime, identify your challenges, and heal your wounds. Dr. Jelusich is able to "see" all aspects of the individual from the mental, emotional, and spiritual states of being, to the functioning of the chakras, and the physical body systems. One-hour sessions in-person or telephone consultations are a combination of intuitive counseling and qualitative energy work, and an *audiotape* is always provided to the client.

Dr. Jelusich may be contacted at:

4389 Mt. Jeffers Ave.
San Diego, CA 92117
Telephone: 760-420-8100
Website: www.lightnews.org
Email: drjelusich@lightnews.org

Cruystal Bowls of Tibet CD

Healing Sounds for Mind, Body, and Spirit

Dr. Jacob Hans, D.C. *and* Dr. Richard Jelusich, Ph.D.

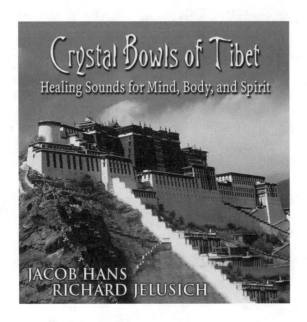

I am pleased to announce that we have finished our new CD, using the healing sounds of Quartz Crystal Bowls. The crystal bowls make one of the purest sounds that can exist, and have been used in healing and energy clearing with very good results.

The Technique

We have positioned the seven bowls in a circle with a special pair of microphones in the middle of the room. One person is stationed at each bowl, and plays in specific patterns on each recorded track. The result varies from one bowl playing alone, to sequences of several bowls playing and fading in and out.

The result is a sound pattern that bathes the central microphones from different directions of the listener's orientation. Listening with headphones very accurately reproduces the sound patterns to the listener. Listening with stereo speakers bathes the room with incredible cascading sounds, and has especially good bass response.

The Recording Method

The special microphones are shaped like the cochlea (inner ear), and are worn by the user on either side of his temples to reproduce the exact environment of hearing related to the ears. The user (Dr. Jelusich) sat in the exact center of the seven bowls, in the plane of their richest sound, to create a highly accurate 3-D reproduction of the crystal bowls. The result is true 3-D recording, because the microphones are separated by the tissue mass of the head, and "hear" in the same way that you do. The sounds were recorded digitally, so no "hiss" will be introduced to the listening experience.

You may order the CD for $16.98 (CA residents add 7.5% tax) plus $3 s/h within the U.S. Foreign orders slightly more shipping cost.

Order by E-Mail to:

drjelusich@lightnews.org or call 760-420-8100

VISA/MasterCard, check/money-order accepted.

Or, mail to:

Crystal Bowls of Tibet
P.O. Box 17035
San Diego, CA 92177

Testimonials

These are only a few of the many testimonials given to Dr. Richard Jelusich for his healing work in private spiritual consultations, healing sessions, and Flower Readings.

****

I had an extraordinary experience that I would like to share with you. I had what is called a "FLOWER READING."

I had heard about this and was very curious about the process. Basically, how it works is that you pick a flower or buy one and you have someone who is an intuitive or psychic (in this case Dr. Richard Jelusich) read the impressions you left on it from your own energy field. The way Dr. Jelusich explains it is, "'You leave an imprint of your soul's history on everything you touch: The history of your past, present and future. What this means is that you have a tremendous potential to make a difference in the world wherever you are and whoever you touch."

Everyone arrived early and put their flowers in a basket. There was no way that Dr. Jelusich saw which flower belonged to whom ... Believe me, I made sure of it! It took about three hours for him to read through all the flowers, **He left us ALL in AWE! It was the consensus of the group that our readings had been 99.9 percent accurate!**

He gave very useful information and details to guide us through upcoming challenges. Personally, I was going through a difficult period in my life and the things that came through the reading made it possible for me to succeed in the challenges I was facing. I was very impressed, to say the least, and I wanted to give all of you the opportunity to experience this.

So, I have invited Dr. Jelusich to Lifesource to do ongoing flower readings. We're going to have a lot of fun and a lot of healing.

Dr. Jacob Hans - Lifesource Chiropractic
3636 4th Ave., San Diego, CA 92103
619-296-4994

****

Hello Richard,

I would like to advise you that I received the tape today from your reading on Aug.17.

I have done some work since then, manifested yesterday, and already received some guidance today. Wow, universe provides this fast!!! I am excited. I feel that we will be celebrating this success when you come to Calgary in October. **You are amazing. Thank you Richard, for the great service you are doing for me and everybody else.**

Let the light and love heal all the wounds in our conscious mind, and let our souls guide us in the place of equality.

With all that I AM.

Sonja
August 2003

****

Dr. Jelusich,

I am blessed to have been able to cross your path. Meeting you has been a true experience for me. **After our private reading session I feel like a new women.** I have been "read" plenty in my past but none compare to the experience of your reading. This is the first time in my life that I have ever physically released the negative that I had been holding within. **All of the things that you said to me were right on track** and who I am, as well as who I am to be, and mostly what I stand for.

You spoke highly of my values on truth, which touched my heart. I could not have said it better myself. You are a blessing and I truly thank you for making time for me. I also thank the Gods for Janice because without her our paths may have never crossed. Thank you, Thank you, Thank you so very much. You will forever be in my prayers.

Continued Blessings,

Theresa Alford
San Diego, CA
February 2003

****

Hi Reverend Rick,

Thank you SO much for yesterday's reading. My thoughts have been "marinating" ever since we got off the phone and I am feeling a rush of energy and inspiration that I haven't felt in quite some time. **Thank you so much for planting seeds, your honesty, guidance, and time. My appreciation is boundless.**

Again, thank you so much. I hope all is well. :)

Ayiko
Los Angeles, CA
May 2003

****

Hi Rick,

I am finally back from Arizona and didn't want to let too much time pass before I thanked you for the exceptionally nice flower reading evening. **All the comments coming to me were full of praise for you & your work.** My sister in particular thought that the readings you did for her adult children were quite accurate and thought they would be pleased as well. The laser show was a wonderful surprise too!

One thing I wanted to comment on—you are very knowledgeable and skillful in your presentations! We all see the impact your work has on our daily lives and think it is much more than special....more like influential with a sensitive touch! **The readings give us permission to heal.** Something that not a lot of others will openly admit they want for the people in their lives. I think the "fear of loss" plays a large role in their resistance.....

So, there you have it — another successful evening — many happy & peaceful people healing in your service.

Sincerely,
Janice Knight
April 2002

****

Hello Rick:

In May 2000, I attended my first Flower Reading session with you. **I was just awed at how you picked up on my family background, and the advice you had for me.** But, what really got my attention was the way you did pick up on my health problems, and preceded to do a healing. My point is that I viewed the healing for a problem I have lived with for years, however, within a month's time it became a very serious problem with my female organs, which had to be removed with the fear of "Cancer." Now Rick and readers, I am not saying that that healing removed the Cancer, but with all the tumors that were found, and the state of my ovaries, well, it hit me like a ton of bricks as to what you truly saw and tried so hard to heal.

I just want to take a few lines to let you and yours know how I believe you did help me.

Thank you and God bless,

Name withheld upon request

****

Hi Rick:

I'm not sure if you remember me, but Shanti brought me to one of your readings a couple of years ago. I asked you if you thought I would be able to have a child with my husband who is HIV+. At that time, I was told by the medical world I would not be able to conceive with my husband's sperm as the risk of infection was too great. I tried using donor sperm and had two very early miscarriages. I was devastated.

You told me that I would be able to have a baby with my husband's sperm and at the time I was so devastated that I did not believe you. Well, one year ago my husband and I were accepted into a program in Boston that helps couples in our situation. In August of 2001 my husband and I did in-vitro fertilization using my husband's individual sperm cells that tested negative for HIV. I am now 7 months pregnant, with my husband's baby! I am due in May and we are having a healthy baby boy. All tests have come back normal and I am completely beside myself with joy.

I thought you would want to know that your prediction was

right. Today, I am a little less skeptical about what a miracle is, and that what I see at any given moment may not be as it really is.

I hope to meet you again someday. All the best,

Name withheld upon request
February 2002

****

Up until the time I called Dr. Jelusich for a life reading, my life had been, at best, mediocre, and at worst, miserable. At the time I called him, I was a live-in, primary caregiver for a terminally ill woman. I was feeling totally drained, emotionally, physically and mentally, and didn't know which way to go with my life.

I won't get into the personal things he told me, but, **the way he read me was nothing short of mind-boggling: and the characteristic I appreciated about him the most was that he had the courage to tell me the Truth about areas in my Life where I needed to work.** This was exactly what I wanted from him. As I told Dr. Jelusich, I didn't want someone who was going to flatter and B.S. me. **He laid it on the line, and it has been the most empowering experience I have had in my life.**

I have a strong metaphysical background — studying astrology, numerology, Runes, card reading, anything to help me understand my life better. I have studied under numerous disciplines and teachers, and I realize that you have to be ready to receive before you can receive anything.

To make a long story short, **Dr. Jelusich has set me on my path to fulfillment**, and I have given up procrastinating. I came to the conclusion some time ago that procrastination was caused from my fear of the unknown, but, now that I know all I have to do is set my intent – it happens. I AM A CREATOR.

My eternal gratitude.

Love and Light,

Penny Phillips
Las Vegas, NV
February 12, 2001

****

I ask great blessings
To be bestowed
On Reverend Doctor Rick
His gaze so sure
Intent most pure
Can read me like a book Life Reading words
Opened up my thoughts
Encouraged and explained
Healing energies received
Revealed hidden keys that
Unlocked the prison of self-doubt
Beginning steps of freedom
A great delight and joy
Bud is opening at last
Words of thanks
Cannot be told
Heart is overwhelmed
God's most exalted
To be yours
Now and evermore.

Solona
Las Vegas, NV
September 2000

****

I first met Rev. Dr. Richard Jelusich at a Phoenix Phyre Bookstore's psychic faire in Southern California. **With absolute certainty, and with respect, he stated information about my core essence, and conducted palpable healing energy.** Subsequent consultations provided accurate readings of situations with their underlying currents, providing clarity by stripping away extraneous concerns to reveal "the bottom line." **Rick is quite direct and concise — what he sees is what he says.**

Las year my adult son was diagnosed as having a tumor in his liver. After many lab tests, and several CT scans and ultrasounds, he was scheduled for biopsy of the tumor to rule out malignancy. The evening before the 7 a.m. scheduled biopsy, I took my son, accompanied by his wife, to Rick for a healing. During that hour, Rick gave my son information about the location and nature of the problem, described in great detail the causal energetic history leading up to the creation of the situation, recommended "exercises" to help prevent its reoccurrence, and performed a healing. My son and his wife were quire impressed.

The next morning the biopsy was performed. It was well over a week until the doctor would return my call about the results of the biopsy. Finally, he explained he hadn't called because he was waiting for further documentation on the results. Why? — because they found no signs of any tumor! He thought perhaps the surgeon had looked in the wrong place (despite the fact that the surgeon had the scans to look at during the procedure)! In any case, there has been no problem since!

Rick's Flower Readings are fun, accurate, entertaining, and certainly give a lot to think about! I've been to two, so far. Each person brings a flower (untouched by anyone else) and, unseen by Rick, places the flower on the table. When all participants are ready, Rick enters the room, sits down, describes how the Flower Readings work, and, holding one flower at a time, with his eyes closed, gives "state of your life now" information and a brief healing. It's a good introduction to Rick's special abilities, and a good reset for your path. Fascinating!

Dr. Jelusich is truly a talented individual.

Susan Katz
08/26/00

※※※※※※※※※※※※※※※※※※※※※※※※

Dear Dr. Jelusich,

What a powerful effect your flower reading has had on my life! The wav you described my traits and personality was 100% on the mark ... you read me like a book. You gave me so many new insights and so much clarity about who I am and what I'm about.

You told me I was a powerful hands-on healer, gave me reasons why I was asleep to the task and stated you were here to awaken me. As I began to explore healing energy per your recommendation, my conservative Roman Catholic upbringing in a traditional medical family (my father an M.D., sister a surgeon, mother an R.N.) left me with the occasional thoughts, "this won't work," and "you can't do this." But I trusted my desire and continued to get my feet wet. I cannot tell you the joy I felt when I actual healed cases of pinkeye, strep throat, my pet's arthritic limping, etc. I continue to explore healing on many levels and I JUST LOVE IT ... thanks to you!

At the end of my flower reading you did the energetic physical healing. You noted a blockage in my back and spine that was preventing a free flow of energy, and worked on that also. (I smiled when you said "'Perhaps from an old injury," because I had a horseback riding fall as a young girl.)

And in the months since then? My posture has effortlessly straightened out, plus I feel physically stronger and more grounded and clear. I am more efficient while being more relaxed and I get more done in less time with less effort. I've also noticed myself breathing more deeply and regularly, as opposed to my previous shallow type of breathing. I find myself listening to and following my intuition more, and in general feel more calm and peaceful with less mental clutter. You see all the ways that 20 minute flower reading has touched my life! I am so very grateful.

I shall encourage my loved ones and friends to attend your flower readings, and I'll be taking advantage of your future lectures and workshops. **I admire you for devoting your life to helping others become empowered. You've been a gift to me ... you are a gift to this planet.**
THANK YOU

Janelle DeCorte
June 2000

* *

Testimonial - June 1, 2000
Oh boy, why did I ever come? I cannot believe this is happening to me. The nerves ... I am getting uncomfortable ... everybody is looking at me. "And now, I would like you all to look at the change in this person's energy field," continues that

voice, relentlessly, mercilessly telling ME that it is time to start taking care of ME.

You guessed it, dear ones. I am attending a Flower Reading with our speaker being no one else but Rev. Dr. Richard Jelusich. It is fun as well as educational to attend a Flower Reading: This is my eighth one. I came because I wanted to hear something about myself, something interesting, something new. I picked a flower in a hurry and spent five minutes (if that) holding it against my chest because I got there late. The flower I picked was a Desert Bird of Paradise. I can tell you that Rev. Dr. Jelusich is not a botanist. When he first saw this flower, he said ...." And we have here a .... *pause* ... flower from Mars ... does anyone know the name of this flower?" Then he proceeds to close his eyes, takes a deep breath, and begins to tell you what he "sees." He does not know who the flower belongs to, and during the reading his eyes remain closed. Did you ever try keeping your eyes closed and talk for ten or twelve minutes?

Understand that when this man does a reading for you, he does so with respect and full integrity. He will scan what comes before him and share with you the things you have to know and hear about in order for you as an individual to stay on your path and grow. Oh yes, he will tell you what you need to hear and not always what you *want* to hear. On the other hand, you may like the information very much.

"It is not important what is said in the reading, but WHAT YOU DO WITH THE INFORMATION!" Many times I heard him say and explain things in a kind and loving way, and sometimes with a "take no prisoners attitude." But each and every time I was able to understand that Dr. Jelusich does what he does only for one reason ... He loves each and every one of us dearly. His Love is so strong that he is willing to tell us in a way that only each individual can understand the real meaning of what is being said. **He conveys the message in the way you NEED to hear it at the time.**

You know by now that there is a reason for everything, and a reason why we came to a Flower Reading. I believe that each individual soul creates such an experience. The information that comes out has been very precise. Oh yes, I find that I still have an ego that gets in the way when I hear certain things. But I also find that once I take the time out to be quiet and look at the information that has been given and compare with what is going on in my life, I always come to the conclusion that **the information is on the button.** (For some of us, that might be a scary thought!) But he is not here to punish you or put you on a pedestal. Whatever you hear, take the time out to analyze and see where and how it fits your life.

Flower readings done by Rev. Dr. Richard Jelusich are all about being given the chance to improve one's growth on this plane, physically, mentally, emotionally, and spiritually.

I for one am grateful that there is such a person available to us. Have you been to a Flower Reading lately? Do it, it's worth it.

Peace, Love and Light,

Donovan Coppenrath

****

On the first day of 1999 I had a session with Rick, the effects of which continue to reverberate in my life. **The healing he facilitated for me has affected me on every level.** Physically, the sciatica, which had become so debilitating that I could not drive my manual transmission car for more than a few miles without experiencing pretty severe pain, disappeared after Rick energetically rotated my right hip back into position. I now drive two to three hours at a time with no discomfort.

This change on the physical level has been reflected on other levels as well. For the first time in my life that I can remember I believe that I have a future, and that that future holds joy and fulfillment for me. As a result, I have taken risks where relationships are concerned, that have led me to a joyful present I would never have thought possible.

Dr. Jelusich was back in Massachusetts in late March 2000. The challenge he left me with this time was about my own psychic abilities, and a commitment to finding ways to communicate what I know to be true. With last year as a reference point, I believe that I can and will do this.

Thank you, Rick, for helping me claim my life as it is meant to be.

Cara Anaam
Marlborough, MA

✱✱✱✱✱✱✱✱✱✱✱✱✱✱✱✱✱✱✱✱✱✱✱✱✱

Rev. Rick:

I wanted to thank you for coming to my home when you were in Washington. The flower reading was so inspiring and helpful. I checked with everyone to get a sense of how they were doing.

The woman with racing thoughts said she really experienced some peace in the days afterwards, which was very beneficial. Another woman who was at the reading has MS and she said her hands are usually numb. She had had an acupuncture treatment sometime before coming to the reading that gave her a little sensation, but she said driving home after the reading she had complete sensations in her hands! That is wonderful for her. We have yet to talk again about any other things that may have happened, but I thought that was truly special.

I have to say my reading really helped me to balance the energy on my head. After I came to realize it was something I had to accept, I began to deeply understand what the Spirit had been trying to convey to me recently. **After your reading I felt completely balanced for several days, which is rare for me.**

Actually for the past 20 years, and that's no exaggeration, I have suffered. It has been tremendously stressful. I've even made decisions to take a less taxing career path because the stress was so great at times. It was wearing me out and sapping all my energy. Now that I understand what was happening, a tremendous load has lifted.

I've been praying a long time for relief and the past few years I wasn't sure that I could bear it any longer. This may be a little hard to understand since you told me what was happening was a gift, something I should accept. But it was only after hearing it that I realized all this time I had been fighting against my purpose and myself! Then so many issues became clear, and I perceived the real root of my disquietude, something I'd known all along, but could never confront. It was always in my peripheral vision but I never quite had the tools to bring it into clear view.

The reading really helped, and I wanted you to know it. I kept thinking about the scripture where Christ healed several people while he was with his disciples and only one came back to offer thanks. He remarked to his disciples that only a few remember to give thanks for the work of the Spirit.

Blessings,

Brenda Jones
Friendship, Maryland
March 2000

* *

Rick has been coming into our home and giving flower readings and private readings since July 1997. In the time I have spent with Rick **he has heightened my awareness and opened me to miracles and the genuine magic of life.** He has gently guided me through the transformational process and has provided me a safe place to heal during private readings.

The word "power" used to have a negative meaning to me, as I feel I had observed people who had abused theirs. Rick has taught me to realize the beauty of my own power, which has given me a huge shift in my consciousness.

The flower readings are truly magical but also provide a place for people to heal, grow and learn more about themselves. All of this has enriched my life more than I can convey on paper. Rick has impacted my life and the lives of my friends and my entire family, and for that I will always be grateful.

Chris Olton
December 1999

* *

I'm not sure if you got my email or not but I'm trying to find out how many spots you have vacant for Richard's *Past Life Workshop* in May (in Vancouver). Please let me know ASAP as I have several people interested in signing up and I'd hate to miss the boat. The Flower Readings, by the way, were a big hit.

I saw my Sho-Tai practitioner a week later and, without me mentioning any symptoms, he treated me for the exact things that Richard talked about in my healing...how about that!

Dana
British Columbia, Canada
February 2003

✳✳✳✳✳✳✳✳✳✳✳✳✳✳✳✳✳✳✳✳✳✳✳✳✳✳✳

Hi Rick,
Tomorrow it will be 4 weeks since the wonderful flower reading at my house. I don't know if you recall a blue rose (with a butterfly attached). It belonged to a lady named Gaye. When she left she gave the flower to me, and guess what — the flower is still very much alive — and not only that, but it's GROW-ING. It has 4 new leaves, and anyone I've mentioned this to has never heard of such a thing. I've kept it in my bedroom and changed the water with plant food 3 times, and I'm just amazed.

Something very magical is happening and although I've looked for answers so far it's eluded me. I've had a blue rose in the past and because of the dye it only lasted a day. Oh by the way I seem to recall that Gaye was coming from a real heart place in her reading. Just thought I should share that with you. Hope you are well Rick.

Yvonne
Alberta, Canada
February 2003

✳✳✳✳✳✳✳✳✳✳✳✳✳✳✳✳✳✳✳✳✳✳✳✳✳✳

Dear Richard,
First off, I'd like to thank you for the amazing Flower Read-ing you did for me on Feb.12 at Gay's home. When you men-tioned that in a previous life I had been a First Nations person **you touched a part of my soul that I have always tried to**

keep suppressed. Whenever I am in a First Nations craft store or at a pow-wow I become so overwhelmed with sadness that it makes me cry, as I did on Feb. 12. Thank you so much.

KL
Vancouver, Canada
February 2003

****

Dear Dr. Rick:

I am Stella, friend of Dora. The reason for this letter is, that after one month from my surgery I want to say thank you and sincerely express to you from the bottom of my heart, "God Bless You, your mind and your hands forever."

Everything went exactly as you forecasted it. The breast cancer wasn't present at surgery time.

One more time I have no more words to say Thank You. Please keep me in your prayers and always remember me, because I will never forget you.

Love, Stella
March 2003

****

Hi Rick,

I just wanted to email you to tell you how informative I found your flower reading.

I had my reading on Feb. 12 of this year and at first...I didn't think that it was valid to who or what I was about. There were some things I could see right off the bat, in the sense I was an impatient person and good with animals, but I didn't understand why I was supposed to learn how to communicate in this lifetime because I do so much of it on a day to day basis, using the phone, emailing, telling people how I feel about things.

I re-visited the reading (via cassette tape) about a month ago and still didn't really get much out of it, but not until something happened just recently did I finally understand what you were talking about. Something had been misunderstood and misinformed and before finding this out, I felt like a broken record when revisiting how I felt about certain issues with certain people, because I thought I had clearly communicated things before, over and over again...so I was getting frustrated at why my point wasn't being understood. Things kept happening that upset me, and I just didn't know what to do.

Now that I know why it happened the way it did, I am now going to look into that book you recommended to me because now that I know...that yes...communication is a problem for me, I need to learn how to do it. I will now appreciate the book more as well as understand more than I did before.

But thanks again for your reading...and even though understanding didn't come to me right away...I'm glad it finally did. :)

Amanda
Pitt Meadows, BC, Canada
March 2003

****

Hi Rick,

Can you believe it is me, Chris out here in cyberspace? Another place I never thought I would journey to. **I think about you so often and the kindness and understanding you gave me during the early stages of my personal growth. You were all about empowering me to realize the gifts that I came here with.** I know now that you could see them, and guess what?? I believe I am beginning to see them as well. It feels so good.

I have been studying the excerpt, *Psychology of the Chakras* that you gave me, and remembering some of the things you told me, both in my readings and in my flower readings. I believe you told me very early on that I was a clairsentient, and at another time, you told me I had a 2-4 disposition, which I also resonate with. In the excerpt I believe you said it was possible to have dominance in this chakra as well as others. "In some cases, individuals with other dominant chakras may have a reference to the sixth; meaning that in addition to their native strength of their dominant chakra's influence, that person also benefits from a reference to the influence of the sixth chakra."

This relieved a little of the confusion that I was feeling at first. I have really enjoyed reading about all of the chakras.

My love, light and peace surround you during this very uncertain time for our earth.

Chris
Los Angeles
March 2003

****

Dear Richard,

I enjoyed the lecture tonight very much. I am listening to my tape daily and have been practicing my exercises. I feel I am lightening up. I know I have good things to give to the universe and also to receive for myself. It's been an arduous prolonged journey to the depths of despair and betrayal that I have experienced. I do finally forgive myself and others who have caused me anger, pain and frustration.

As I keep listening to the tape I feel an ok-ness with you about my stuff. I believe my acceptance of you is because **you do have a real sense of my intensity, passion and vastness of emotion.** It was significant for me you had a sense of my qualities and you are a man to boot! The closest description of me by a man was still waters run deep, and that's not accurate.

With Love,
Name withheld upon request
San Diego
March 2003

****

Richard,

Just a quick note of appreciation for the February 1st Flower Reading – **I resonated with everything you said.**

Coming into the reading, I had been struggling with a respiratory virus for 7 weeks. Had also recognized depression was playing a significant factor in its resilience. As you started the healing energy, my ears, throat and chest eased in pain and continued to cool down as we sat in circle. Truly grateful for your help and the exercise provided.

Respectfully,

AL
Canada
April 2003

✳✳✳✳✳✳✳✳✳✳✳✳✳✳✳✳✳✳✳✳✳✳✳✳

I was fortunate to have been invited to Yvonne's flower reading during your recent visit, and was overwhelmed by your presence and your insight. You mentioned the importance of validation and I would like to share my thoughts on the experience.

I was amazed at the accuracy and detail of your readings and the fact that you could zero in on 1998 as being a turning point in my life. As you indicated, it was a time when I did leave a very comfortable life to rebuild and renew my spirit; a process that is ongoing and will, I hope, continue always. **You spoke many truths and I feel honored to have met you.** I am grateful to Yvonne for inviting me and look forward to your next visit.

May you continue to bring enlightenment and encouragement to all of us who seek guidance and direction on our journey.

Sincerely,

Bonnie Moore
Calgary
March 2003

✳✳✳✳✳✳✳✳✳✳✳✳✳✳✳✳✳✳✳✳✳✳✳✳

Dr. Jelusich,

I just want you to know that before I went to your flower reading I had a problem with my throat — when it came to swallowing dry foods, they would get stuck real easy. I don't want to get into the details about it but **the good thing is that after the reading the problem is gone.**

So I just want you to know........Thank you, Thank you and Thank you :-)

Robert Moore
April 2002

＊＊＊＊＊＊＊＊＊＊＊＊＊＊＊＊＊＊＊＊＊＊＊＊＊＊

Hi Rick!

Last summer you did a life reading for me in Calgary, a few days before I left for my year's sabbatical in Mexico.

At the time, my energy was very scattered and I listened to the tape a couple of times down here. The one thing you said that stuck in my mind was that I needed to stay in my body and be grounded all the time, and I have been doing a much better job with it than ever before in my life. I hadn't listened to the tape since August!

A few days ago, I was suddenly inspired to pull out the tape again and continue transcribing your words. WOW!! It was like it was a completely different tape!! I had forgotten most of what was on the tape and/or didn't get it or remember it. But the whole thing about *Grounding and Staying in My Body*, was engrained in me. I never really got that it made a big difference in my life, until finishing transcribing the tape the other night and then it brought back the memory of some challenging experiences here in Mexico. **Here's an example of how the whole grounding thing saved me from a great deal of trauma and possibly even saved my life!**

I've been working as a Nanny in an affluent original part of Puerto Vallarta. One afternoon at about 4:00pm, I was walking to work and noticed a young man walking ahead of me. We were both walking up a narrow cobblestone road. He turned around a couple of times, smiled and made eye contact. I was hot and tired and really didn't pay much attention to him.

Then he slowed down and started to look around at the doorways. I assumed he was looking for an address and was going to ask him if he was lost, as I caught up to him. (I realize now that he was likely looking around to make sure that there would be no witnesses!) He suddenly turned around, grabbed my right arm, and uttered some words in Spanish that don't warrant repeating. I pulled my arm away and he grabbed my left arm, while trying to pull down his shorts with his right hand, with full intention of raping me. I had a canvas bag over my shoulder that contained a few heavy things including a hard-cover book. I calmly but forcefully hit him in the side of the head with the bag, which caught him off guard and "rang his bell"!

He loosened his grip and I was able to get away. As I left him, I uttered a few comments of my own and turned and walked away with determination. I didn't run, I didn't look back, I merely walked to work! I was more annoyed than anything and never experienced the panic, trauma, nightmare, panic attacks etc. etc., that other women I know who have survived similar experiences often live with for days, months or years.

I guess that's what you meant by how essential it was to stay in my body!! In the tape you used the analogy of a lightning rod and how if I was grounded, the negatives would go right through me as if my body were a lightning rod. I didn't melt down when I was "hit by lightning!!"

When I thought back about the experience, I realize that it was my groundedness, calmness and conviction that saved me! The man outweighed me by at least 100lbs. and was half my age and had I been in an ungrounded victim space, I fear I would be telling a different story.

Another thing you mentioned in my tape is that I am a very powerful woman and that powerful people have powerful experiences and challenges. I certainly don't want to have to any more similar experiences in my life, but know if I can handle an attempted rape I can handle anything life has to throw at my as I continue to live and learn.

Thanks again for your insights! I think you probably said in your tape at least 15 times - STAY GROUNDED! STAY IN YOUR BODY! I didn't get it then, but I do now! THANKS!

Cindy
May 2003

****

Dear Dr. Rick,

I attended your Flower Reading, with the Iris, on May 14th. Thank you for your explanation of why I needed to be in nature more often and to just "be" without expectations. Other therapists, trying to help me, have told me that I "think too much" and "stay out of your head" but when it is a part of who you are, that is a difficult task.

With your insight, my logical side has been satisfied and I understand the importance of my behavior change. Now I have the reason I can give to my family when I head out for a walk, dig in my garden or just cuddle with my cats. **I truly feel you have given me a crucial piece of information to allow me to find the peace I need to live my life in the richness of the present, while still being open to what life offers.**

I know you chuckled over my efforts to get to that flower reading, and I laughed myself at the apparent "extreme" measures to get there. After hearing about the readings in a casual conversation a couple months ago, I made a spontaneous phone call and filled the last space for that evening. I felt privileged to be there and I wasn't going to have my family or myself sabotage this for me, as has happened before. Getting what I feel I need, while being part of a family who don't really "get" what I am doing, and who "humor" me, is a challenge. I know I need to be responsible for my own needs.

I appreciated your insight, guidance and healing. I can see hope in getting off thyroid medication after 30 years. I know it can be done. It was interesting also to hear about my counter-clockwise third chakra, as the illness that put me on to this journey was related to the feminine/masculine energies within me. I have had to re-work many conditioned beliefs about being female to balance the two. From your comments, I now know that discounting the masculine energy is not to my benefit either, as it seems to be inherently part of who I am.

A *fascinating evening.* I hope to have the opportunity to share in such an evening again, as there were words of wisdom from each reading that could be applied to me. Funny, I'm even "thinking," only a little bit, about when would be the best time to do it again. Imagine that.

Namaste,
Ginger Wilson
May 18, 2003

＊＊＊＊＊＊＊＊＊＊＊＊＊＊＊＊＊＊＊＊＊＊＊＊＊＊＊

For Dr. Rick—

I've been listening to all my tapes of our sessions & the flower readings that you've done for me. Thank you so much for all your energy, love and support. **You've always been so gentle and caring with me, and you always say the things that I really need to hear in order to keep making my world more balanced and beautiful.**

The last year was extremely painful. I felt so horrible that I couldn't listen to any of my tapes. But as I've begun to feel better, I came to a recent flower reading — and the most miraculous thing happened. You told me the EXACT same things that you said to me in my very first flower reading with you more than two years ago! You couldn't see me but my jaw was in my lap.

You told me that, as a defender of those who cannot defend themselves, I see in others and resonate the qualities of Truth and Innocence. I suppose I had a really difficult time believing your words, as it seems I've been spending the last while and a great deal of energy trying to disprove it all to myself!

With your ability to stay within your heart and be so open, focused and tuned in to all those around you, you gave me a powerful and loving gift that I will never forget. If you could see those things in me, and more than once, then it's about time for me to take an honest, loving look for myself.

Thank you, Rick, for helping me to see the Innocence again, in myself and others, and as well, to reclaim my voice of Truth. I joyously receive and cherish your gift to me, and I promise that I will always remember it, and that I will live it as well.

Love,
Chantal
Calgary
May 2003

****

Hi Dr. Rick,

I just wanted to take a moment to thank you for the flower reading I received this weekend. Before attending your reading, I was plagued with feelings of being in the wrong place, in spite of a good position that provides my family with a relatively decent measure of security. Somehow it seemed wrong however, and to make matters more difficult, I had been experiencing a series of dreams that seemed to be prompting me to take a step that made no logical sense (at least in the short term). I found your website after an extensive search on the Internet and decide to attend one of your flower readings.

You began my reading by noting that the flower I had brought was not my first choice, and accurately identified the type of flower that I would have otherwise brought. It was absolutely amazing that you were able to pick that up, not only for the content, but also for the fact that **it was the kind of miraculous validation that I would need to make the tough decisions ahead.** I believe in the kind of abilities that you possess, but maintain a cautious skepticism of anyone who claims to possess them. It was exactly the kind of sign that I needed to take action on the words that would come.

I have begun a series of steps towards a future I was once frightened to pursue, and though I do not know what that future will bring, I now pursue it without fear.

Thank you very much!

Tim
June 2003

Hi Rick,

It's me, Chief Talkalot. I just had to express my deep appreciation once again for the wonderful workshop on Sunday. I've hesitated in the past from taking other trainings in healing and didn't know why until I attended yours. **The principle behind your training truly resonates with what I've been seeking.**

It's also good to know that if I ever want to, I can attend whichever level I'm at in other cities. As I briefly mentioned to you, I live temporarily at my parent's here in AZ. I haven't felt drawn to any particular city as of yet but do know that I will be going on to wherever I feel "called" - I've been considering moving to Las Vegas as I attend your training. I just have to let you in on a little secret: one of my guides had prophesied to me back in 1999 that I would meet a "fatherly" figure who's a teacher, someone who would guide, teach, help, work and walk with me - I suppose like a mentor. *And that I would meet this teacher in Las Vegas.* Imagine my surprise when I heard that you moved to L.V. because back then you were in S.D. I have been considering your training since back then! As you know, divine timing is everything.

I could go on & on but you're a busy teacher and **I just wanted you to know my sincere gratitude for assisting all of us on this journey through life.**

Until we meet again!

Namaste,

Kathy
June 2003

****

Valhallasun (Regd.) Kennels
Box 1535
Okotoks, Alberta, Canada
T1S 1B5
www.norrbottenspets.net
e-mail valhallasun@norrbottenspets.net

To whom it may concern:

On Jan 30, 2003 I had a reading with Dr. Richard Jelusich, Ph.D. One of my main concerns was which of our four Canadian Champions to enter in the World Show in Dortmund, Germany.

One dog was a 4-time World Champion, now 10 years old. Dr. Rick reviewed all the photos and without hesitation chose Valhallasun Thorer, a 3-year-old male from a totally different line than our existing World Champion. My husband and I knew we already had a 4-time winner, but Dr. Richard Jelusich, without question said "THIS ONE WILL WIN!"

Four months later Valhallasun Thorer became the new WORLD Champion 2003, Competition at the World Show level is competing with 20,000 of the best dogs on the planet.

Thank You Dr. Richard Jelusich Ph.D. You sure know how to pick a WINNER!

See you at the next Healers Course — already signed up
Most Sincerely,

Inger & Zale Colins
Calgary, Alberta, Canada
July 1, 2003

****

Rick,

I had a very interesting experience the other day, and felt that I should share it with you. **The flower reading I received a month and a half ago from you has set a off a series of life-changing events and attitudes.** After spending that time in a very energized state I began to experience some frustration that the changes I am trying to make would not come quickly enough. The bottom line however, was that I needed to regain my momentum.

As I prepared to sleep, I attempted to place myself in a meditative state, and to implant a suggestion that my dreams would show me selected pieces of the future that would encourage and revive and me. Scarcely had a drifted into sleep (or so it seems) that a very strange thing began to occur. I was completely aware of my environment and my place within it (but not in the manner that it is perceived by the physical eye). Things appeared in the form of energy patterns, void like, as though floating in space and very peaceful. It was in many ways as though I was existing in two very different planes of existence simultaneously, with a sensory awareness of each.

Of particular interest was my own body, which I saw as a series of blue/white energy patterns. I studied the environment briefly with a childlike sense of curiosity. At this point *your voice* instructed me to remain still, and explained that my energy patterns were very pliable in this state, and it was much easier to work. I remained still as you began to conduct your energy work. Suddenly I felt energy coursing through me, first outward in a way that felt very cleansing, and finally a great inward surge that felt very empowering. **The power, the invigoration, and the incredible sense of well-being were like nothing I have ever experienced.**

The logical mind would summarize it as a nice dream, and it may have been. But the sheer power of the experience, and the positive effect of it upon me, leave me loath to accept such a simple explanation. I cannot help but feel that I owe you my thanks.

Thank you again for your work, and for your service,

Tim
San Diego
June 2003

* *

"How Does Your Garden Grow?"

A stem of Sweet William and one Daffodil proved valuable beyond their typical aesthetic appeal when I had the privilege of attending two "Flower Readings" conducted by Dr. Richard Jelusich in Redding, California.

So gifted is Dr. Jelusich, that he is able to apply his own soul's grace, empathy, intuition and humor in a "reading" of flowers that meets each individual's comfort level, cognitive level, level of wisdom, and spiritual growth, as well as penetrating any compromise of the mind/body/spirit, by applying specific, personalized healing in the moment.

A good time is indeed had by all, whether one is simply looking for an interesting introduction to the delights that metaphysics delivers, or whether one is solidly on his or her spiritual path and is seeking the extraordinary healing, and intuited information that only Richard can provide.

I truly believe the best of Prophets are blessed with sense of humor—one comes away from the flower readings resonating to the blessing as well as to the sheer fun of it all.

With my own readings, I listen to the tapes frequently, absorbing the healing, while exploring the life lessons Richard has described, thus maximizing the experience and taking my understanding and personal growth to the next level.

It may well be that "A rose is a rose is a rose..." That is, until Dr. Richard Jelusich gets his hands on one!

KJ
Redding, California
June 2003

****

Hi Richard,
   I wrote a poem for you:

   You are a being of light and love
   Sent to us from the heavens above
   All in the name of "Love"
   You have been a guiding light
   Like a shining star in the night
   You've made such a difference in my life
   You've shown me my magnificence
   That I now can sense
   You've helped me heal so much
   To release and feel peace
   I had to do my part
   To let go
   So I may grow

Behold the glow
I now hold
Shades of gold
I've been told
Although no longer a wife
I get a chance at a new life
To be me
Whomever that may be...

Much Love,
Lynn Schafer, LV, NV
8/1/03

* *

Dear Richard,

Thank you again for the time you gave me at my house on Monday. **I so appreciate and receive your gift.** I have dived into a lot of recapitulation and the gifts keep flowing from it. I am very grateful. I have been directing people your way and I would like to stay in touch.

Many blessings to you,

Kovida
August 2003

* *

Rick, **I have come to know over the years that your work is notably inspiring and appreciated.**

I had a wonderful epiphany last April when you were here. I realized that my life was exactly what I hoped it would be. I had finally become the person I wanted to be. I had been a wife & mother for so long that I had forgotten "me." And quite frankly, I was afraid to be alone when those relationships began to change (my children grew up and my marriage dissolved).

Your last reading, interestingly enough, reflected the progress, yet I had not felt it in my heart till that night. Such a freedom of spirit has come over me. One more fear conquered! So, I recommend you to my friends with great sincerity.

Janice
San Diego, CA
March 2003

∗∗∗∗∗∗∗∗∗∗∗∗∗∗∗∗∗∗∗∗∗∗∗∗∗

Dear Richard,

I attended your flower reading, never realizing how it might change my life. I have read *The Power Of Now* many times, and it sits by my bedside for swift reference if I need it, which I often do. I found so much need to heal.

More and more souls are beginning the process of remembering the truth of who they are. Your email came at a very dark time for me, and while reading it, I was uplifted, and at the same time chastened, because I realized how I had fallen asleep again and not even known it. I will have to take full and complete responsibility, stay awake, and find the riches of more awareness.

I thank you for coming into my life; there is nothing random in the universe. I am going to take your healing workshops, and look forward to meeting with you again.

Joan
March 2003

∗∗∗∗∗∗∗∗∗∗∗∗∗∗∗∗∗∗∗∗∗∗∗∗∗

Dear Richard,

Thank you for replying so quickly. **Your words of wisdom mean the world to me.**

I'm sure you are probably already aware of this, but I was awoken from a sleep this evening and when I left my bedroom, the rest of the house was completely enveloped in a haze. I just knew that you had sent your message to me. My computer is downstairs, and when I finished reading your message and went back upstairs, the haze had dissipated.

Thank you again for taking the time to point me in the right direction. I will spend time asking plenty of questions. (I'm glad I started with you.)

Maple Ridge
BC, Canada
March 2003

* *

Dear Dr. Rick:
I am Stella friend of Dora. The reason of this letter is, that after one month from my surgery I want to say thank you and sincerely express to you from the bottom of my heart ,"God Bless You, your mind and your hands "for ever.
Everything went the very same way exactly as you forecasted it. The breast cancer wasn't present at the surgery time.
One more time I have no more words to say Thank You. Please keep me in your prayers and always remember me, because I will never forget you.

Love, Stella
March, 2003

* *

Richard -
Just a quick note of appreciation for the February 1st Flower Reading - resonated with_everything_ you said.
Coming into the reading, I had been struggling with a respiratory virus for 7 weeks. Had also recognised depression was playing a significant factor in its resilience. As you started the healing energy, my ears, throat and chest eased in pain and continued to cool down as we sat in circle. Truly grateful for your help and the exercise provided.

Respectfully
AL, Canada
April 2003

* *

I was fortunate to have been invited to Yvonne's flower reading during your recent visit, and was overwhelmed by your presence and your insight. You mentioned the importance of validation and I would like to share my thoughts on the experience.

I was amazed at the accuracy and detail of your readings and the fact that you could zero in on 1998 as being a turning point in my life. As you indicated, it was a time when I did leave a very comfortable life to rebuild and renew my spirit; a process that is ongoing and will, I hope, continue always. You spoke many truths and I feel honoured to have met you. I am grateful to Yvonne for inviting me and look forward to your next visit.

May you continue to bring enlightenment and encouragement to all of us who seek guidance and direction on our journey.

Sincerely,

Bonnie Moore
Calgary
March 2003

****

Hi Dr. Rick,

I just wanted to take a moment to thank you for the flower reading I received this weekend. Before attending your reading, I was plagued with feelings of being in the wrong place, in spite of a good position that provides my family with a relatively decent measure of security. Somehow it seemed wrong however, and to make matters more difficult, I had been experiencing a series of dreams that seemed to be prompting me to take a step that made no logical sense (at least in the short term). I found your website after an extensive search on the Internet and decide to attend one of your flower readings.

You began my reading by noting that the flower I had brought was not my first choice, and accurately identified the type of flower that I would have otherwise brought. It was absolutely amazing that you were able to pick that up, not only for the content, but for the fact that it was the kind of miraculous validation that I would need to make the tough decisions ahead. I believe in the kind of abilities that you possess, but maintain a cautious skepticism of anyone that claims to possess them. It was exactly the kind of sign that I needed to take action on the words that would come.

I have began a series of steps towards a future I was once frightened to pursue, and though I do not know what that future will bring, I pursue it without fear.

Thank you very much!

Tim
June 2003

✳✳✳✳✳✳✳✳✳✳✳✳✳✳✳✳✳✳✳✳✳✳✳✳✳

To Whom it may concern

On Jan 30th 2003 I had a reading with Dr. Richard Jelusich Ph.D.

One of my main concerns was which of four of our Canadian Champions to enter in the World Show in Dortmund Germany.

One was a 4 time World Champion, now 10 years old. He reviewed all the photos and without hesitation chose Valhallasun Thorer a 3 year old male, from a totally different line than our existing World Champion. My husband & I knew we already had a 4 time winner, but Dr. Richard Jelusich, without question said "THIS ONE WILL WIN!"

Four months later Valhallasun Thorer became the new WORLD Champion 2003, Competition at the World Show level is competing with 20,000 of the best dogs on the planet.

Thank You Dr. Richard Jelusich Ph.D. You sure know how to pick a WINNER!

See you at the next Healers Course, already signed up

Most Sincerely,

Inger & Zale Colins
Calgary, Alberta
Canada
June 2003

✳✳✳✳✳✳✳✳✳✳✳✳✳✳✳✳✳✳✳✳✳✳✳✳✳

About a year ago my wife came home and told me that she had made an appointment with Dr. Rick for an hour session. At that time there was just no way that I would consider participating in that spiritual intuitive nonsense. I was a dental specialist with six years of postgraduate training immersed in scientific evidence based therapy. There was just no possibility that there was any validity to this man and his intuitive processes. I refused to go and my son visited Dr. Rick instead.

Last spring I was diagnosed with a pituitary tumor called a prolactinoma (a benign growth of 1 cm). The tumor would compress my eye nerves if it continued to grow and I could suffer permanent blindness .Well I had to mobilize to solve this problem. Fortunately within four weeks time I was able to see my doctor, get a cat scan and have an appointment with an endocrinologist. Truly a major feat accomplished within the Canadian Medicare system. I learned from the endocrinologist that a small pill taken twice a day could shrink the tumor. Within 2 weeks it was almost gone. This was determined by a blood test that showed an almost normal level of hormone prolactin.

However along with the pituitary shrinkage I felt that I was hit by a bolt of spiritual lightening. Did my sixth Chakra open? I wasn't even aware of Chakra's at that time. I had opened the door to the universe and just was in awe.

I began to experience some interesting visions and intuitive senses. When I heard that Dr. Rick was going to be in Calgary I knew that I had to try attending his flower reading. At the last moment a cancellation (not a coincidence I am now convinced) came up and my wife and I were able to attend.

Well my flower wasn't picked till the end. Dr. Rick you knew exactly why I came, "to soak up all the spiritual juice of the flower reading". Your accuracy was uncanny not just about me and why I was there but pretty well about all the participants. When you picked up on my eye problem (contact lens irritation) as you sent the healing energy my way at the end of reading that just blew me away.

So much for scientific evidence. I knew then that my being there was not an accident. The next night I attended your Psychology of the Chakra's lecture with my wife and a close friend.

You picked up exactly on why our friend's relationship and marriage were struggling. You knew her essence, her soul, and sensed that all three of us were on this "aggressively moving foreword" spiritual journey. How right you are!

Also as you mentioned in my flower reading be careful for what you ask for when traveling the spiritual pathways. Well I am interested in taking your healing classes and I do have a meeting set up with you in Jan/04 when you visit Calgary. I am hoping to get the guidance and knowledge about the journey I am facing. My heart has opened. I have walked through the door and there is no turning back. Thank you, Dr. Rick

Albert

****

Dear Rick,

I have been intending to write to you for some time now, and am just now getting around to doing it.

You did a phone conference with me in December of '99, and I want to tell you that out of all the reading, consciousness expansion groups, churches, etc. that I have done in my 30 years of conscious "truth seeking", you have helped me to find the Truth of myself, more than anyone or anything else.

I realize you don't remember me, but, you "diagnosed" me as having a powerful third chakra dominance, and the analyzation of me and what my trials and purpose here was, was incredible. I have done everything possible to be true to that reading, and as a result, I believe God has brought into my Life my True Spiritual partner. I have recommended you so highly, he is interested in having a phone conference with you, and will be taking some time off starting Monday, March 29. Would you be available during that week for a phone conference, and if so, when?

Please let me know asap. Thank you for all you are doing, and for being who you are.

In Love and Light,

Penny Phillips
March 2004

****

Hi Richard!

I don't know if you remember me and Tenaya, my partner. We lived at the Village Green and received a couple of readings from you. One at the Green and one at your place down near San Diego. We were certainly in a bad way back then.

We pressed you to give us a clue as to where in the world we should be since it wasn't LA. You gave some clues... "Pines"....other things. You said you and I knew each other as Druids and that this life was my recapitulation life.

Well, a couple years ago we received some insight, and inheritance, and moved here to Clearwater, Florida. We live on a pine-lined street called "Pineview." It's just off Druid Street. We laughed when we realized all your clues were showing up in our new location.

Anyway, we'd like to know how you are doing. We are thriving here and like you also predicted, my music blew out the top since leaving LA and I speak with people all over the world via the internet, collaborating on music and a new online music production business. And my CD release, <u>Magnificent Obsession</u>, even won a major award for which I had to travel to New York... (http://www.tareywolf.com) So we have been doing very well and thank you for your much needed guidance when things were so rough back there, a couple years ago.

Nice talking with you and hope to hear from you soon.

Tarey Wolf
Tampa, FL
August 2004

Herbs and other natural health products and information are often available at natural food stores or metaphysical bookstores. If you cannot find what you need locally, you can contact one of the following sources of supply.

Sources of Supply:

The following companies have an extensive selection of useful products and a long track-record of fulfillment. They have natural body care, aromatherapy, flower essences, crystals and tumbled stones, homeopathy, herbal products, vitamins and supplements, videos, books, audio tapes, candles, incense and bulk herbs, teas, massage tools and products and numerous alternative health items across a wide range of categories.

WHOLESALE:

Wholesale suppliers sell to stores and practitioners, not to individual consumers buying for their own personal use. Individual consumers should contact the RETAIL supplier listed below. Wholesale accounts should contact with business name, resale number or practitioner license in order to obtain a wholesale catalog and set up an account.

Lotus Light Enterprises, Inc.
PO Box 1008 EL
Silver Lake, WI 53170 USA
262 889 8501 (phone)
262 889 8591 (fax)
800 548 3824 (toll free order line)

RETAIL:

Retail suppliers provide products by mail order direct to consumers for their personal use. Stores or practitioners should contact the wholesale supplier listed above.

Internatural
PO Box 489 EL
Twin Lakes, WI 53181 USA
800 643 4221 (toll free order line)
262 889 8581 office phone
EMAIL: internatural@internatural.com
WEB SITE: www.internatural.com

Web site includes an extensive annotated catalog of more than 14,000 items that can be ordered "on line" for your convenience 24 hours a day, 7 days a week.

Yoga & Ayurveda

Self-Healing and Self-Realization
by Dr. David Frawley

Yoga and Ayurveda together form a complete
approach for optimal health, vitality and
higher awareness. YOGA & AYURVEDA
reveals to us the secret powers of the body,
breath, senses, mind and chakras. More
importantly, it unfolds transformational
methods to work on them through diet,
herbs, asana, pranayama and meditation.
This is the first book published in the West
on these two extraordinary subjects and
their interface. It has the power to change
the lives of those who read and apply it.

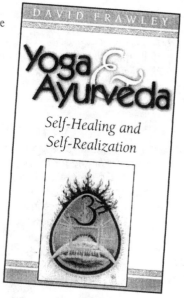

Dr. David Frawley (Vamadeva Shastri) is
recognized both in India and the West for
his knowledge of Vedic teachings, which
include Ayurveda, Vedic Astrology, and
Yoga. He is the author of twenty books
published over the last twenty years, including Ayurveda and the Mind,
Yoga of Herbs, Ayurvedic Healing and Astrology of the Seers. His Vedic translations and
historical studies on ancient India have received much acclaim, as have his journalistic
works on modern India.

| Trade Paper | ISBN 0-914955-81-0 | 360 pp | $19.95 |

Available through your local bookseller or direct from:
Lotus Press, P O Box 325, Dept. EL, Twin Lakes, WI 53181 USA
262-889-8561 (office phone)   262-889-2461 (office fax)   800-824-6396 (toll free order line)
email: lotuspress@lotuspress.com   web site: www.lotuspress.com

To Order send $19.95 plus $2.50 shipping/handling ($.75 for each additional copy) to
Lotus Press.

Lotus Press is the publisher of a wide range of books in the field of alternative health, including
Ayurveda, Chinese medicine, herbology, reiki, aromatherapy, and energetic healing modalities.
Request our free book catalog.